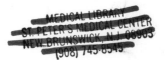

Neurological Complications of Renal Disease

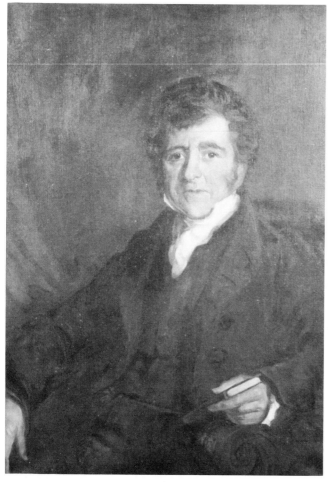

This portrait of Richard Bright hangs in Guy's Hospital, London, England.

Richard Bright, M.D. (1789–1858) made his historic discoveries on renal disease in Guy's Hospital during the first half of the nineteenth century. He associated the clinical features of renal failure, elevation of urea in the blood, and proteinuria with renal pathology at autopsy. He described the clinical course of patients with glomerulonephritis and estimated the prevalence of acute attacks.

Bright was as much a neurologist as a nephrologist. In 1831 he published a two-volume work on the nervous system, and later described the clinical and pathological features of the brain in uremia. In the days before effective therapy, he noted "the peculiar train of cerebral symptoms" which underlined "the insidious nature of this malady and its fatal tendency."

Neurological Complications of Renal Disease

Charles F. Bolton, M.D., C.M., F.R.C.P.(C)

Professor of Neurology, Department of Clinical Neurological Sciences, University of Western Ontario; Director, EMG Laboratory, and Consultant Neurologist, Victoria Hospital, London, Ontario

G. Bryan Young, M.D., F.R.C.P.(C)

Associate Professor of Neurology, Department of Clinical Neurological Sciences, and Chairman, Department of the History of Medicine and Science, University of Western Ontario; Director, EEG Laboratory, Victoria Hospital, London, Ontario

Butterworths

Boston London Singapore Sydney Toronto Wellington

Every effort has been made to ensure the drug dosage schedules within this text are
accurate and conform to standards accepted at time of publication. However, as
treatment recommendations vary in the light of continuing research and clinical
experience, the reader is advised to verify drug dosage schedules herein with
information found on product information sheets. This is especially true in cases of
new or infrequently used drugs.

Library of Congress Cataloging-in-Publication Data

Bolton, Charles Francis, 1932–
    Neurologic complications of renal disease / Charles F. Bolton, G. Bryan
Young.
        p.   cm.
    Includes bibliographies and index.
    ISBN 0–409–95139–0
    1. Nervous system—Diseases.   2. Chronic renal failure—Complications and
sequelae.   3. Uremia—Complications and sequelae.   4. Hemodialysis—
Complications and sequelae.   I. Young, G. Bryan (Gordon Bryan)
II. Title.
    [DNLM: 1. Nervous System Diseases—etiology.   2. Uremia—
complications. WJ 348 B694n]
    RC346.B63   1989
    616.8'0471—dc20
    DNLM/DLC
    for Library of Congress   89–15690
                                                                           CIP

British Library Cataloguing in Publication Data
Bolton, Charles F.
    Neurological complications of renal disease.
    1. Man. Kidneys. Diseases. Neurological aspects
    I. Title   II. Young, G. Bryan
    616.6'1

    ISBN 0–409–95139–0

Butterworth Publishers
80 Montvale Avenue
Stoneham, MA 02180

10 9 8 7 6 5 4 3 2 1

Printed in the United States of America

Contents

Preface

Renal disease is an important component of health care management. In the United States in 1985, over 100,000 persons were being treated for end-stage renal disease, 80 percent by various forms of dialysis and the rest by transplantation. Nervous system complications are common occurrences in these very ill patients.

Encephalopathy almost invariably accompanies acute uremia and is a significant problem throughout the stages of chronic renal failure; peripheral neuropathy occurs in at least 50 percent of patients with end-stage renal disease. Both conditions are due to the toxic effects of renal failure. In addition, a large group of associated conditions, such as diabetes mellitus, affect both the nervous system and the kidney by the same process. Various complications may also arise from the treatment itself, notably, dialysis and renal transplantation. Yet, we know of no other book that deals with this subject.

In discussing the various disease manifestations and how they should be managed, we thought it important to include descriptions that would be understandable not just to nephrologists and neurologists, but also to medical personnel not necessarily expert in those specialities. Because we are both neurologists, we particularly hope we have been successful insofar as the nervous system is concerned. Conversely, we felt it inappropriate to attempt to be authoritative in the area of kidney dis-

ease. Fortunately, many fine textbooks on this subject are available. Throughout, we have sought to portray the illnesses as the physician would see them at the bedside and then offer rational suggestions for appropriate investigation and treatment.

We were impressed during our research by the many fine publications in the scientific literature. Not all appear in the reference lists, but we have included, and often discussed in detail, those we consider the most important. In the course of the volume, we have tried to present observations and ideas as they developed chronologically. Of special value have been the writings of Asbury, Funck–Brentano, Dobblestein, Tyler, Tenckhoff, Jebsen, Dyck, Thomas, Nielsen, Jennekins, Bergstrom, Alfrey, Arieff, and Massry.

We hope this book will be a valuable source of information for all medical staff involved in the care of patients who suffer from kidney disease. The list is long and includes not only nephrologists and neurologists, but also the internists who must deal with illnesses affecting multiple organ systems in these patients, the physiatrists who manage their rehabilitation, the surgeons involved in postoperative care following transplantation, and family physicians who may supervise the care of patients on home dialysis. Nurses and other health care workers are involved in every stage of renal disease.

The neurological complications of renal disease have preoccupied the authors for some time. Both of us are clinical neurologists, C.F.B. specializing in electromyography and G.B.Y. in electroencephalography. Initially we worked at the University Hospital in Saskatoon, Saskatchewan, where nephrologists Mark and Richard Baltzan established one of the earliest and most successful hemodialysis and transplant programs. By 1970, more than 100 procedures had been performed, and it was there that the remarkable recovery from severe uremic neuropathy following successful renal transplantation was first observed. Ultimately, we moved to Victoria Hospital in London, Ontario, where a major chronic hemodialysis program is directed by nephrologists Adam Linton, Robert Lindsay, and William Clark. Besides this collaboration, important links were also established with Anthony Hodsman, nephrologist at St. Joseph's Hospital, London, who is particularly interested in aluminum toxicity as a complication of dialysis. Thus, over the years, we have observed renal patients in a variety of clinical settings.

It is impossible to achieve all of one's objectives in writing a book, and users of this volume will undoubtedly find omissions, areas of overemphasis, and so forth. Consequently, we invite readers to send us their comments. Whether favorable or not, they will further enrich us in our involvement with this absorbing subject.

C.F.B.
G.B.Y.

Acknowledgments

Charles Bolton expresses gratitude to his parents, Frank and Grace Bolton, who were his best teachers; to his wife Margaret for encouraging him to enter and then supporting him in the specialty of neurology; to his children, David, Katherine, and Nancy, whose achievements have given him his greatest satisfaction; to the people of his home province, Saskatchewan, who continue to demonstrate how to conquer adversity; to Queens University, Kingston, Ontario, for teaching him to be a doctor; to clinicians at the University of Saskatchewan and the Mayo Clinic who taught him neurology; to Henry Barnett for asking him to come to London, Ontario; to his colleagues in the Department of Clinical Neurological Sciences at the University of Western Ontario, who continue to educate him in the science of neurology and neurosurgery; to Tony Parkes in the Electromyography Laboratory; and to his admired friend and collaborator in this work, Bryan Young, without whose talents the book would not have been possible. Finally, it was Richard Baltzan, nephrologist at University Hospital, Saskatoon, who, in 1966, over coffee in the surgeon's lounge, suggested to Charles Bolton that he systematically study the peripheral nervous system of uremic patients.

Bryan Young thanks Charles Bolton, who invited him to share in this project. He also thanks his wife Christine for her encouragement and support, his family, who tolerated him throughout the writing, and the following individuals who offered help, criticism, and suggestions: Warren T. Blume (his EEG mentor), Alistair Buchan, A. (Tony) Hodsman, John Kreeft, and Stephen Oppenheimer.

Both authors are particularly grateful to Betsy Toth, who not only was entirely responsible for the preparation of the manuscript but assisted in many other important ways. David, Katherine and Nancy Bolton assisted in literature searches as part of summer research projects. William Brown, Tom Feasby, Angelika Hahn, and Richard Baltzan critically read portions of the manuscript. Peter Dyck and Art Asbury provided invaluable discussions on uremic neuropathy. Mr. David Bragg, Director of Audiovisual Services at Guy's Hospital, London, England, kindly supplied a color transparency of the portrait of Richard Bright. Nancy Megley of Butterworths has cheerfully given sound advice, and her colleagues have always been helpful.

Neurological Complications of Renal Disease

Chapter 1

Historical Introduction

Contents

Early descriptions of the uremic syndrome and specific concepts of renal disease are presented chronologically, followed by a section dealing selectively with neurological complications.

Early Descriptions

The writings of Aretaeus, the Cappadocian, date to between 81 and 138 A.D. In these, he chiefly describes renal stones and the obstruction of urine flow. He probably gives one of the earliest descriptions of the uremic syndrome, including dropsy, or the accumulation of water in the tissues or cavities of the body.

> Certain persons pass bloody urine periodically: this affliction resembles that from hemorrhoids, and the constitution of the body is alike; they are very pale, inert, sluggish, without appetite, without digestion; and if the discharge has taken place, they are languid and relaxed in their limbs, but light and agile in their head. But if the periodical evacuations do not take place, they are afflicted with headache; their eyes become dim, dull and rolling: hence many become epileptic; others are swollen, misty, dropsical; and others again are filled with melancholy and paralysis. (Adams, 1836)

Aretaeus appears even to have deduced the role of the kidney in detoxifying the blood: "These complaints are the offspring of the stoppage of a customary discharge of blood" (circa 1210–1280).

De Saliceto described "durities in renibus," or sclerosis of the kidneys, as well as renal abscess. He linked hardness of the kidneys to dropsy:

> Signs of hardness of the kidneys are that the quantity of urine is diminished, and there is a heaviness of the kidneys and of the spine with some pain: and the belly begins to swell up after a time and dropsy is produced the second day. (De Saliceto, translated by Major, 1945)

Frederik Dekkers (1695) described the presence of protein in the urine of patients with renal tuberculosis. He also described a method for detecting albuminuria that was unsurpassed for nearly 300 years:

> I cannot pass by that the urines in phthisics and those afflicted with consumption are limpid and clear. Indeed I have observed these placed over a flame too soon become milky, indeed to smell like milk and to have the savor of sweet milk, indeed if a drop or so of acetic acid be added and is exposed the cold air, soon a white coagulum falls to the bottom without doubt cheesy particles, and oily, or buttery particles swim on the top, and now deprived of the said particles all but resembles serum and which all observers agree with me: wherefore we should conclude it to be not so much as chyle finely dissolved or aqueous and usually to on that account to grant the men a brief life. (De Saliceto, translated by Major, 1945)

Domenico Cotugno, a professor of anatomy in Naples, again confirmed albuminuria in dropsy in 1775 (Cotugno, translated by Dock, 1922): "for with two pints of urine exposed to the fire, when scarcely half evaporated, the remainder made a white mass, already loosely coagulated like egg albumen." Further, he noted the effect on mental function: "there was but little urine, and he was wholly cast down in mind."

In 1812, William Charles Wells confirmed the presence of blood protein (albumin) in dropsical urine, noted the edema to occur in the upper parts of the body, and described convulsive seizures in association with renal dropsy.

Richard Bright and Renal Disease

The most comprehensive early work on uremia is that of Richard Bright (1789–1858), who established the connection of systemic illness, including neurological manifestations, with "albuminous urine." At postmortem examination, he uniformly found pathology in the kidneys. The protein was detected by heating the urine in a spoon and looking for coagulation as a milky precipitate. Pathological examinations at the time of his early work in the 1820s and 1830s antedated the microscope. His gross descriptions and the paintings he commissioned for his 1827 book are without comparison. Some of the original kidneys from his cases have been preserved in the museum of

Guy's Hospital in London. These have been recently examined histologically and found to show the same spectrum of diseases as we encounter today: proliferative glomerulonephritis, amyloidosis, etc. Details of Bright's contributions to neurological nephrology are given under History of the Neurological Manifestations in this chapter.

From a survey of a number of cases, Bright deduced the existence of what we now know as poststreptococcal glomerulonephritis, the generalized edema related to proteinuria, the elevation of urea in the blood, and the fluctuating course:

A child, or an adult, is affected with scarlatina, or some other acute disease . . . he is exposed to some casual cause or habitual source of suppressed perspiration, or he discovers his urine is tinged with blood: or without having made any such observation, he awakens in the morning with his face swollen, his ankles puffy or his legs oedematous. If he happens in this condition to fall under the care of a practitioner who suspects the nature of his disease, it is found, that already his urine contains a notable quantity of albumen: his pulse is full and hard, his skin dry, he often has headache, and sometimes without any treatment, the most obvious and distressing of these symptoms disappear; the swelling, whether casual or constant, is no longer observed; the urine ceases to give evidence of any red particle; and according to the degree of importance that has been attached to these symptoms, they are gradually lost sight of, or are absolutely forgotten. Nevertheless, from time to time the countenance becomes bloated; the skin is dry; headaches occur with unusual frequency; or the calls to micturition disturb the night's repose. After a time the healthy color of the countenance fades; a sense of weakness or pain in the loins increases; headaches, often accompanied by vomiting, add greatly to the general want of comfort; and a sense of lassitude, of weariness, and of depression, gradually steal over the bodily and mental frame. . . . If the disease is not suspected, the liver, the stomach, or the brain divide the care of the practitioner, sometimes drawing him away entirely from the important seat of the disease. . . . Again the patient is restored to tolerable health; again he enters on his active duties: or he is perhaps, less fortunate;—the swelling increases, the urine becomes scanty, the powers of life seem to yield, the lungs become oedematous, and, in a state of asphyxia or coma, he sinks into the grave. . . . Should he, however, have resumed the avocations of life, he is usually subject to the constant recurrence of

his symptoms; or again, almost dismissing the recollection of his ailment, he is suddenly seized with an acute attack of pericarditis, or with a still more acute attack of peritonitis, which, without any renewed warning, deprives him in eight and forty hours, of his life. (Bright, 1836)

Early Epidemiology

Bright realized that his initial observations of cases of renal disease underestimated the prevalence of the disorder. He therefore investigated the matter further:

In the winter of 1828–9, I instituted a series of experiments, by taking the patients promiscuously, as they lay on the wards, and trying the effects of heat upon the urine of each, and at the same time employing other re-agents. The whole number I took amounted to 130; out of which no less than eighteen proved to have urine decidedly coagulable by heat . . . and it is worth noting, that in every instance, where the result allowed us to ascertain the state of the kidneys (by post-mortem examination), it corresponded to the (clinical) diagnosis. Those who had albuminous urine were found to have more or less of this disease in the kidneys; whilst those whose urine did not coagulate by heat had kidneys without disease.

The average number of cases with the disease under consideration varies much, as might be expected in different trials . . . it still remains as an incontrovertible fact, that the disease, in its various stages, from its earliest functional derangement to the continued confirmed malady is one of the most frequent, as well as of most fatal occurrence: and I think I am borne out in the estimate . . . that not less than 500 deaths annually occur in this metropolis, from this single disease. (Bright, 1836)

Postmortem Findings

A major component of Bright's monumental work on the association of renal disease with the uremic syndrome is his descriptions and illustrations of the gross anatomical pathology of the kidney.

As part of the general pathology associated with uremia, Bright noted left ventricular hypertrophy of the heart and peritoneal adhesions.

The Concept of Renal Failure

Although the uremic syndrome was produced experimentally by bilateral nephrectomy (Prevot and Dumar, 1821), the concept arose that the uremic syndrome was due to toxins or "nephrolysins" released from the diseased kidney, which acted on the central nervous system (Ascoli, 1903). However, the concept of uremia as an intoxication due to retained metabolites, especially urea, again prevailed. This was strengthened by the development of the chronic uremia model produced by a 75 percent nephrectomy by Bradford in 1892. Renal insufficiency became the accepted mechanism for the uremic syndrome. Subsequently, however, the observations of Pearce (1908) that experimental uremia was associated with increased protein catabolism and that there was an imbalance of renal excretory capacity and exogenous nitrogen intake and nitrogen from catabolism led to a more dynamic concept of renal failure. The functional derangement was elucidated further by Jeghers and Bakst (1938), who described prerenal azotemia. Ditman and Welker (1909) proposed inadequate oxidation by the kidney of various metabolic end products. It became apparent that uremia was not equivalent to just the addition of urine to the blood.

Further refinements of the concept of renal failure came first of all with the separation of hypertensive encephalopathy from the uremic syndrome per se by Oppenheimer and Fishberg in 1928. Peters (1932) clarified altered electrolyte and water metabolism in renal failure.

There then followed a period when attempts were made to treat renal failure in an aggressive and imaginative way, notably dialysis and renal transplantation.

Peritoneal Dialysis

A comprehensive account of peritoneal dialysis for the treatment of renal failure has been provided by Drukker (1983). The first description of the experimental use of peritoneal dialysis in uremia was by Ganter in 1923.

For a number of years, it was used effectively to treat acute renal failure. A stylette-type catheter was used to perform peritoneal lavage for 24 to 72 hours. The catheter was then removed, but the procedure might be repeated if necessary. Long-term treatment by this method was first reported by Boen et al. in 1962. The introduction of the Tenckhoff catheter (Tenckhoff and Schecter, 1963) and closed, continuous-cycle dialysate delivery equipment allowed continuous chronic peritoneal dialysis. The method, however, did not gain much favor until the development, in 1976, of continuous ambulatory peritoneal dialysis (Popovich et al., 1976). This differs from intermittent peritoneal dialysis in that patients instill fluid in their own peritoneal cavity, seal the catheter, are then able to ambulate and every six hours empty the peritoneal cavity and replace the dialysate. Two-liter containers of dialysate are utilized, but other dialysis equipment is not necessary. In the United Kingdom, approximately one-third of all dialysis patients are now treated by this method (Gokal, 1987).

Hemodialysis

The term *dialysis* was coined by Thomas Graham, a Scottish chemist who demonstrated that a vegetable membrane coated with albumin acted as a semipermeable membrane (1861). He also showed that certain crystalloids, particularly urea, passed through the membrane. He even predicted that some of his findings might be applied to medicine. Abel, Rountree, and Turner (1914) first used the term *artificial kidney* when they performed hemodialysis on experimental animals using celloidin tubes and hirudin, a thrombin inactivator found in the salivary glands of leeches, as an anticoagulant. The blood passed through an arterial cannula into the dialysis tubing and was returned to a vein via another cannula.

George Haas (1928) was the first to perform successful hemodialysis in human uremia. His apparatus consisted of a series of celloidin tubes through which the blood circulated in a bath of Ringer's solution. For the anticoagulant he used purified hirudin. Several such dialyses were carried out on patients in the terminal stages of uremia. He achieved modest success in one case but, in general, the dialysis periods were too short and a maximum of 600 mL of blood was dialyzed. The practical development of hemodialysis awaited the use of heparin and the invention of cellophane. This was first attempted using these materials in a uremic dog model by Thalhimer in 1937.

Willem Johan Kolff (1947) was the first to develop a practicable technique of hemodialysis in treating human uremia. Along with J. Berk, he developed an effective dialyzer. The blood was carried in a long cellophane tube that wound around a large drum, which in turn rotated horizontally in a bath of dialysate. The heparinized blood passed from the radial artery into the tubing and was pumped back into an antecubital vein. Heparinization of the blood proved extremely helpful in allowing this development. Kolff did much to promote the use of this treatment around the world.

It was thus possible to successfully treat many patients in acute renal failure. However, access to the arteriovenous system for dialysis was a major problem. In 1960, Quinton and colleagues in Seattle accomplished a major breakthrough with an exteriorized Teflon arteriovenous shunt. It helped reduce the frequency of local infection, septicemia, recurrent clottings, and pulmonary embolism, although such problems continued to occur. In the meantime, workers in Seattle successfully modified the Kiil dialyzing unit, originally invented in Oslo, Norway. Utilizing a cuprophan membrane, they were able to carry out dialysis for longer periods over larger membrane surfaces (Drukker, 1983). It was this same group that was to successfully begin chronic hemodialysis. The first patient they treated, Mr. Clyde Shields, ultimately survived for 11 years, dying at the age of 50 of a myocardial infarction.

Further refinements of hemodialysis have since occurred. A system of home dialysis was first developed in Japan. In 1966, the Cimino-Brescia fistula, an internal connection in the forearm between artery and vein, proved to be a remarkably successful method of hemo-

dialysis access, largely eliminating problems of recurrent clotting and infection (Brescia et al., 1983). This method is extensively used at the present time.

Scribner and colleagues introduced the concept that removal of middle molecules, as opposed to molecules of lower molecular weight, might better control the uremic syndrome (Scribner, 1965; Babb et al., 1973). This has resulted in a number of different types of dialysis machines and dialysis procedures (Drukker, 1983). The most recent advances have included the use of bicarbonate instead of acetate in the dialysis fluid. Hemofiltration is now being tried, the principle being the removal of solutes by convection, a process that mimics the performance of the human kidney. Small and large molecules are moved at the same rate. One drawback may be that smaller molecules, urea and creatinine, are removed somewhat less efficiently. However, it offers the advantage that peripheral nerve function may be better (Drukker, 1983). Finally, knowledge that dialyzers with a cuprophan membrane may eventually induce amyloidosis has prompted a switch to other types of membranes (Chanard et al., 1986).

Renal Transplantation

The first experimental autotransplantation of kidneys in dogs was performed by Ullmann in 1902. In 1908, Alexis Carrel transplanted the kidney from one animal to another.

The first human kidney transplant, from an unrelated donor, was performed by Lawler et al. (1950), in Chicago. Unfortunately, there was evidence of chronic rejection—immunosuppression was not used—although the patient lived for four years after the procedure. The first successful transplantation of the human kidney between identical twins was reported by Merrill et al. (1956). The kidney survived permanently, signs of advanced renal failure and malignant hypertension disappearing.

In 1960, Merrill et al. reported the transplantation of a kidney between nonidentical twins without the use of immunosuppressive drugs and only 450 rads of irradiation to the torso of the recipient. Although a skin graft from the recipient of the kidney to his donor-brother was abruptly rejected, the skin transplant from the kidney donor to the recipient showed a reduced and delayed rejection. The technique has since become so successful that approximately 8,000 operations are now performed every year in the United States.

History of the Neurological Manifestations

As we expressed at the beginning of this chapter, it was recognized during the Christian era that renal failure had important effects on the nervous system. Aretaeus used the following terms with respect to patients with renal failure: sluggish, languid, relaxed, headache, epileptic, melancholy and paralysis (Adams, 1836).

Richard Bright (1827; 1836) described the association of renal disease with the following: headache and lassitude (prominent early symptoms); intermittent confusion; multifocal myoclonus; seizures (both generalized convulsions, which sometimes terminated fatally, and focal seizures); amaurosis and visual blurring (usually transient); tinnitus and decreased hearing; and stupor and coma, which often terminated in death. Some patients developed hemiplegia or apoplexy.

From a series of 100 patients, Bright (1836) traced the course to death in 70 and found "that no less than thirty . . . have died of well-marked symptoms of cerebral derangements, noted under the titles of 'coma,' 'convulsion,' and 'epilepsy'."

However, Bright was not alone in his investigations. James Arthur Wilson (1832–1833), from observations of patients at St. George's Hospital in London, declared "the well-known fact of coma supervening upon retention of urine was adduced as showing the extent to which the brain was influenced by the kidneys—an influence held by the learned author to be produced upon it through the medium of the blood rather than by "nervous sympathy."

Bright's colleague Addison (1839), building on Bright's work at Guy's Hospital, elucidated a set of clinical signs and symptoms that point to a renal etiology for neurological dysfunction: cerebral symptoms (quiet stupor, coma, convulsions, "dullness of intellect, sluggishness of manner and drowsiness, often preceded by giddiness, dimness of sight and pain in the head"), pallor, and hyperventilation: "from the first, [breathing is] much more hurried than is observed in the coma of ordinary apoplexy."

Perhaps one of the best descriptions of renal failure, one that has stood the test of time, is Osler's (1892). These were based on his own observations and those of "French writers." He divided the chief manifestations of renal failure into cerebral, dyspneic, and gastrointestinal. The cerebral manifestations consisted of mania, in which the patient would be noisy, talkative, restless, sleepless, and occasionally violent. The name *delusional insanity* (folie Brightique) was applied to patients who exhibited delusions of persecution or profound melancholia that might end in suicide. Convulsions might occur in a generalized fashion or be "local or Jacksonian." He noted that the "fits may recur rapidly" and, if too rapidly, consciousness was not regained in the interval. However, he stressed that in other instances, unconsciousness would "develop gradually without any convulsive seizures." This state of coma was frequently preceded by headache, and the patient would become "dull and apathetic." "Twitching of the muscles occur, particularly in the face and hands." Finally, there might be "local palsies," which were manifest as hemiplegia or monoplegia. He also emphasized that unless the urine was examined, the nature of the mental disorder might be overlooked. Osler observed that subsequent autopsy might show "no gross lesion of the brain" but only "a localized or diffuse edema."

These observations by Osler remained the definitive statement on the subject until interest in all aspects of renal failure was renewed in the late 1950s by the advent of chronic hemodialysis. At that time, Schreiner (1959) provided a detailed documentation of the various disturbances of mental function in chronic renal failure.

While it was not until the classic paper by Asbury et al. (1963) that it became generally recognized that the peripheral nervous system could be significantly affected in the form of peripheral neuropathy, there were earlier descriptions, although tentative. Kussmaul (1864) described fatty degeneration of the myelin sheath in the sciatic nerve of a uremic patient who suffered from paresis of the legs. In Charcot's 1880 lectures on diseases of the nervous system, he indicated "that the weakness of the limbs observed in the course of urinary disease depends not on a spinal affection but on a lesion of the nerves of the sacral plexus directly produced, as it were, by gradual propagation of the morbid process." In 1887, Lanceraux attributed sensory symptoms to "polynévrite urémique." Once again, in Osler's classic textbook (1892) in a single statement he noted that "other nervous symptoms of uremia are intense itching of the skin, numbness and tingling of the fingers and cramps in the muscles of the calves, particularly at night."

All of these nervous system manifestations at that time, and even now, are presumed to be the result of "uremic toxicity." However, with the advent of modern, aggressive, and often successful forms of treatment, such as dialysis and renal transplantation, a variety of nervous system diseases have arisen that are direct complications of the treatment itself. Thus, as will be seen in the various chapters of this book, diseases of the nervous system in renal failure have now become remarkably complex and varied.

References

Abel JJ, Rountree LB, Turner BB. On the removal of diffusible substances from the circulating blood of living animals by dialysis. J Pharmacol Exp Ther 1914;5:275–316.

Adams F. The extant works of Araetus, the Cappadocian. London: The Sydenham Society, 1836:340–343.

Addison T. Disorders of the brain connected with diseased kidneys. Guys Hosp Rep 1839;4:1–7.

Asbury AK, Victor M, Adama RD. Uremic polyneuropathy. Arch Neurol 1963;8:413–428.

Ascoli G. Vorlesungen über Urämie. Jena; Fischer, 1903:296.

Babb AL, Johansen PJ, Strand MJ, et al. Bi-directional permeability of the human peritoneum to middle molecules. Proc Eur Dial Transplant Assoc. 1973;10:247.

Boen ST, Mulinari AS, Dillard DH, Scribner BH. Periodic peritoneal dialysis in the management of chronic uraemia. Trans Am Soc Artif Intern Organs 1962;8:256–265.

Bradford JR. The influence of the kidney on metabolism. Philos Trans Soc Lond 1892;51:25–40.

Brescia MJ, Cimino JE, Appel K, Hurwicz BJ. Replacement of renal function by dialysis. In: Drukker W, Parsons FM, Maher JF, eds. A textbook of dialysis. New York: Martinus Nijhoff, 1983: 410–439.

Bright R. Reports of medical cases selected with a view of illustrating the symptoms and cure of disease by a reference to morbid anatomy. London: Longman, 1827: 1–88.

Bright R. Cases and observations illustrative of renal disease accompanied by the secretion of albuminous urine. Guys Hosp Rep 1836;1:338–400.

Carrel A. Transplantation in mass of the kidneys. J Exp Med 1908;10:98–140.

Chanard J, Lavaud S, Toupance O, et al. B₂-Microglobulin-associated amyloidosis in chronic haemodialysis patients. Lancet 1986;1:1212.

Charcot JM. Des paraplégies urinaires. In: Bourneville DM, ed. Leçons sur les maladies du système nerveux. 3rd ed. Paris: Delahaye, 1880:295.

Cotugno D. De ischiade nervosa commentarius. Naples and Bologna: St. Thomas Aquinam 1775, 27. In: Dock W, transl. Annals. of medical history. Vol 4. New York: Paul B. Hoeber, 1922:288.

Dekkers F. Exercitationes medicae practicae circa medendi methodum. Leyden: Boutesteyn, 1695: 338.

De Saliceto G. Liber in scientia medicinali: de duritie in renibus. In: Major RH, ed. Classic descriptions of disease. 3rd ed. Springfield: Charles C. Thomas, 1945:526–527.

Ditman NE, Welker WH. Deficient oxidation and its relation to the etiology, pathology and treatment of nephritis. NY J Med 1909;89:1000–1006.

Drukker W. Hemodialysis: a historical review. Replacement of renal function by dialysis. In: Drukker W, Parsons FM, Maher JF, eds. A textbook of dialysis. New York: Martinus Nijhoff Publishers, 1983:24–29; 34–37.

Ganter G. Ueber die Beseitigung giftiger Stoffe aus dem Blute durch Dialyse. MMW 1923;70:1478–1480.

Gokal R. Continuous ambulatory peritoneal dialysis

(CAPD)—ten years on. Q J Med (New Series 63) 1987;242:465–472.

Graham T. Liquid diffusion applied to dialysis. Philos Trans R Soc Lond 1861;151:183–224.

Haas G. Ueber Blutwaschung. Klin Wochenschr 1928;7:1356.

Jeghers H, Bakst HJ. Syndrome of extrarenal azotemia. Ann Intern Med 1938;11:1861–1899.

Kolff WJ. New ways of treating uremia; the artificial kidney, peritoneal lavage, intestinal lavage. London: Churchill, 1947.

Kussmaul A. Beitrage zur Anatomie und Pathologie des Harnapparats. VI. Zur Lehre von der Paraplegia urinaria. Wurzburg Med Z 1864;4:24–72.

Lanceraux E. Les troubles nerveux de l'urémie. Union Med 1887;43:413–418.

Lawler RH, West JW, McNulty PH, et al. Homotransplantation of the kidney in the human. JAMA 1950;144:844–845.

Major RH. Classical descriptions of disease. 3rd ed. 1945.

Merrill JP, Murray JE, Harrison JH. Successful homotransplantation of the human kidney between identical twins. JAMA 1956;160:277–282.

Merrill JP, Murray JE, Harrison JH, et al. Successful homotransplantation of the kidney between nonidentical twins. N Engl J Med 1960;262:1251–1260.

Oppenheimer BS, Fishberg AM. Hypertensive encephalopathy. Arch Intern Med 1928;41:264–278.

Osler W. The principles and practice of medicine. London: Appleton, 1892:737–741.

Pearce RM. The influence of the reduction of kidney substance upon nitrogenous metabolism. J Exp Med 1908;10:632–644.

Peters JP. Salt and water metabolism in nephritis. Medicine 1932;11:435–535.

Popovich RP, Moncrief JW, Decherd JF, et al. The definition of a novel portable-wearable equilibrium dialysis technique. Abstracts of Annual Meeting of Am Soc Artif Intern Organs 1976;5:64.

Prevot JL, Dumas JA. Examen du sang et de son action dans divers phénomènes de la vie. Ann Chim Physique (second series) 1821;23:90–104.

Quinton W, Dillard D, Scribner BH. Cannulation of blood vessels for prolonged hemodialysis. Trans Am Soc Artif Intern Organs 1960;6:104–113.

Schreiner GE. Mental and personality changes in the uremic syndrome. Med Ann DC 1959;28:316–323.

Scribner BH. Discussion. Trans Am Soc Artif Intern Organs 1965; 11:29.

Tenckhoff H, Schecter H. A bacteriologically safe peritoneal access device. Trans Am Soc Artif Intern Organs 1968;14:181–187.

Thalhimer W. Experimental exchange transfusion for reducing azotemia. Use of the artificial kidney for this purpose. Proc Soc Exp Biol Med 1937/38;37:641–643.

Ullmann E. Experimentelle Nierentransplantation. Vorläufige Mitteilung. Wien Klin Wochenschr 1902;15:281–282.

Wells WC. On the presence of red matter and serum of blood in the urine of dropsy, which has not originated from scarlet fever. Trans Soc Improve Med Chir Knowl 1812;3:194–240.

Wilson JA. London Medical Gazette 1832/1833;2:777.

Wilson JA. On fits and sudden death, in connexion with disease of the kidneys. London Medical Gazette 1832/33;11:777–779.

PART ONE

Scientific Background and Critical Approach

Chapter 2

Uremic Neurotoxins and the Biochemical Basis of Neurological Dysfunction in Uremia

Contents

Acronyms

5-HIAA	5-Hydroxyindoleacetic acid
2,4-DHBA	2,4-dihydroxybenzoic acid
3,4-DHBA	3,4-dihydroxybenzoic acid
ATP	adenosine triphosphate
BCAA	branched-chain amino acid
C	carboxy
CNS	central nervous system
CSF	cerebrospinal fluid
EEG	electroencephalogram
GABA	γ-aminobutyric acid
MAO	monoamine oxidase
MG	methylguanidine
N	amino
Na-K-ATPase	sodium-potassium adenosine triphosphatase
NADPH	reduced nicotinamide adenine dinucleotide phosphate
PTH	parathyroid hormone
TPTX	thyroparathyroidectomy

Richard Bright (1831) deduced that in uremia there was an accumulation of substances in the blood that caused neurological dysfunction. The term *uremia* (literally "urine in the blood") was coined by Piorry and l'Hertier (1840) to reflect the same concept.

Bright found the blood contained increased amounts of urea (1831). He astutely considered that urea "may be but in part a cause of the general derangement of the system." Since then, numerous other chemicals have been discovered that accumulate in uremia and that are differentially affected by different treatment modalities. There is as yet no consensus on which is *the* uremic neurotoxin, or which chemicals, in combination, best explain the altered nervous function in uremia.

In this chapter, we shall review the potential neurotoxins and then discuss the altered physiology produced by the toxins.

Proposed Uremic Neurotoxins

The following substances have been found to accumulate in uremia and are discussed in turn, not necessarily in order of importance: urea, creatinine, guanidine and related compounds, uric and oxalic acids, phenols and conjugates of phenol, organic acids of the tricarboxylic acid cycle, aliphatic amines, *myo*-inositol, parathyroid hormone, "middle molecules," and β_2-microglobulin. The roles of amino acid balance in the plasma and brain and of neurotransmitters are also addressed.

Before discussing these substances, it is helpful to consider what qualifications a substance should have in order to be a neurotoxin. It shall be seen that no substance thus far fully meets all of these criteria. Further, there is controversy in some cases over which criteria are met for the various chemicals. These criteria (Hanicki, 1985; Massry, 1985) are similar to those proposed by Koch (1876) for proving the causative role of a bacterium for an infection. These postulates are:

1. The substance must be identifiable, and its chemical structure must be known.

2. The substance should be elevated in the blood of patients with uremia. Furthermore, a direct, positive, linear relationship should be shown between the degree of encephalopathy or neuropathy and the blood level of the proposed chemical.

3. The substance should be capable of causing encephalopathy/neuropathy when given to experimental animals in doses that produce blood levels similar to those encountered in human uremic encephalopathy/neuropathy. There should be a correlation of plasma and/or nervous tissue levels with specific symptoms.

4. Removal of the substance from the blood of affected humans and experimental animals should improve cerebral or peripheral nerve function.

Urea

Urea is formed by the liver as an end product of protein metabolism (Figure 2.1), whether the protein is from food or from the catabolism of proteins in the body. Elevation of urea in the blood and tissues is one of the most striking abnormalities in uremia. Urea enters the brain and cerebrospinal fluid (CSF) at rates slower than it penetrates systemic tissues (Kleeman et al., 1962). This causes dehydration in the

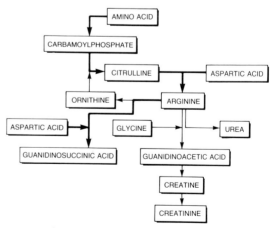

Figure 2.1. The urea cycle is shown. The pathway leading to guanidinosuccinic acid is shown with bold arrows (redrawn from Cohen, 1970).

brain and spinal cord when urea is infused acutely. When equilibrated, the concentration of urea is higher in gray than in white matter. The concentration ultimately is higher in the central nervous system (CNS) than in plasma. It is possible that urea attaches to intracellular proteins in a dissociable fashion. In acute uremia, there is a good correlation between the severity of illness and the serum urea level. In chronic renal failure, the creatinine level correlates better with severity of illness.

Urea could act as an enzyme inhibitor. In concentrations comparable to those found in uremia (0.05 to 0.2 M), urea significantly inhibits monoamine oxidase (MAO) (Giordano et al., 1962). Interestingly, inhibition did not occur at higher or lower concentrations. There are implications for effects of urea on brain amines (especially serotonin), which are degraded by MAO. Lascelles and Taylor (1966) tested several individual chemical substances known to accumulate in uremic plasma for their effect on the oxygen uptake of brain slices. They found that urea at 500 mg/dL, but not at 200 mg/dL, inhibited oxygen uptake. However, ultrafiltrates of plasma from seven patients in uremic coma, with urea concentrations ranging from 310 to 530 mg/dL, produced no significant inhibition of oxygen metabolism. They therefore proposed an inhibitor substance in uremic plasma that prevents urea's effect on oxidative metabolism. Their findings suggest that in clinical uremia, urea is not responsible for reduced brain oxidative metabolism.

Urea administration to patients on chronic hemodialysis induces carbohydrate intolerance (Hutchings et al., 1966). Urea and creatinine each inhibit glucose uptake and utilization in rat diaphragm *in vitro;* together the effect is additive (Bakestru et al., 1982). It is possible that the effects of urea on enzyme activity and glucose metabolism could contribute to altered brain metabolism in uremia, but the contribution appears to be a minor one.

Some early studies on experimental animals suggested that urea may play an important role in the production of lethargy, stupor, and coma, as well as in the manifestations of neuronal excitability, including myoclonus and seizures.

Grollman and Grollman (1959) used different amounts of urea in the dialysate in dogs maintained on peritoneal dialysis for 4 to 10 days after bilateral nephrectomies. The study lacked a control group of nephrectomized animals treated with peritoneal dialysis without urea added to the dialysate. Thus, it is difficult to attribute the retching, vomiting, and decrease in conscious level in their animals to urea alone. Furthermore, the serum levels of urea ranged from 5.4 to 15.6 g/L, levels considerably higher than those encountered even in the most severe cases of acute uremia.

Stevenson et al. (1959) studied the effects of intravenous urea infusions into cats following bilateral ureteric ligation. The study was uncontrolled. Spontaneous epileptiform activity occurred in the cerebral cortex, but there was no consistent relation of nonprotein nitrogen level to epileptiform activity on the electrocorticogram. In one cat, epileptiform activity was seen only with nonprotein nitrogen blood levels of 290 mg/dL or greater. There was no abnormality found in somatosensory evoked responses or in thalamic or midbrain periaqueductal gray matter activity. There were no abnormalities in serum electrolytes or serum ammonia.

Zuckerman and Glaser (1972) studied cats during infusions of urea and other osmotic substances (mannitol, sucrose, and sodium chloride). Abnormalities were found only with urea infusions. After a delay of more than 60 minutes, epileptiform activity in the form of paroxysmal depolarization shifts occurred in neurons of the nucleus reticularis gigantocellularis and the nucleus reticularis caudalis of the medulla. This was associated with myoclonic jerking. The reticular epileptiform activity could be abolished by sectioning the spinal cord or by inducing muscular paralysis with curare. The latter indicated an interaction of sensory systems, at least from muscle afferents, on the nucleus reticularis gigantocellularis. This study was performed without ureteric ligation or nephrectomies, so the effects could be attributed to the urea itself. The cellular mechanism is uncertain; the 60-minute lag time begs the question of an indirect action of the urea.

In this acute model, urea was found to have a specific effect on a CNS structure known to be important in the generation of myoclonus in other experimental models and probably in some clinical types of myoclonus in humans (Halliday, 1986). The type of myoclonus encountered in humans with acute uremia resembles reticular reflex myoclonus induced experimentally by urea infusions (Chadwick and French, 1979). It is still unclear, however, whether this acute urea infusion model has clinical relevance.

It is unlikely that urea plays a significant role in the neurotoxicity of chronic uremia. Merrill et al. (1953) dialyzed chronically uremic patients against solutions of high urea concentrations and noted clinical improvement, even though the serum urea levels were unaltered.

Creatinine

Creatinine is formed as an anhydride of creatine. Creatine synthesis is initiated in the kidney by the formation of guanidosuccinic acid and is completed in the liver by the coupling with *S*-adenosylhomocysteine. Creatinine is an end product of the metabolism of amino acids, which involves the process of transamidation. Creatinine production is directly proportional to lean body mass; normally, its excretion is also affected by age (Cockcroft and Gault, 1976). Creatinine production and excretion is reduced in chronic renal failure (Mitch et al., 1980), but its serum level still roughly reflects the severity of the renal dysfunction.

Creatinine has a tranquilizing effect when administered to healthy rats (Lis and Bijan, 1970). However, there is no hard clinical or experimental evidence that creatinine acts as a neurotoxin. Acute administration of creatinine to dogs with a single nephrectomy produced serum levels of 18 to 38 mg/dL (Giovanetti et al., 1969). These animals did not show any clinical neurological manifestations. In concentrations of 50 mg/dL, creatinine had no effect on metabolism of rat cortical slices (Lascelles and Taylor, 1966).

Guanidine and Related Compounds

There are several guanidine compounds that either are produced in greater than normal amounts or accumulate in the blood or tissues in uremia. These are methylguanidine, guanidinoacetic acid, and guanidinosuccinic acid.

Methylguanidine (MG) is closely related to creatine (methylguanidoacetic acid). In uremia, MG is increased in the serum and is excreted in the urine in increased quantities (Stein et al., 1971). In fact, the metabolic production of MG is increased above normal in uremia (Giovanetti et al., 1973). This may be due to conversion of creatinine to MG and possibly accounts for the decreased creatinine production in advanced uremia (Mitch et al., 1980; Giovanetti et al., 1973). In the anuric dog model, MG is increased to about eight times control values in liver and skeletal muscle (Giovanetti et al., 1969) Giovanetti and Barsotti (1975) argue that MG is mainly intracellular and exerts its toxic effect by enzyme inhibition, although these statements have yet to be justified. Its concentration in brain, sciatic nerve, and CSF is about one-eighth the concentration in other organs in both controls and experimental animals, but brain MG is increased by the same factor as for other organs. Sciatic nerve MG increased to only three times control values in uremia.

Giovanetti et al. (1969) acutely intoxicated dogs with MG, producing serum levels within the range encountered in human uremic patients. The dogs had a single nephrectomy prior to receiving MG injections. Maximum survival time was 19 days. The animals became anorexic and required intravenous fluid, electrolyte, and glucose administration. Red blood cells survival and production were reduced; platelet counts dropped. Gastric erosions and pulmonary edema and hemorrhages occurred. The dogs showed ataxia, tremors, myoclonic twitching, and convulsions. Motor nerve conduction was slowed. At postmortem, regional swellings, fragmentation, and disruption were found in axons in peripheral nerve, dorsal columns of the spinal cord, and cerebral cortex. Foci of demyelination were also found in peripheral nerve. Although confounding issues included the anorexic state, with the probability of disturbed nutrition and fluid and electrolyte balance, this experiment provides suggestive evidence that MG can be acutely toxic and produce systemic as well as neurological abnormalities that are seen in clinical uremia.

Further studies of MG by Giovanetti et al. (1973) showed that when used alone in normal dogs in a more chronic model, MG produced encephalopathic features, such as hypertonicity and myoclonic twitches, only with advanced intoxication. Similarly, nerve conduction slowed only when serum MG levels rose to about four times those achieved in dogs with ureteric ligation.

MG administration to dogs causes a flattening of the glucose tolerance curve, likely related to facilitated glucose uptake in tissues (Balestri et al., 1972).

Minkoff et al. (1972) produced inhibition of brain sodium-potassium (N-K) ATPase *in vitro* by adding MG in a concentration equal to 1:20 that found in uremic plasma (see Sodium and Potassium Transport, Acid-Base Balance, and Permeability Changes in Uremia, below).

Felgate and Taylor (1972), using MG concentrations more than four times those encountered in uremic plasma, failed to produce any alterations in oxygen uptake by cerebral cortical, liver, or kidney slices. This argues against any significant depressant metabolic effect and against MG accounting for uremic coma, in which depressed cerebral oxygen uptake occurs.

Guanidinoacetic acid is a product of the urea cycle and a precursor of creatine and thus of creatinine. It is increased in uremic plasma to levels about three times normal, as a result of decreased creatinine clearance. Increases in guanidinoacetic acid levels lead to preferential shunting of the amidine group of arginine to aspartate, causing increased formation of guanidinosuccinic acid (see Figure 2.1) (Cohen, 1970). This reduces the amount of guanidinoacetic acid, which would otherwise accumulate in greater amounts in uremia.

Guanidinosuccinic acid has been proposed

as a more likely neurotoxin than the other guanidine compounds (Cohen, 1970). It clearly does increase in uremic plasma and CSF (Stein et al., 1969), as a "preferred" product of arginine metabolism (see Figure 2.1). However, there is no evidence that it has any toxic effect on the brain or other organ systems when given to experimental animals, either acutely or chronically (Dobbelstein et al., 1971). Although *in vitro* guanidinosuccinic acid decreases platelet factor III function (Stein et al., 1968; Stein et al., 1971), no increased bleeding tendency was found in experimental animals by Dobbelstein et al. (1971). Lonergan et al. (1970) found that guanidinosuccinic acid produced significant inhibition of erythrocyte transketolase. Whether this is important as a cause of neurological dysfunction is uncertain, as guanidinosuccinic acid is dialyzable (see Transketolase Function, below).

Guanidine, itself, when administered to humans for treatment of myasthenic syndrome, can produce anorexia, gastric discomfort, nausea, vomiting, pruritus, paresthesias, and muscle fasciculations (Giovanetti and Barsotti, 1975), likely by facilitating release of acetylcholine from nerve terminals.

Guanidine causes inhibition of oxygen uptake in kidney but not in cerebral slices (Lascelles and Taylor, 1966). This occurred only at concentrations higher than those found in uremic plasma. A mixture of guanidine, MG, and guanidinosuccinic acid produce an increase in glucose uptake by isolated rat diaphragm (Balestri et al., 1972); guanidine may play an additive role in the production of uremic hypoglycemia.

Even in severe renal failure, the concentration of guanidine in the plasma or tissues is too low to exert significant toxicity by itself (Giovanetti and Barsotti, 1975).

Uric and Oxalic Acids

Both uric and oxalic acids accumulate in uremia (Wills, 1985). Uric acid retention does not parallel that of creatinine because of reduced tubular reabsorption in the kidney and uricolysis in the gastrointestinal tract in uremia. This appears to be an adaptive mechanism in uremia. There is no known neurotoxic effect of uric acid, although it may play a role in uremic pericarditis (Clarkson, 1966).

Oxalic acid can accumulate in crystalline form in the myocardium and kidney tissues in uremia (Wills, 1985). It is possible that the functioning of these organs could be affected if such accumulation is extensive. Further, oxalate can act as an enzyme inhibitor, especially for lactate dehydrogenase isoenzymes 1 and 2 (Emerson and Wilkinson, 1965). There is no evidence of direct or indirect neurotoxicity, however.

Phenols, Aromatic Hydroxyacids, and Indican

These substances are increased in body fluids in uremia. Phenols are elevated in conjugated, but not in free, form (Schmidt et al., 1950). Conjugated phenols have little, if any, toxicity (Schmidt et al., 1950; Dunn et al., 1958). However, it has been proposed that phenols may exist intracellularly in the unconjugated state (Kramer et al., 1968) and thus act as toxins.

A number of aromatic acids have been assessed for their ability to inhibit respiration and the activity of several brain enzymes. These have been tested on rat brain slices in free, rather than conjugated, form at concentrations of over 100 times those found in uremic plasma (Hicks et al., 1964). Those experiments showed that cinnamic acid inhibited oxygen consumption and activities of MAO, glutamic acid decarboxylase (involved in synthesis of γ-aminobutyric acid, an inhibitory neurotransmitter), and aromatic acid decarboxylase (involved in the synthesis of dopamine and serotonin). Phenylacetic acid inhibited glutamic acid decarboxylase and aromatic acid decarboxylase. The relevance of these experiments to clinical uremia is suspect. There is a possibility that the same chemicals, present over a longer time at lower concentrations, could exert a depressant effect on enzyme function, or there may be an additive effect with other metabolic poisons. This is speculative and completely unproven.

In rats with bilateral ureteric ligation, Record et al. (1969) administered 150 μmol/100 g body weight of 3,4-dihydroxybenzoic acid (3,4-DHBA), 2,4-dihydroxybenzoic acid (2,4-DHBA), or saline. Rats with 3,4-DHBA injections had shorter survival times and showed decreased motor activity compared to saline controls. Myoclonic jerks, grand mal seizures, and paroxysmal bursts of generalized epileptiform activity on electroencephalogram (EEG) were also more common in animals treated with 3,4-DHBA than in those treated with 2,4-DHBA or saline, although numbers in each group (four, four, and six, respectively) were too small for statistical treatment. In this study, there is suggestive evidence that 3,4-DHBA is more toxic than 2,4-DHBA or saline. However, the chemical was injected in large bolus doses to rats that were acutely uremic. There was no measurement of plasma levels of the chemical. The relevance to uremia of the huge, pharmacological doses of the free form of a compound (that is normally present mainly in conjugated form) used in this model is dubious. It is of interest, however, that 3,4-DHBA, which bears stronger chemical resemblance to dopamine and catecholamines than its isomer 2,4-DHBA, is more toxic than 2,4-DHBA.

Several aromatic acids (hippurate, m-hydroxyhippurate, p-hydroxyhippurate, and p-hydroxybenzoic acids) have been identified in the dialysate of uremic patients by Kramer et al. (1965). Hippuric acid was found in concentrations 11 to 87 times those of the other compounds. The question of toxicity was not addressed, however.

A strong blow against significant toxicity of indican, major phenols, and aromatic hydroxyacids, was rendered by Giovanetti and Barsotti (1975), who administered these substances to healthy dogs over a three-week period. Plasma levels ranged from those observed in uremic patients to 10 times higher. No neurological or behavioral symptoms appeared.

Amines

Both aliphatic (Simenoff et al., 1963) and aromatic (Morgan and Morgan, 1966) amines are elevated in plasma of uremic patients. There has been speculation that amines may cause neurotoxicity, similar to the effect in hepatic encephalopathy (Simenoff et al., 1963). However, intravenous administration of methylamine, dimethylamine, and ethanolamine to healthy dogs to increase plasma concentration to 10 times those found in uremic plasma failed to have any toxic effect (Giovanetti and Barsotti, 1975).

myo-*Inositol*

myo-Inositol is a cyclic hexitol that acts as a substrate in phospholipid, especially phosphatidylinositol, metabolism. The latter system acts as a "second messenger" in those cells that do not use cyclic adenosine monophosphate. Phosphatidylinositols form a component of myelin in both central and peripheral nervous systems. There is also evidence that they may play a role in ion channels (Hawthorne and Kai, 1970).

myo-Inositol is deficient in tissues and blood of diabetics, but accumulates in uremic patients' plasma, probably as a result of decreased renal catabolism (Clements et al., 1973). In uremia, hemodialysis reduces plasma levels from an initial average of 17 times to about seven times the upper limit of normal (Blumberg et al., 1978). In uremic patients, levels of *myo*-inositol in CSF are about 3.5 times higher than normal (Blumberg et al., 1978).

Clements et al. (1973) found that hyper-*myo*-inositolemia from oral loading in rats produced significant reduction in motor nerve conduction velocity. On this basis, it was proposed that *myo*-inositol may act as a neurotoxin in uremia, contributing to progressive peripheral neuropathy. Reznek et al. (1971) studied plasma *myo*-inositol, creatinine clearance, motor and sensory (sural) nerve conduction velocity, and clinical features in conservatively managed and chronically hemodialyzed uremic patients. There was a correlation between plasma *myo*-inositol levels and creatinine clearance and between the logarithm of sensory conduction velocity in the sural nerve and *myo*-inositol levels in the con-

servatively treated patients. However, there was no correlation of plasma *myo*-inositol concentration with motor nerve conduction velocity in either group, with clinical evidence of peripheral neuropathy in either group, or with sensory conduction velocity in the hemodialyzed group. Blumberg et al. (1978) were unable to find any correlation of plasma or CSF *myo*-inositol levels with nerve conduction velocity or qualitatively graded EEG changes in a group of 28 uremic patients. One patient who had stupor, asterixis, and seizures, which resolved with increased dialysis, had only moderately elevated CSF *myo*-inositol during the acute illness (Blumberg et al., 1978).

At most, *myo*-inositol may slow conduction velocity in peripheral nerves, but the evidence is against it being a major clinical neurotoxin for either the central or peripheral nervous system.

Middle Molecules

A Seattle research group noted that polyneuropathy occurred less frequently in patients on intermittent peritoneal dialysis than in uremics on hemodialysis. In patients on hemodialysis therapy, peripheral neuropathy decreased when dialysis time was prolonged (Scribner and Babb, 1978). This led them to propose that the peritoneal membrane was more permeable to some uremic toxins than was artificial dialysis membrane. The latter clears lower molecular weight solutes more efficiently than peritoneal membrane, and such clearance is dependent on plasma and dialysis flow rates and dialysis time. On the other hand, clearance of some substances of somewhat higher molecular weight is more dependent on the membrane characteristics and surface area of the membrane, as well as on the amount of time for dialysis. This led to the formal "square meter–hour hypothesis" (Babb et al., 1971) and the "middle-molecule" concept (Babb et al., 1972).

The molecular size of the more slowly cleared toxic substances was first stated to be from 2,000 to 5,000 daltons (Babb et al., 1971), but the range of "middle molecules" was subsequently lowered to 500 to 2,000 daltons (Babb et al., 1972).

Early studies suggested that peak 7 was the most important middle-molecule fraction (Furst et al., 1975) in that these compounds impaired glucose utilization and amino acid transport *in vitro* (Frohling et al., 1982). This same fraction correlated with levels of parathyroid hormone (PTH) (See Parathyroid Hormone and Calcium Metabolism, below) and decreased after parathyroidectomy. It should be pointed out that this middle-molecule fraction is not equivalent to PTH (molecular weight, 9,000d) or its fragments (molecular weight, > 3,000d). A major component of the peak 7c has been identified as glucuronidated *o*-hydroxybenzoylglycine (Zimmerman et al., 1981), but its functional role has not been studied. The identity of peak 7 needs to be clarified, as does any regulatory role of PTH over the fraction. Toxicity of the individual chemicals then should be assessed.

The end point of peripheral neuropathy is a somewhat imprecise basis for studying a dose effect of such presumed chemical substances. Central nervous signs and symptoms form an equally imprecise basis for quantitative comparison with plasma levels of middle molecules (Valek et al., 1986). However, the clinical status of the central and peripheral nervous systems has been regarded as an important method of assessing uremic toxicity in biological terms. Thus far, plasma concentrations of middle molecules have not correlated well with such clinical measurements (Valek et al., 1986).

The separation and identification of candidate chemicals has been a monumentally difficult task. There has been great effort to develop techniques that differentiate uremic from nonuremic plasma and to specify potentially toxic middle molecules. If a quantitative approach is used, there are logistic problems in that there is not a reproducible relationship between the elution volumes of the standards and their molecular weights (Brunner and Mann, 1985). Also, many middle molecules are small peptides whose amino acid side chains interact with the gel matrix (Brunner and Mann, 1985). It has been very difficult to adequately separate different substances using gels and chromatograhic techniques. Some

combinations have been moderately successful, such as the combined use of high-speed gel filtration and subsequent gradient elution chromatography using a diethylominoethyl cellulose Sephadex microcolumn (Furst et al., 1975).

Several middle molecules have been identified in plasma and CSF (Sperschneider et al., 1982), but their specific neurotoxicity awaits confirmation. These include a dipeptide (Akibo et al., 1978a), a basic tripeptide (Akibo et al., 1978c), an acidic tripeptide (Akibo et al., 1980), a pentapeptide containing tryptophan and showing inhibitory effects on rosette formation of sheep erythrocytes (Akibo et al., 1979), a heptapeptide corresponding to the 13 through 19 amino acid sequence of β_2-microglobulin (Akibo et al., 1978b), a hexapeptide (Bovermann et al., 1982), glucuronidated *o*-hydroxybenzoylglycine (Zimmerman et al., 1981), and a glucuronide (Brunner and Mann, 1985).

The use of alternate methods of separation according to molecular shape, polarity, and complexing techniques, as well as refinements of electrical charge separation (such as isotachophoresis and ion-pair chromatography) may hold promise (Brunner and Mann, 1985).

Thus far, it apears that the number of potential neurotoxins in the middle-molecule range has exceeded expectation (Brunner and Mann, 1985). The middle-molecule hypothesis is still alive, but remains a hypothesis until considerably more work is done. The status of some middle molecules has been likened to the Loch Ness monster, which, although it may have been seen, needs to be further validated (Hanicki, 1985). A positive outcome of the middle-molecule hypothesis has been the careful examination of hemodialysis techniques, not only dialysis time and frequency, but the dialysis membrane itself. New membranes have been and are still being developed that have different spectra of separation characteristics.

β_2-*Microglobulin*

β_2-Microglobulin is a low molecular weight protein (11,800d) that is present in small amounts in serum and other body fluids of healthy humans (Berggard and Bearn, 1968). It has been found to accumulate in the plasma of patients who have been on hemodialysis for many years, probably because conventional hemodialysis does not remove this molecule. Geyjo et al. (1986) found that the amyloid present in the flexor retinacula of four patients on chronic hemodialysis with carpal tunnel syndrome was composed of β_2-microglobulin units. The authors postulate that amyloid fibrils are formed from plasma β_2-microglobulin and are deposited in the region of the carpal tunnel. Whether there is a more systemic effect of this newly described form of amyloidosis is not yet settled.

Parathyroid Hormone and Calcium Metabolism

PTH is an 84–amino acid peptide that is present in the circulation in three forms: as the intact hormone and as carboxy (C)- and amino (N)-terminal fragments. PTH plays an important role in calcium and phosphate homeostasis by increasing phosphate exertion in renal tubules and promoting calcium and phosphate resorption from bone. In uremia, plasma phosphate elevation causes a decrease in ionized calcium concentration, which stimulates release of PTH. There is also a relative resistance to PTH at its sites of action in uremia. A sustained output of PTH leads to hyperplasia of the parathyroid glands. Furthermore, the reduction of renal mass in uremia impairs the renal degradation of PTH, especially the C-terminal fragment. Most of the biological actions of PTH lie with the N- rather than the C-terminal fragment, however (Slatopolsky et al., 1980). It is unknown whether the C-terminal fragment in high concentrations has any toxic effect.

A careful prospective clinical study was performed by Avram et al. (1979) on uremic patients on hemodialysis programs. Group I consisted of four patients with normal or moderately elevated PTH levels. Group II contained five patients with markedly increased plasma PTH concentrations. Group III comprised two patients who underwent parathy-

roidectomy. Group II patients had more striking EEG abnormalities and lower nerve conduction velocities than did group I patients. Group III patients showed improved nerve conduction velocities after parathyroidectomy. This initial study was encouraging, but numbers were small. Further, it was difficult to control for age and duration on dialysis.

Parathyroidectomy has also been shown to improve the EEG in humans with primary hyperparathyroidism (Berggard and Bearn, 1968). In acute uremia in humans, the EEG abnormalities occur in association with elevated levels of the N-terminal PTH fragment (Cooper et al., 1978; Goldstein et al., 1980).

Further evidence of a neurotoxic role for PTH comes from experimental literature. Akmal et al. (1984) performed a study on partially nephrectomized dogs (a model for chronic uremia). Seven dogs had thyroparathyroidectomies (TPTX) and seven did not. Those without TPTX had a significantly higher percentage of EEG frequencies under 7 Hz than did those with TPTX. Furthermore, brain calcium levels were increased in both groups compared to nonuremic controls but were significantly higher in those without, than in those with, TPTX. Mahoney et al. (1983) found that the calcium increase was mainly in the cerebral cortex and the hypothalamus.

Similar effects of TPTX on prevention of nerve conduction slowing and excessive calcium accumulation in peripheral nerves in an acute uremia model (bilateral ureteric ligation) were shown by Massry (1983). Mahoney et al. (1983) used a bilateral nephrectomy model in the dog to study acute renal failure and a partial nephrectomy model to study chronic renal failure. These workers did not find any slowing of motor nerve conduction velocity in either group. Although these authors found brain calcium to be elevated, peripheral nerve calcium was decreased in acute renal failure and was low normal in chronic renal failure. There was no effect of prior TPTX on nerve calcium in their model. It should be noted, however, that their uremic model did not produce even electrophysiologic evidence of neuropathy. Since peripheral neuropathy is not a feature of hyperparathyroidism, it seems unlikely that PTH plays a significant role in the pathogenesis of uremic neuropathy. The role of PTH on peripheral nerve function is thus unsettled.

The mechanism for the putative neurotoxicity of PTH is uncertain. One possibility is an increase in brain calcium, which has been found in experimental animals (Akmal et al., 1984; Mahoney et al., 1983; Goldstein and Massry, 1978; Fraser et al., 1985b). Fraser et al. (1985b), using an acute uremia model, found evidence that the increase was due to entry of calcium into synaptosomes (membrane vesicles formed from presynaptic terminals from the brain) in uremia. This entry appeared to be due to an enduring change in permeability to calcium, which was energy dependent. Such a change of membrane behavior was observed *in vitro* without PTH being present. It is possible that PTH induced some effect on the membrane that persisted, however. Such changes in brain calcium transport could alter neuronal function, especially neurotransmission. At the present time, the role of PTH in the increased brain calcium content is unsettled.

Adler and Berlyne (1985) have challenged the significance of increased PTH and the role of increased brain calcium in uremic encephalopathy. Using a chronic uremia model, they found that brain mitochondrial calcium content, which they maintain reflects intracellular calcium, is not increased, although there is an increase in total brain calcium. These authors did not find any correlation of brain calcium content with PTH levels. They also propose that in uremia increased PTH levels may be necessary to maintain normal brain calcium levels. The extra brain calcium, they propose, is membrane or protein bound.

Although the issue is still unsettled, PTH, or one of its degradation products, comes closer than any potential toxin studied thus far in satisfying the criteria for a neurotoxin. Whether PTH can account for the neuropathy, the severe degrees of encephalopathy, or the full spectrum of encephalopathic features seems unlikely. There may be other potential mechanisms by which PTH operates; for example, alteration of phospholipid metabolism, Na-K-ATPase function, neurotransmitter release (via altered intracellular-extracellular calcium ratio), or membrane permeability or integrity.

Amino Acids and Neurotransmitters

It has been shown that uremia is associated with abnormal concentrations of various amino acids in plasma (Alvestrand et al., 1982). Plasma levels of the branched-chain amino acids (BCAAs) leucine, isoleucine, and valine, as well as taurine, threonine, tyrosine, phenylalanine, and lysine are reduced, while citrulline and L-methylhistidine are increased. The skeletal muscle pool of amino acids is also altered; the amino acid imbalance does not entirely reflect that found in plasma. For example, tyrosine is deficient in muscle, but not in plasma. Some of these changes are due to uremia itself, and others are due to nutritional factors. The low levels of BCAAs may relate to increased insulin secretion in uremia; although there is resistance to insulin's effects in general, BCAA metabolism retains its sensitivity to insulin. Reduced tyrosine concentration in plasma may be due to decreased phenylalanine hydroxylase or to increased tyrosine aminotransferase (Alvestrand et al., 1982). Different modes of dialysis affect plasma amino acid concentrations differently (Biasoli et al., 1983). Hemodialysis alters concentrations more than intermittent peritoneal dialysis, when pre- and posttreatment states are compared. Biasoli et al. (1983) have noted alterations in plasma to CSF amino acid ratios for several amino acids (especially the BCAAs) as a result of hemodialysis. However, there was little change in absolute CSF amino acid concentrations, except a reduction in aspartic acid and citrulline. Pye et al. (1979) studied patients with chronic renal failure who were fairly stable but who had never been dialyzed. They found significant differences between these patients and controls in CSF concentrations of the following amino acids: phosphoserine, phosphoethanolamine, glycine, valine, tyrosine, ornithine, and lysine. Hemodialysis lowers CSF concentrations of the following amino acids: phosphoserine, taurine, phosphoethanolamine, threonine, valine, ornithine, and lysine (McGale et al., 1979). There is a lag in clearance of CSF compared to plasma.

Biasioli et al. (1986) have found that CSF ratios of glycine to BCAAs and phenylalanine to tyrosine are increased in chronic uremia compared to controls. The CSF to plasma ratio of glutamine was also increased. Jeppson et al. (1982) studied acute and chronic uremic animal models and did not find any essential differences between them in regard to brain and plasma levels of amino acids. Despite the reduction of BCAA levels in plasma, they were not reduced in brain. Some neutral amino acids were, however, taken up more readily than basic amino acids. Their findings suggest a blood-brain barrier alteration in uremia, but the importance is unknown; it is uncertain whether these findings would account for a neurotransmitter imbalance in the CNS. The significance of variations in CSF levels of amino acids is unclear, as is the ratio of plasma to CSF amino acid levels. McGale et al. (1977) found that in healthy individuals there was no correlation between plasma and CSF levels of the following amino acids: taurine, serine, valine, isoleucine, asparagine, phosphoserine, and phosphoethanolamine. Many other amino acids do show a strong correlation between the plasma and CSF levels, but there are other factors that alter CSF amino acid composition in healthy individuals, including age and sex (Massry, 1983). Furthermore, even in healthy persons there are fairly large standard deviations for CSF concentrations of most amino acids (Massry, 1983). These factors do not appear to have been adequately considered in the studies on uremic patients.

Competing amino acids play a role in transport across the blood-brain barrier for tryptophan, which is important in serotonin synthesis. Uremic rats fed 18 percent casein diets had lower brain serotonin levels than those fed an 11 percent casein diet (Siassi et al., 1977).

There is some evidence for altered neurotransmitter function in uremia. Biasioli et al. (1986) found increased CSF levels of homovanillic acid, a product of dopamine. Jellinger et al. (1978) found brain dopamine to be reduced in a patient dying of uremic coma. Ksiazek (1982) found dopamine and norepinephrine turnover and MAO activity, which is involved in their breakdown, to be decreased in the brain in uremia.

Sullivan et al. (1980) did not find any difference in CSF levels of the serotonin precursor tryptophan between uremic patients and controls but found elevated levels of 5-hydroxyindoleacetic acid (5-HIAA) in uremic patients, as did Biasioli et al. (1986). Jellinger et al. (1978) found increased 5-HIAA levels in the brains, especially in the midbrain region, of three patients dying of uremic coma. Patients who died of hepatic encephalopathy had similar findings (Jellinger et al., 1978). Free, or unbound, plasma tryptophan levels are elevated in uremia and are reduced by hemodialysis (Sullivan et al., 1980), an effect which is at least partly due to increased plasma protein binding. Serotonin concentration and turnover were increased in most brain regions in the acutely uremic rat model (Ksiazek, 1982). Serotonin has been implicated in several CNS functions: sleep and other body rhythms, thermoregulation, memory, anterior pituitary regulation, appetite, eating and drinking behavior, respiration, blood pressure and heart rate control, and pain regulation.

Taurine accumulates in plasma in renal failure (Alvestrand et al., 1982). It was shown to be increased, along with γ-aminobutyric acid (GABA) in the brain cortex of experimental animals (Michalk et al., 1982). Taurine is thought to be a neuromodulator in the CNS. (Neuromodulators alter the response of a neuron to a neurotransmitter either by altering transmitter release or by modulating the postsynaptic receptor function.) Although taurine facilitates the influx of calcium into neurons, potassium influx also increases, and the resting membrane potential appears to be stabilized (Durelli et al., 1982). It has potent antiepileptic properties in experimental models of epilepsy (Huxtable, 1981). GABA serves mainly as an inhibitory neurotransmitter in the CNS (McGeer and McGeer, 1981) that acts principally by hyperpolarizing the neuron through opening chloride channels. Michalk et al. (1982), using experimental animals with chronic uremia, found that brain taurine levels are increased out of proportion to concentrations in other organs and that the taurine levels are lowered (but still above normal) if dietary methionine is reduced. The observation that GABA and taurine levels are increased in chronic but not in acute renal failure (Michalk et al., 1982) may explain, in part at least, why convulsions are less common in chronic than in acute renal failure. These authors propose that the increase in these chemicals is a compensatory mechanism adapted by the brain to counteract increased neuronal excitability, which occurs in uremia.

The role of the possible "false neurotransmitter" octopamine has yet to be fully evaluated in uremia. Octopamine, or p-hydroxy-β-phenylethanolamine, is probably formed as a byproduct in the formation of catecholamines. It is present in plasma of healthy individuals in concentrations between 0 and 1.91 ng/mL, with a mean of 0.24 ng/mL (Kinniburgh and Boyd, 1979). Its physiological role, if any, remains to be defined. It can be taken up, stored, and released by central nerve terminals (Baldessarini, 1971; Baldessarini and Vogt, 1971), and it may block the actions of putative neurotransmitters at postsynaptic receptors. Octopamine has been found to accumulate in plasma in hepatic failure (Lam et al., 1973; Fischer, 1974). It is increased to a lesser extent in plasma in primary renal failure (Lam et al., 1973). It may be, at least in part, synthesized by bacteria in the gut, as plasma levels are reduced when animals with hepatic failure are given neomycin (Fischer, 1974). A possible alternative mechanism for increased production is related to amino acid imbalance. In hepatic and renal failure, there is accumulation of phenylalanine and tyrosine. Tyrosine hydroxylase, which converts tyrosine to dopa (dihydroxyphenylalanine, the precursor of dopamine), has significant rate limitations, and is inhibited by end products of catecholamine metabolism (Kaufman and Friedman, 1965). If this were to occur in hepatic or renal failure, phenylalanine and its hydroxylated product, tyrosine, might be metabolized by an alternative pathway to tyramine and then to octopamine by dopa decarboxylase and dopamine β-hydroxylase, respectively.

A role for octopamine in uremic encephalopathy has to be viewed with caution. The plasma levels are elevated, but only moderately compared with those in hepatic failure. Paradoxically, plasma octopamine levels are higher after than before hemodialysis (Kinni-

burgh and Boyd, 1979). This may occur because of the increased release of transmitters from sympathetic nerve terminals during the stress of dialysis. However, since dialysis is helpful in preventing uremic encephalopathy, this finding raises serious doubts about octopamine's potential role as a uremic neurotoxin.

Major Theories of Pathogenesis

This section discusses the major theories by which the presumed uremic toxin(s) affects brain function. These are listed separately, not necessarily in order of likelihood.

The Trade-off Hypothesis

Bricker (1972) has proposed that the systemic side effects of homeostatic mechanisms in renal failure may constitute a trade-off for such homeostasis. The argument is as follows: In renal failure, there is a net reduction in renal function. Surviving nephrons, even if they are diseased, have to increase their activity to compensate for the reduction in the number of functioning nephrons. Such increase in function has to be regulated by a mechanism in the body that senses altered function, for example, the accumulation of a solute. In the case of solute regulation, this is likely to be a hormone. The increased level of hormone in the blood may have adverse effects on other organ systems, such as the nervous system. The hormone then constitutes a uremic neurotoxin.

Bricker uses the example of a secondary hyperparathyroidism in renal failure. However, other regulatory hormones, such as natriuretic factor, are also candidates.

Transketolase Function

Transketolase is an enzyme involved in the pentose phosphate shunt (Figure 2.2). The pentose phosphate shunt is active in the brain and probably accounts for 5 to 8 percent of glucose metabolism in the CNS (Hostetler et

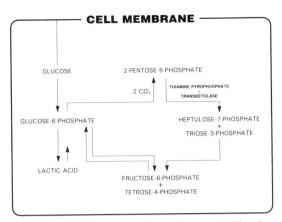

Figure 2.2. The "pentose phosphate shunt." The site of action of transketolase and thiamine pyrophosphate is shown.

al., 1970). The shunt's main function in the CNS is to provide the reduced form of nicotinamide adenine dinucleotide phosphate (NADPH) required for the reductive processes necessary for lipid synthesis. The activity of the shunt is depressed if transketolase activity is deficient. Transketolase activity is dependent on thiamine pyrophosphate as a cofactor, as well as on magnesium.

Lonergan et al. (1970) found that erythrocyte transketolase activity in uremic subjects was depressed, especially in those with clinical neuropathy. Further, they found that uremic plasma inhibited transketolase activity in erythrocytes from nonuremic subjects. The inhibitory substance had a molecular weight of under 500 daltons. The addition of thiamine did not correct the impaired transketolase activity when due to uremia, but hemodialysis did. These authors propose that transketolase deficiency may be an important mechanism for uremic neuropathy. Since the enzyme is present in the CNS as well, CNS dysfunction, especially problems with myelin maintenance, might be expected. It has yet to be substantiated that there is deficient transketolase activity in the central or peripheral nervous system in uremia. This depends on the hypothesized toxin crossing the blood-brain and blood-nerve barriers. Furthermore, some patients may have neuropathy or encephalopathy despite continued hemodialysis.

Disturbed Energy Metabolism

Unless uremic patients have significant vascular disease, total cerebral blood flow is normal (Heyman et al., 1951; Scheinberg, 1954). Brain glucose and oxygen uptake are reduced (Heyman et al., 1961; Scheinberg, 1954). Levels of adenosine triphosphate (ATP), phosphocreatine, and glucose are normal to increased in acutely and chronically uremic experimental rats (Van den Noort, 1967; Van den Noort et al., 1968; Van den Noort et al., 1970; Mahoney et al., 1984). In uremia, brain levels of adenine, adenine monophosphate, adenine diphosphate, and lactate were lower than normal. (Van den Noort et al., 1970; Mahoney et al., 1984). The brain energy charge potential, a measure of high-energy phosphate content, was normal (Mahoney et al., 1984). Mild hypoxia failed to alter these values (Mahoney et al., 1984), but severe acute ischemia (30 seconds after decapitation before freezing) showed uremic rats to have decreased utilization of high-energy phosphate stores compared to controls (Van den Noort et al., 1970). These findings are similar to those observed with anesthesia (Lowry, et al., 1964). Adenosine itself does not appear to be responsible for the abnormal response to ischemia; although it increases brain ATP and phosphocreatine, there is normal utilization of high-energy phosphate and glucose in the face of anoxic-ischemic insult (Van den Noort et al., 1968).

Sodium and Potassium Transport, Acid-Base Balance, and Permeability Changes in Uremia

Sodium and potassium transport across the cell membrane is dependent on a specific adenosine triphosphatase enzyme. An early study by Welt et al. (1964) reported elevated levels of sodium in erythrocytes in severely uremic patients. In rats with acute uremia (bilateral nephrectomy), Minkoff et al. (1972) found decreased brain Na-K-ATPase when assayed either in the presence of ouabain, an inhibitor of the sodium-potassium membrane pump, or by the deletion of potassium from extracellular fluid. Animals were sacrificed in the extreme terminal phase of the uremic illness. These findings are in conflict with those of Van den Noort et al. (1970), who found normal levels of Na-K-ATPase in their acutely and chronically uremic rat models, but the latter group did find other evidence of defective ATP utilization (see Disturbed Energy Metabolism, above). In an *in vitro* experiment, Minkoff et al. (1972) found that MG and inorganic phosphate each caused inhibition of Na-K-ATPase.

Fraser et al. (1985a) studied sodium transport in synaptosomes, membrane vesicles from the synaptic regions of the brain. They found that sodium-potassium transport in brains from acutely uremic rats was normal in the "resting" state. However, when the ATPase enzyme was stimulated by veratridine, brain sodium transport was decreased in uremic rats compared to controls. This was shown to be due to reduced activity of the ouabain-sensitive sodium-potassium pump. Since this assay was done *in vitro*, not in the presence of uremic plasma, it appears that the alteration of Na-K-ATPase function is an enduring functional change in neuronal membrane produced by uremia.

It is not clear just how the reduction of stimulated, as opposed to resting, Na-K-ATPase activity would affect brain function in uremia. Presumably at high levels of synaptic activity, there could be problems in sodium and potassium handling and a delay in restoring the membrane potential from a depolarized state. If there is deficient Na-K-ATPase function, what is causing it? Izumo et al. (1984) have found the inhibitory substance to be dialyzable. Whether it could be MG remains to be determined.

Using erythrocytes, Welt (1969) confirmed that the ouabain-sensitive sodium-potassium pump is defective in uremia. He also showed that another component of the sodium-potassium pump, known as pump II, which is inhibited by ethacrynic acid, also shows reduced activity in uremia. Whether this has physiological significance to the brain is uncertain.

The chemical environment of the brain or extracellular fluid is reflected in the composition of the CSF. Brennan and Plum (1971) showed that CSF from severely uremic patients, when infused into the cerebral ventricles of healthy cats, caused an encephalopathy, as measured by disturbed behavior. There is evidence of altered blood-brain barrier function in uremia. Freeman et al. (1962) showed that there is increased penetration of bromide into the CSF of uremic patients and that this increased permeability was reversed by dialysis. Fishman and Raskin (1967) and Fishman (1970), using the acutely uremic rat model, demonstrated increased permeability of the blood-brain barrier to insulin and sucrose. The effect was greater with sucrose, probably because of its smaller molecular size. Penicillin entry was at first slowed for two hours, then increased. There was decreased flux of sodium and increased entry of potassium from plasma to brain, but the authors did not determine which compartment (extracellular fluid space versus parenchyma) was affected. Net sodium and potassium content were increased in the brain.

Despite these changes, there appear to be powerful homeostatic mechanisms in the brain. Brain water content is not increased (Fishman, 1970), and the extracellular fluid (sulfate) space is normal (Fishman and Raskin, 1967). Potassium concentration in CSF does increase, but the rate of rise is less than in plasma, probably because of increased sodium-potassium pump activity by the choroid plexus (Hise and Johanson, 1979). A rise in potassium concentration in the extracellular fluid of the brain could produce depolarization of neurons and increased excitability (Somjen et al., 1986). However, glia have uptake mechanisms to prevent potassium concentration elevations in the brain parenchyma (Katzman and Pappius, 1973). The actual mean level of interstitial brain potassium concentration in uremia is not known. Brain parenchyma does show a small, steady increase with progressive worsening of acute uremia (Hise and Johanson, 1979). Cerebrospinal fluid production is reduced by about 25 percent in uremia, but CSF electrolyte and acid-base balance are quite well maintained, even in advanced uremia (Posner et al., 1965). Posner et al. (1965) showed that CSF pH in uremia remained normal or was slightly alkalotic in all their uremic patients. This was confirmed by Arieff et al. (1976), who also found that brain intracellular pH was normal in uremia. Hemodialysis was associated with a rise in plasma pH but a fall in CSF pH. As expected, this was more marked with rapid, as opposed to slow, hemodialysis. Brain parenchyma pH remained normal with slow hemodialysis but fell significantly with rapid hemodialysis. Such changes are transient and are restored after equilibrium is reestablished. It has been proposed this may account for the acute encephalopathy accompanying hemodialysis (see Chapter 7B).

Although homeostatic mechanisms undoubtedly prevent encephalopathy from alterations of commonly measured electrolytes and pH changes, the increased blood-brain and blood-nerve permeability may contribute to the entry of certain uremic toxins that are not routinely measured.

The Role of Aluminum, Calcium, and Other Minerals

There is good evidence that aluminum plays an important role in dialytic encephalopathy, or dialysis dementia (see Chapter 7A). However, it may also play a role in uremic encephalopathy, if one considers aluminum to cause a spectrum of neurological impairment, with mild (uremic) encephalopathy at one end and full-blown dialytic encephalopathy at the other end.

Calcium has been discussed above (see Parathyroid Hormone and Calcium Metabolism). It should be mentioned that calcium homeostasis is also regulated by 1,25-dihydroxyvitamin D_3. This vitamin is dependent for its synthesis (hydroxylation of 25-hydroxyvitamin D_3) on the kidney. Furthermore, 1,25-dihydroxyvitamin D_3 has effects on the CNS and may be antagonistic to PTH (Ritz and Merke, 1986). This could have implications for uremic encephalopathy, but much more work is needed.

Fraser et al. (1985b) showed that there is increased calcium uptake into uremic rat brain synaptosomes. This could lead to augmented neurotransmitter release and increased lysosomal enzyme release. This could have impli-

cations for uremic encephalopathy and possibly for neuropathy.

The role of magnesium in uremic encephalopathy is largely unexplored. Magnesium depletion could occur from poor nutritional intake, impaired absorption from the gut, vomiting, or diarrhea (Lim et al., 1969). Intracellular magnesium depletion in skeletal muscle is not rare in uremic patients, but whether this has clinical importance is not known (Lim et al., 1969). Theoretically, intracellular magnesium deficiency could alter the function of several enzyme systems, including those involved in the breakdown of ATP (which has a role in axoplasmic transport and other functions), transketolase (see Transketolase Function, above), and catecholamine o-methyltransferase, CO, which is involved in catecholamine metabolism (Coyle and Snyder, 1981). Adler and Berlyne (1985) found in their chronically uremic rat model that brain magnesium was depressed. These same authors, however, also found brain calcium to be reduced, in contrast to reports of others. Magnesium accumulation is more common, probably because of impaired renal excretion (Lindeman, 1986). This is usually mild, but more serious hypermagnesemia may occur if the patient receives a large oral load that cannot be excreted. Hypermagnesemia can cause encephalopathy, respiratory failure, muscle weakness, and areflexia. More subtle effects on the brain, notably on learning and memory, could theoretically result from excess magnesium. Memory is likely dependent on an electrophysiological phenomenon known as long-term potentiation, which is dependent on activation of N-methyl-D-aspartate receptors on neurons. The ion channels for this receptor are blocked by elevated extracellular magnesium concentrations (Ascher and Nowak, 1987).

Altered Neurotransmitter and Synaptic Function

Evidence for altered concentrations of various putative neurotransmitters has been discussed above (see Amino Acids and Neurotransmitters). In addition to imbalance of various neurotransmitters and altered neurotransmitter function, altered function of neuromodulators such as peptides, including neurohormones, has not been adequately addressed. Further work is needed regarding toxins that interfere with normal synaptic function, including false neurotransmitters such as octopamine, and substances in the extracellular fluid. The latter could interfere with synaptic function by altering neurotransmitter release (e.g., by acting on or blocking autoreceptors on nerve terminals), by acting on or blocking receptors on postsynaptic membrane, or by interfering with ion channel function. Neurotoxins could also alter the effects of synaptic activity by interfering with "second messenger" physiology after receptor activation.

Enzyme Inhibition

Wills (1985) proposed that several of the potential neurotoxins discussed above (urea, creatinine, phenols and other aromatic compounds, and amines) could act together to cause neuronal failure because of multiple enzyme inhibitions. Individual enzyme inhibitions by the various chemicals are minor, but combined effects could produce more significant consequences.

Axonal Transport

Brauger et al (1986) showed *in vitro* that the 2.5 fraction of middle molecules from uremic patients has an inhibitory effect on tubulin 6S polymerization. The mechanism of this inhibition was different from the action of Vinca alkaloids and colchicine, previously recognized inhibitors of tubulin polymerization. The authors propose a similar phenomenon could account for uremic polyneuropathy.

Conclusion

As can be deduced from the above discussion, the "uremic neurotoxin" has not been positively identified. Some conclusions are possible, however.

1. The toxin(s) is (are), for the most part, dialyzable and removed fairly well by thrice weekly hemodialysis. This largely prevents uremic neuropathy and encephalopathy. These conditions may persist to a mild degree in some patients, however.
2. It is possible to exclude as toxins, or to reduce to a minor role, some chemicals that accumulate in the blood in uremia. These include: urea, creatinine, guanidinoacetic acid, guanine, uric and oxalic acids, phenols, indican, aromatic hydroxyacids, methylamine, dimethylamine, ethanolamine, and *myo*-inositol.
3. Most neurotoxin candidates have not been sufficiently investigated or characterized, or there is conflicting information about them. These are still in the running, but unproven: methylguanidine, middle molecules, PTH, amino acid imbalance, and false neurotransmitters.
4. It seems naive to think that one chemical could be solely responsible for all the neurotoxic phenomena in uremia. Even if the effects of one chemical predominate, the combined or additive role of other chemicals is quite likely.
5. It is entirely possible that other neurotoxins, some of which could be very important, have not yet been identified in the "chemical wasteland" of uremia.

In terms of the mechanisms by which the uremic neurotoxin may exert its effects, a number of possibilities were put forward: a trade-off such that a hormone exerts an effect in return for maximal nephron function; transketolase deficiency and decreased NADPH and myelin synthesis; impaired energy metabolism; altered sodium, potassium, calcium, or magnesium handling; problems with microtubule formation and distal axonopathy; altered synaptic physiology; and enzyme inhibition.

It is clear that there are powerful homeostatic mechanisms in the nervous system that must be overcome for toxins to exert their effect. There does not appear to be a problem with high energy levels in the nervous system, with water content of the nervous system, or with acid-base balance.

Altered synaptic function in the CNS undoubtedly accompanies uremic encephalopathy, but the factors that produce this altered physiology are not fully identified. Altered sodium and calcium transport and abnormal neurotransmitter and neuromodulator functions seem likely candidates. The role of altered intracellular functions needs to be considered as well. This may be especially important in the neuron's response to acute stress regarding the utilization of high-energy phosphate stores and the handling of intracellular calcium, free radicals, and other chemicals capable of damaging the intracellular structures. Microtubule formation and problems in axoplasmic transport could especially affect neurons with long axons.

References

Adler AJ, Berlyne GM. Effect of chronic uremia in the rat on cerebral mitochondrial calcium concentrations. Kidney Int 1985;27:523–529.

Akibo T, Kumikawa M, Dazai S, et al. Studies on uraemic toxins; structure-activity correlation in H-Asp(Gly)-OH. Biochem Biophys Res Commun 1978a;82:707.

Akibo T, Kumikawa M, Higuchi H, Sekino H. Identification and synthesis of a heptapeptide in uremic fluid. Biochem Biophys Res Commun 1978b;84:184–194.

Akibo T, Kumikawa M, Ishazaki M, et al. Identification and synthesis of a tripeptide in ECUM fluid of a uremic patient. Biochem Biophys Res Commun 1978c;83:357–364.

Akibo T, Onodera I, Sekino H. Isolation, structure and biological activity of the Trp-containing pentapeptide from uremic fluid. Biochem Biophys Res Commun 1979;89:813–821.

Akibo T, Onodera I, Sekino H. Characterization of an aciditic tripeptide in neurotoxide dialysate. Chem Pharm Bull (Tokyo) 1980;28:1629–1633.

Akmal M, Goldstein DA, Multani S, Masry SG. Role of uremia, brain calcium and parathyroid hormone on changes in electroencephalogram in chronic renal failure. Am J Physiol 1984;246:F585–F589.

Alvestrand A, Furst P, Bergstrom J. Plasma and muscle free amino acids in uremia: influence of nutrition with amino acids. Clin Nephrol 1982;18:297–305.

Arieff AI, Guisado R, Massry SG, Lazarowitz VC. Central nervous system pH in uremia and the effects of hemodialysis. J Clin Invest 1976;58:306–311.

Ascher P, Nowak L. Electrophysiological studies of NMDA receptors. TINS 1987;10:284–288.

Avram MM, Iancu M, Morrow D, et al. Uremic syndrome in man: new evidence for parathormone as a multisystem neurotoxin. Clin Nephrol 1979;11:59–62.

Babb AL, Farrell PC, Urelli DA, Scribner BH. Hemodialyzer evaluation by examination of solute molecular spectra. Trans Am Soc Artif Intern Organs 1972;18:98–105.

Babb AL, Popovich RP, Christopher TG, Scribner BH. The genesis of the square meter–hour hypothesis. Trans Am Soc Artif Intern Organs 1971;17:81–91.

Baldessarini RJ. Release of aromatic amines from brain tissues of the rat in vitro. J Neurochem 1971;18:2509–2518.

Baldessarini RJ, Vogt M. Uptake and subcellular distribution of aromatic amines in the brain of the cat. J Neurochem 1971;18:2519–2533.

Balestri PL, Rindi P, Biagini M, Giovanetti S. Effects of uremic serum, urea, creatinine and methylguanidine on glucose metabolism. Clin Sci 1972;42:395–404.

Berggard I, Bearn AG. Isolation and properties of a low molecular weight β-2 globulin occurring in human biological fluids. J Biol Chem 1968;243:4095–4103.

Biasoli S, Chiaramonte S, Fabris A, et al. Neurotransmitter imbalance in plasma and cerebrospinal fluid during dialytic treatment. Trans Am Soc Artif Intern Organs 1983;29:44–49.

Biasoli S, D'Andrea G, Feriani M. et al. Uremic encephalopathy: an updating. Clin Nephrol 1986;25:57–63.

Blumberg A, Esslen E, Burgi W. *myo*-Inositol—a uremic neurotoxin? Nephron 1978;21:186–191.

Bovermann G, Rautenstrauch H, Seybold G, Jung G. Isolierung, Strukturaufklärung und Synthese eines Hexapeptide aus dem Hämodialysat urämischer Patienten. Hoppe Seylers Z Physiol Chem 1982; 363:1187–1202.

Braguer D, Gallice P, Monti JP et al. Inhibition of microtubule formation by uremic toxins: action mechanism and hypothesis about the active component. Clin Nephrol 1986;25:212–218.

Brennan RW, Plum F. A cerebrospinal fluid transfer model for hepatic and uremic encephalopathies. Trans Am Neurol Assoc 1971;96:210–211.

Bricker NS. On the pathogenesis of the uremic state: an exposition of the "trade-off hypothesis." N Engl J Med 1972;296:1093–1099.

Bright R. Reports of medical cases with a view of illustrating the symptoms and cure of disease by reference to morbid anatomy. Vol 2. Longman, Rees, Orme, Brown and Green, London, 1831.

Brunner H, Mann H. What remains of the "middle molecule" hypothesis today? Contrib Nephrol 1985;44:14–39.

Chadwick D, French AT. Uraemic myoclonus: an example of reticular reflex myoclonus? J Neurol Neurosurg Psychiatry 1979;42:52–55.

Clarkson BA. Uric acid related to uremic symptoms. Proc Eur Dial Transplant Assoc 1966;3:3–7.

Clements RS Jr, De Jesus PV Jr, Winegrad AI. Raised plasma myo-inositol levels in uremia and experimental neuropathy. Lancet 1973;1:1137–1141.

Cockcroft DW, Gault MH. Prediction of creatinine clearance from serum creatinine. Nephron 1976;16:31–41.

Cohen BD. Guanidosuccinic acid in uremia. Arch Intern Med 1970;126:846–850.

Cooper JD, Lazarowitz VC, Arieff AI. Neurodiagnostic abnormalities in patients with acute renal failure. Evidence for neurotoxicity of parathyroid hormone. J Clin Invest 1978;61:1448–1455.

Coyle JT, Snyder SH. Catecholamines. In: Siegel GJ, Albers RW, Agranoff BW, Katzman R. Basic neurochemistry. Boston: Little, Brown, 1981;205–217.

Dobbelstein H, Grunst J, Schubert G, Edel HH. Guanidinbernsteinsäure und Urämie. II. Tierexperimentelle Befunde. Klin Wschr 1971;49:1077–1083.

Dunn I, Weinstein IM, Maxwell MH, Jutzler GA. Significance of circulating phenols in anemia of renal disease. Proc Soc Exp Biol Med 1958;99:86–88.

Durelli L, Mutani R, Fassio F, et al. Taurine and hyperexcitable human muscle: effects of taurine on potassium-induced hyperexcitability of dystrophic myotonic and normal muscles. Ann Neurol 1982;11:258–265.

Emerson PM, Wilkinson JH. Urea and oxalate inhibition of the serum lactate dehydrogenase. J Clin Pathol 1965;18:803–807.

Felgate RA, Taylor WH. The effects of methylguanidine on glucose metabolism. Clin Sci 1972;42:395–404.

Fischer J. False neurotransmitters and hepatic coma. In: Plum F, ed. Brain dysfunction in metabolic disorders. Res Publ Assoc Res Nerve Ment Dis 1974;63:53–73.

Fishman RA. Permeability changes in experimental uremic encephalopathy. Arch Intern Med 1970;126:835–837.

Fishman RA, Raskin NH. Experimental uremic encephalopathy. Arch Neurol 1967;17:10–20.

Fraser CL, Sarnacki P, Arieff AI. Abnormal sodium transport in synaptosomes from brain of uremic rats. J Clin Invest 1985a;75:2014–2023.

Fraser CL, Sarnacki P, Arieff AI. Calcium transport abnormality in uremia brain synaptosomes. J Clin Invest 1985b;76:1778–1795.

Freeman RB, Sheff MF, Maher JF, Schreiner GE. The blood-cerebrospinal fluid barrier in uremia. Ann Intern Med 1962;56:233–240.

Frohling PT, Kokot F, Cernacek P, et al. Relation between middle molecules and parathyroid hormone in patients with chronic renal failure. Miner Electrolyte Metab 1982;7:48–53.

Furst R, Bergstrom J, Gordon A, et al. Separation of middle molecule peptides from uremic patients. Kidney Int 1975;7:272–275.

Gejyo F, Odani S, Yamada T, et al. β-2 microglobulin: a new form of amyloid protein associated with chronic hemodialysis. Kidney Int 1986;30:385–390.

Giordano C, Bloom J, Merrill JP. Effects of urea on physiological systems. 1. Studies on monamine oxidase activity. J Lab Clin Med 1962;59:396–400.

Giovanetti S, Baigini M, Balestri PL, et al. Uremia-like syndrome in dogs chronically intoxicated with methylguanidine and creatinine. Clin Sci 1969;36:445–452.

Giovanetti S, Balestri PL, Barsotti G. Methylguanidine in uremia. Arch Intern Med 1973;131:709–713.

Giovanetti S, Barsotti G, Uremic intoxication. Nephron 1975;14:123–133.

Goldstein DA, Feinstein EI, Chiu LA, et al. The relationship between the abnormalities in the electroencephalogram and blood levels of parathyroid hormone in dialysis patients. J Clin Endocrinol Metab 1980;51:130–134.

Goldstein DA, Massry SG. Effects of parathyroid hormone and its withdrawal on brain calcium and electroencephalogram. Miner Electrolyte Metab 1978;1:84–91.

Grollman EF, Grollman A. Toxicity of urea and its role in the pathogenesis of uremia. J Clin Invest 1959;38:749–754.

Halliday AM. Evolving ideas on the neurophysiology of myoclonus. In: Fahn S, Marsden CD, Van Woert M, eds. Advances in neurology. Vol. 43. Myoclonus. New York: Raven Press, 1986;339–355.

Hanicki Z. Middle molecules, myth or reality? Mater Med Pol 1985;17:51–55.

Hawthorne JN, Kai M. Metabolism of the phosphoinositides. In: Lajtha A, ed. Handbook of neurochemistry. Vol. 3. New York: Plenum Publishers, 1970:491–507.

Heyman A, Patterson JL, Jones RW Jr. Cerebral circulation and metabolism in uremia. Circulation 1951;3:558–563.

Hicks JM, Young DS, Wootton ID. The effect of uraemic blood constituents on certain cerebral enzymes. Clin Chim Acta 1964;9:228–235.

Hise MA, Johanson CE. The sink action of cerebrospinal fluid in uremia. Eur Neurol 1979;18:328–337.

Hostetler KY, Landau BR, White RJ, et al. Contribution of the pentose cycle to the metabolism of glucose in the isolated perfused brain of the monkey. J Neurochem 1970;17:33–39.

Hutchings RM, Hegstrom RM, Scribner BH. Glucose intolerance in patients on long-term intermittent dialysis. Ann Intern Med 1966;65:275–285.

Huxtable RJ. Insight on function: metabolism and pharmacology of taurine in the brain. In: Lombardine JB, Kenny A, eds. The role of peptides and amino acids as neurotransmitters. New York: Alan R. Liss, 1981:53.

Izumo H, Izumo S, DeLuise M, Flier JS. Erythrocyte Na-K ATPase pump in uremia. Acute correction of a transport defect by dialysis. J Clin Invest 1984;74:581–588.

Jellinger K, Reiderer P, Kleinberger G, et al. Brain monoamines in human hepatic encephalopathy. Acta Neuropathol 1978;43:63–68.

Jeppson B, Freund HR, Gimmon Z, et al. Fischer JE. Blood-brain barrier derangement in uremic encephalopathy. Surgery 1982;92:30–35.

Katzman R, Pappius HM. Brain electrolytes and fluid metabolism. Baltimore: Williams & Wilkins, 1973.

Kaufman S, Friedman S. Dopamine β-hydroxylase. Pharmacol Rev 1965;17:71–100.

Kinniburgh DW, Boyd ND. Determination of plasma octopamine and its level in renal disease. Clin Biochem 1979;12:27–32.

Kleeman CR, Davson H, Levin E. Urea transport in the central nervous system. Am J Physiol 1962;203:739–747.

Koch R. Die Aetiologie der Milzbrand-Krankheit begründet auf die Entwick—lungsgeschichte des Bacillus antracis. Beitr Biol Pflanzen 1876;2:277–310.

Kramer B, Seligson H, Baltrush H, Seligson D. The isolation of several aromatic acids from the hemodialysis fluids of uremic patients. Clin Chim Acta 1965;11:363–371.

Kramer HJ, Keller HE, Kramer HK, Jutzler GA. Studies on concentrations of single phenolic compounds in serum of patients treated with chronic intermittent hemodialysis. Proc Eur Dial Transplant Assoc 1968;5:213–218.

Ksiazek A. Brain serotonin and catecholamine turnover in uremic rats. Nephron 1982;31:270–272.

Lam KC, Tall AR, Goldstein GB, Mistilis S. Role of a false neurotransmitter, octopamine, in the pathogenesis of hepatic and renal encephalopathy. Scand J Gastroenterol 1973;8:465–472.

Lascelles PT, Taylor WH. The effect upon tissue respiration *in vitro* of metabolites which accumulate in uraemic coma. Clin Sci 1966;31:403–413.

Lim P, Dong S, Khoo OT. Intracellular magnesium depletion in chronic renal failure. N Engl J Med 1969;280:981–984.

Lindeman RD. Chronic renal failure and magnesium metabolism. Magnesium 1986;5:293–300.

Lis AW, Bijan R. The function of creatinine. Physiol Chem Phys 1970;2:293–299.

Lonergan ET, Semar M, Lange K. Transketolase activity in uremia. Arch Intern Med 1970;126:851–854.

Lowry OH, Passonneau JV, Hassellberger FX, Schulz DW. Effect of ischemia on known substrates and cofactors of the glycolytic pathway in brain. J Biol Chem 1964;239:18–30.

Mahoney CA, Arieff AI, Leach WJ, Lazarowitz VC. Central and peripheral nervous system effects of chronic renal failure. Kidney Int 1983;24:170–177.

Mahoney CA, Sarnacki P, Arieff AI. Uremic encephalopathy: role of brain energy metabolism. Am J Physiol 1984;247 (Renal Fluid Electrolyte Physiol 16): F527–F532.

Massry SG. The toxic effects of parathyroid hormones in uremia. Semin Nephrol 1983;3:306–328.

Massry SG. Current status of the role of parathyroid hormone in uremic toxicity. Contrib Nephrol 1985;49:1–11.

McGale AHF, Pye IF, Corston R, et al. The effect of haemodialysis on cerebrospinal fluid and plasma amino acids. Clin Chim Acta 1979;92:73–80.

McGale AHF, Pye IF, Stonier C, et al. Studies of the inter-relationship between cerebrospinal fluid and plasma amino acid concentrations in normal individuals. J Neurochem 1977;29:291–297.

McGeer PL, McGeer EG. Amino acid neurotransmitters. In: Siegel GL, Albers RW, Agranoff BW, Katzman R, eds. Basic Neurochemistry. Boston: Little, Brown, 1981:233–253.

Merrill JP, Legrain M, Hoigne R. Observations on the role of urea in uremia. Am J Med 1953;14:519–520.

Michalk DV, Essich H-J, Bohles HJ, Scharer K. Taurine and hyperexcitable human muscle: effects of taurine on potassium-induced hyperexcitability of dystrophic myotonic and normal muscles. Ann Neurol 1982;11:258–265.

Minkoff L, Gaertner G, Manoochehr D, et al. Inhibition of brain sodium-potassium ATPase in uremic rats. J Lab Clin Med 1972;80:71–78.

Mitch WE, Collier VU, Walser M. Creatinine metabolism in chronic renal failure. Clin Sci 1980;58:327–335.

Morgan RE, Morgan JM. Plasma levels of aromatic amines in renal failure. Metabolism 1966;15:479–481.

Piorry PA, l'Hertier D. Traité des alterations du sang. Paris: Ballière, 1840.

Posner JB, Swanson AG, Plum F. Acid-base balance in cerebrospinal fluid. Arch Neurol 1965;12:479–496.

Pye LF, McGale AHF, Stonier C, et al. Studies of cerebrospinal fluid and plasma amino acids in patients with steady state chronic renal failure. Clin Chim Acta 1979;92:65–72.

Record NB, Prichard JW, Gallagher BB, Seligson D. Phenolic acids in experimental uremia. Arch Neurol 1969;21:387–394.

Reznek RH, Salway JG, Thomas PK. Plasma myo-inositol concentration in uraemic neuropathy. Lancet 1971;1:675–676.

Ritz A, Merke J. Recent findings in 1,25 (OH)$_2$ vitamin D$_3$ may provide new concepts for understanding the pathogenesis of uremia. Contrib Nephrol 1986; 50: 109–118.

Scheinberg P. Effects of uremia on cerebral blood flow and metabolism. Neurology 1954;4:101–105.

Schmidt EG, McElvain NF, Bowen JJ. Plasma amino acids and ether-soluble phenols in uremia. Am J Clin Pathol 1950;20:253–261.

Scribner BH, Babb AL. Retrospective support for the middle molecule hypothesis. Proceedings of the Seventh International Congress on Nephrology. Basel: Karger, 1978:663–667.

Siassi F, Wang M, Koppe JD, Swendseid ME. Plasma tryptophan levels and brain serotonin metabolism in chronically uremic rats. J Nutr 1977;107:840–845.

Simenoff ML, Asatoor AM, Milne MD, Silva JF. Retention of aliphatic amines in auremia. Clin Sci 1963;25:65–77.

Slatopolsky E, Martin K, Hruska K. Parathyroid hormone metabolism and its potential as a uremic toxin. Am J Physiol 1980;239 (Renal Fluid Electrolyte Physiol 8):F1–F12.

Somjen GG, Aitken PG, Giacchino JL, McNamara JO. Interstitial ion concentrations and paroxysmal discharges in hippocampal formation and spinal cord. In: Delgado-Escueta AV, Ward AA, Woodbury DM, Porter RJ, eds. Advances in neurology. Vol. 44. Basic mechanisms of the epilepsies: Molecular and cellular approaches. New York: Raven Press, 1986:663–680.

Sperschneider H, Spustova V, Stein G, Dzurik R. Middle molecular weight substances in the cerebrospinal fluid of uremic patients. Clin Nephrol 1982;17:298–302.

Stein IM, Cohen BD, Horowitz HI. Guanidosuccinic acid: "X" factor on uremic bleeding? Clin Res 1968;16:397.

Stein IM, Cohen BD, Kornhauser RS. Guanidinosuccinic acid in renal failure, experimental azotemia and inborn errors of the urea cycle. N Engl J Med 1969;280:926–930.

Stein IM, Perez G, Johnson R, Cummings NB. Serum levels and excretion of methylguanidine in chronic renal failure. J Lab Clin Med 1971;77:1020–1024.

Stevenson GC, Jacobs RC, Ross MW, et al. Effect of urea on central nervous system activity in the cat. Am J Physiol 1959;197:141–144.

Sullivan PA, Murnaghan D, Callaghan N, et al. Effect of dialysis on plasma and CSF tryptophan and CSF 5-hydroxyindoleacetic acid in advanced renal disease. J Neurol Neurosurg Psychiatry 1980;43:730–743.

Valek A, Spustova V, Lopot F, et al. Can plasma concentration of middle molecules contribute to assessment of adequate dialysis treatment. Artif Organs 1986;19:37–44.

Van den Noort S. Brain nucleotides in experimental uremia. Neurology 1967;17:303.

Van den Noort S, Eckel RE, Brine K, Hrdlicka JT. Brain metabolism in uremic and adenosine-infused rats. J Clin Invest 1968;47:2133–2142.

Van den Noort S, Eckel RE, Brine K, Hrdlicka JT. Brain metabolism in experimental uremia. Arch Intern Med 1970;126:831–834.

Welt LG. A further evaluation of erythrocyte sodium transport in control subjects and patients with uremia. Nephron 1969;6:406–417.

Welt LG, Sachs JR, McManus TJ. An ion transport defect in erythrocytes from uremic patients. Trans Assoc Am Physicians 1964;169–181.

Wills MR. Uremic toxins, and their effect on intermediary metabolism. Clin Chem 1985;31:5–13.

Zimmerman L, Jornvall H, Bergstrom J, et al. Characterization of a double conjugate in uremic body fluids. FEBS Lett 1981;129:237–240.

Zuckerman EG, Glaser G. Urea-induced myoclonic seizures. Arch Neurol 1972;27:14–28.

Chapter 3

Approach to the Nervous System in Renal Disease

Contents

Acronyms

CNS   central nervous system
CT   computed tomography
EEG   electroencephalogram
MRI   magnetic resonance imaging

The Central Nervous System

The chief central nervous system (CNS) complications of renal disease (Table 3.1) are roughly grouped into three divisions: those found prior to specific treatment of the uremic condition or with conservative therapy, those associated with dialysis, and those that follow renal transplantation. Some disorders, such as chronic encephalopathy and stroke, may fit into more than one of these three divisions.

Acute and chronic uremic encephalopathies are thought to be due to neurotoxins that accumulate in renal failure. These are largely but incompletely cleared by dialysis and completely corrected by successful renal transplantation.

Certain conditions affecting the CNS are not directly related to uremic neurotoxins but to complications of renal disease, such as stroke related to hypertension, hyperlipidemia, or coagulation problems. The failure of the kidneys to properly regulate hormonal balance causes a number of endocrinological problems, some of which have a neurological aspect. Also, when the kidney fails in its role in fluid and electrolyte homeostasis, the stage is set for certain conditions such as hyponatremia. If not carefully managed, this can lead to serious neurological complications such as seizures, coma, and central pontine myelinolysis.

Some conditions are directly or indirectly the result of treatment combined with the renal disorder. An example is dialysis dysequilibrium, in which the shifts of fluid and electrolytes are related to the dialysis procedure in the face of accumulated osmotic substances in renal failure and the absence of normal homeostatic mechanisms for regulating fluid, electrolyte, and osmotic balances. Dialytic encephalopathy appears to be due to an increased aluminum content in the brain: aluminum gets into the body through treatment either from the dialysate, oral phosphate binders containing aluminum, or both; the burden cannot be eliminated, again because of the lack of renal homeostatic control. The effects of altered drug handling in uremia, along with the resultant neurological complications, are discussed in Chapter 9. In the broad picture, these could be regarded as CNS complications associated with uremia, as the drugs would not have been given in the first place had it not been for the uremia; their altered pharmacodynamics are due to the uremia and its treatment.

Undoubtedly, some diseases are directly and solely related to the treatment of renal disease. These arise as risks attendant upon immunosuppression for renal transplantation, upon the transplantation itself (e.g., rejection encephalopathy), or perhaps upon altered physiology created by the transplanted kidney in a body previously affected by uremia and its vascular complications.

There are a number of disease entities or syndromes, discussed in Chapter 6B, in which the brain and kidney are commonly independently affected. In these conditions, the CNS is sometimes doubly affected: by the particular disease process itself and, indirectly, because of the renal dysfunction due to the same disease.

The etiology and pathogenesis of some conditions, e.g., uremic encephalopathy itself and dialytic encephalopathy, are incompletely understood. It is hoped that in the attempt to clarify aspects of these diseases, the biases of

Table 3.1. Syndrome Classification in Various Treatment Modalities

Conservative Management	Dialysis	Post–Renal Transplantation
Acute uremic encephalopathy	Dialysis dysequilibrium	Opportunistic infections
Chronic uremic encephalopathy	Dialytic encephalopathy	Malignancy
	Subdural hematoma	Rejection encephalopathy
	Vitamin deficiencies	Central pontine myelinolysis
	Dialysis headache	Complications of drugs (including cyclosporine)
	Chronic encephalopathy (?)	
	Stroke (hemorrhage)	Augmented atherosclerosis (ischemic stroke)

the authors and certain dogmas of contemporary thought will not too seriously distort the picture.

The Bedside Approach

Any physician who treats patients with renal diseases or systemic conditions that affect the kidney will soon discover the advantage of having some skill at assessing central nervous function. The increasing subspecialization of medicine puts internists, nephrologists, and urologists at risk of neglecting neurological aspects of the diseases they encounter. Awareness of the initial manifestations of the various CNS problems described below is essential for the early recognition, investigation, and treatment of these diseases.

History

The history is usually the most crucial step towards making the diagnosis. In neurology, the history must be precise in the description of symptoms and order of appearance. For conditions that affect the mental status, including dementing illnesses or discrete episodes of altered consciousness, it is necessary to have information from a witness, usually a family member or friend. The time course of the symptoms and overall illness can suggest diagnostic categories or specific conditions; e.g., steady progression with tumors, oppor-

tunistic infections, and degenerative diseases; abrupt, stepwise addition of symptoms with strokes; fluctuations or remissions and exacerbations with some metabolic diseases and subdural hematoma; or brief, intermittent problems that completely clear, such as epileptic seizures or transient ischemic attacks.

Of course, the neurological history should not be considered in isolation from the medical history in making the diagnosis. The nature of the underlying systemic disease, the severity of the renal disease, complications of the renal disease such as hypertension, and treatment modalities used for the systemic and renal disease usually are relevant.

Mental Status Examination

The first step of the neurological examination is observation of behavior. The patient's appearance, conduct, and speech are noted during the history. Any impairment in level of consciousness is particularly noted. It is best to describe what the patient does rather than use a term that lacks uniform meaning. For example, it is better to state that the patient is inactive and sleeps unless stimulated, at which time he obeys only simple commands, rather than to write, "The patient was obtunded." The Glasgow Coma Scale (Jeannett and Teasdale, 1981) can be used to supplement the written report (Table 3.2). This is a standardized assessment of level of consciousness, which, although lacking in much detail, can be

Table 3.2. Glasgow Coma Scale

Category of Response	Response	Score
Eye opening	Spontaneous	4
	To speech	3
	To pain	2
	Nil	1
Best verbal response	Oriented	5
	Confused conversation	4
	Inappropriate words	3
	Incomprehensible	2
	Nil	1
Best motor response	Obeys	6
	Localizes	5
	Withdraws	4
	Abnormal flexion (decorticate)	3
	Extends (decerebrate)	2
	Nil	1

used to follow the trend of consciousness in an acutely ill patient.

Attention and concentration can be assessed by simple digit repetition. There are a number of standardized bedside tests, but this is conveniently performed as part of the Mini-Mental State Examination (Folstein et al., 1975) (Table 3.3).

An assessment of language function should clearly differentiate dysarthria, which is a disorder of articulation of speech, from aphasia. Aphasia is a true disorder of language per se; the defect is in higher integrative processing of linguistic function. Errors may be in fluency, comprehension, repetition, naming, or various combinations of these that constitute specific aphasic syndromes (Kertesz, 1979). Alexia refers to loss of previously acquired reading ability. Agraphia is an impairment of writing skills. Each of these can be seen separately with specific lesions or in nonstructural brain dysfunction (Kertesz, 1979).

Memory function can be divided into immediate, short term, and long term. The immediate and short term are of particular value in assessment of patients with metabolic disorders. This can again be fitted into the Mini-Mental State Examination.

Constructional ability and higher cognitive functions, such as mathematical ability and other dominant and nondominant cortical functions, can be individually assessed (Strub and Black, 1985). Again, simple constructive visual spatial function can be assessed as part of the Mini-Mental State Examination.

Other Aspects of the Neurological Examination

Details of the technique for other aspects of the examination of the CNS can be found in a number of manuals of neurological examination. We recommend *Clinical Examinations in Neurology* (Mayo Clinic, 1981).

Important aspects for patients suffering from renal disease include inspection for signs of metabolic encephalopathy (see Chapter 4), cranial nerve examination, examination for upper motor neuron signs, and tests to bring out asterixis and tremor.

Electroencephalography and Evoked Responses

The electroencephalogram (EEG) is a sensitive test of cerebral function. In the standard EEG, disk-shaped electrodes are attached in a standardized fashion to the scalp, and the

Table 3.3. Mini-Mental State Examination

Maximum Score	Test
	Orientation
5	What is the (year) (season) (date) (day) (month)?
5	Where are we? (state/province) (country) (city) (hospital) (floor)
	Registration
3	Name 3 objects (1 second to say each), then ask the patient to repeat all 3. Give 1 point for each correct answer. Repeat until the patient learns all 3. Count trials and record.
	Attention and calculation
5	Serial 7s (counting backwards by 7 from 100). Stop after 5 answers. Alternatively, spell "world" backwards.
	Recall
3	Ask for the 3 objects repeated above. Give 1 point for each correct answer.
	Language
9	Name a pencil and a watch (2 points). Repeat the following: "No ifs, ands or buts" (1 point). Follow a 3-stage command: "Take a paper in your right hand, fold it in half and put it on the floor" (3 points).
	Read and obey: "Close your eyes" (1 point). Write (not copy) a sentence (1 point). Copy a design (1 point).

change in electrical potential between pairs of electrodes or between an "active" electrode and a reference electrode or collection of electrodes is amplified and then recorded on moving paper. The EEG records activity related to synchronous synaptic potentials of large aggregates of neurons in the cerebral cortex.

One of the main applications is for epileptic seizures, which usually arise from the cerebral cortex. Using the EEG along with clinical information, the seizure can be classified into generalized or partial (focally originating). In the latter, the site of the seizure activity can often be determined from interictal findings, even if the seizure, itself, is not recorded. The EEG is also very sensitive to level of consciousness, especially in metabolic encephalopathies, and is helpful in differentiating these from psychological and psychiatric conditions such as depression. The EEG may be useful in following the severity of the encephalopathy and may help establish certain specific diagnoses, e.g., dialytic encephalopathy (see Chapter 7A).

Certain limitations of the EEG should be borne in mind. Although the EEG may be sensitive to lesions affecting the cerebrum or subcortical structures that alter the function of the reticular activating system, it lacks specificity. If a structural lesion is considered, it is better to go directly to a neuroimaging test, as discussed in the next section. The EEG is seldom of much help in headache or in psychiatric disturbances, except in differentiating the latter from organic brain conditions.

The contribution of individual frequency bands to the EEG signal has had some application in renal disease. The various quantitative methods and their advantages and limitations are discussed in Chapter 4B.

Event-related potentials are EEG signals that have been enhanced by an averaging computer. The object is to determine the presence or absence and the timing of CNS signals that are time-related to a particular event, usually a sensory stimulus. In some paradigms, the stimulus of interest may be a "novel" one that depends on the attention of the subject. In this case, there is a cognitive component that is sought. In other paradigms, the particular sensory pathway can be examined. Computer technology thus allows the electroencephalographer to physiologically look below the cortex at the generators of "far field potentials" and in detail at "near field potentials" generated in the cortex. Standard sensory-evoked response tests include visual, auditory, and somatosensory stimuli. Relevant event-related potentials are discussed in more detail in Chapters 4B and 5A.

Neuroimaging

Conventional radiological and nuclear imaging of the nervous system is rapidly giving way to computerized tomography (CT) and magnetic resonance imaging (MRI). In CT, the attenuation coefficients to x-rays of different structures in the head and spine are determined by computers that generate images as if slices were taken through these structures. When these slices are performed sequentially, an analysis of the whole brain can be obtained.

MRI uses computer technology similar to that used in CT to construct images, but instead of x-rays, pulsed magnetic fields cause photons of energy to be given off from water molecules as they change their polar orientations. These photons are detected, and images are generated. Advantages of MRI over CT include absence of ionizing radiation, creation of images of greater detail, better gray–white matter contrast with less artifact from bone, and increased sensitivity to white-matter lesions. In addition, there is more versatility in imaging in various planes; coronal and sagittal images are easily obtained in MRI in addition to the standard transaxial images of CT.

Mention should be made of cerebral angiography, which, unlike pneumoencephalography and myelography, is not likely to be completely replaced by CT and MRI. Angiography is performed by injecting contrast material into the artery to the brain, or, in digital intravenous angiography, into a peripheral vein, and watching for its appearance in the arteries to the brain. The technique is very helpful in showing the details of vascular pathology: atherosclerosis, embolic arterial occlusion, some vasculitides, and other abnormalities of blood vessels, such as berry aneurysms and arteriovenous malformations.

Laboratory Investigations

The appropriate biochemical, endocrinological, pharmacological, and microbiological tests are discussed in relevant chapters. Most of these tests are available in large hospitals. Special emphasis on aluminum assays is given in Chapter 7A.

Brain Biopsy

Brain biopsy is sometimes necessary to establish the diagnosis in certain neoplasms and infections. This is particularly relevant to the posttransplant patient who, because of immunosuppression, is prone to infection by opportunistic organisms and development of certain neoplasms that may only affect the nervous system (see Chapter 8).

The Peripheral Nervous System

The type of neuromuscular disorder associated with renal disease (Table 3.4) depends largely on which stage of renal failure is being managed: during conservative treatment, during hemodialysis, or after renal transplantation. Most of these conditions are caused by uremic toxicity, arise as complications of methods used to treat this toxicity, or are a result of an associated disease, that is, a disease that is primarily affecting both the kidney and at the same time the peripheral nervous system, such as diabetes mellitus. Those conditions due to uremic toxicity, such as polyneuropathy, occur only on chronic exposure to the as-yet-unknown uremic toxins. Acute renal failure appears to have little effect on the peripheral nervous system, other than muscle weakness induced by acute water and electrolyte disturbances.

When taken together, these various peripheral nervous system conditions form a significant component of the uremic syndrome. Peripheral neuropathy of some degree, usually only mild, occurs in approximately 60 percent of patients who reach end-stage renal failure; this incidence persists during chronic hemodialysis, reversing only after successful renal transplantation. Another common condition, amyloid-induced carpal tunnel syndrome, will appear in the majority of patients once they have been on hemodialysis for more than 10 years, provided it is being performed by a dialyzer using a Cuprophan membrane. On the other hand, the modern procedure of hemodialysis and successful renal transplantation, while achieving the obvious goal of prolonging life in many patients who would have otherwise died, has almost eliminated instances of severe uremic polyneuropathy and cachectic myopathy, which were particularly common before these procedures had been adequately developed.

After having performed a history or physical examination, the physician will often be reasonably certain of the correct nature of the

Table 3.4. The Main Disorders of the Peripheral Nervous System in Uremia

During Conservative Management	During Dialysis	After Renal Transplantation
Developing uremic polyneuropathy	Stabilizing uremic polyneuropathy	Recovery from uremic polyneuropathy
Diabetic mononeuropathy and polyneuropathy	Persisting diabetic neuropathy	Persisting diabetic neuropathy
Pressure palsies and cachexia	Carpal tunnel syndrome and amyloidosis	
Cachectic myopathy	Ischemic neuropathy and shunts or fistulas	
	Primary myopathy and bone disease	

peripheral nervous system disease, but in other instances it will be necessary to carry out further investigations, particularly electromyography and nerve conduction studies, and occasionally, muscle and/or nerve biopsy.

The Bedside Approach

In many instances the patients' own descriptions of his or her symptoms are diagnostic. For example, the early sensory symptoms of neuropathy are characteristically not only numbness and tingling, but a tight or bandlike feeling about the ankles, a sensation on the soles of the feet as if one is wearing tight socks, and more rarely, pain or burning. The restless leg syndrome, which may or may not be associated with peripheral neuropathy, is often an indescribably unpleasant sensation in the legs that is relieved only by movement of the legs. One should systematically ask about muscle weakness or fatigue, muscle cramps, the degree of sweating in the hands and feet, sexual drive, sexual performance, bowel and bladder control, and problems in standing or walking.

In making general observations, the overall state of nutrition should be noted. Muscle wasting may be difficult to detect if there is generalized edema of the subcutaneous tissues. Observe surgical scars, particularly at sites of current and past access to hemodialysis, most commonly in the upper limbs. Observe any abnormal motor activity, such as focal or multifocal myoclonus or fasciculations (fasciculations have been extremely rare in uremia in our experience). Examine the joints for range of movement, pain, localized areas of tenderness, and thickening of the joint capsules or tendons. Severe muscle wasting may occur entirely on the basis of underlying joint or bone disease. In this circumstance, the muscle wasting is most likely to occur proximally in the lower limbs but occasionally occurs in the upper limbs (see Chapter 6, Figure 6.2). In polyneuropathy, the distal lower limb muscles are the first to become atrophic. In carpal tunnel syndrome, the proximal portion of the thenar eminence becomes atrophied only when

this condition has reached an advanced stage. Some uremic patients tend to be frail, particularly if elderly, and vigorous testing of muscle strength should be avoided.

In testing deep tendon reflexes, use a hammer that is of sufficient length and carries enough weight to effectively move the tendon but has a soft enough rubber not to cause undue discomfort. The ankle jerks are usually the earliest to be reduced in polyneuropathy, and these can usually be reinforced while the patient is recumbent or sitting, simply by having the patient partially contract the calf muscles.

The most important information obtained in examination of the sensory system is simply to ask the patient to outline with his index finger areas of sensory loss. Then, these can be formally tested with a Kleenex for light touch and with a sharp piece of splinter from a tongue depressor for pain. (This splinter should be disposed of and not used on another patient for fear of transmitting a potentially infecting agent.) Vibratory sensation should be tested with a 128 cycle/second tuning fork. Position sense is impaired when the patient cannot detect even the smallest movement of a distal joint. Two-point discrimination, tested with an instrument that has two well-defined but not excessively sharp points, will be abnormal if the values are greater than 3 mm in the fingertips in persons of all ages, greater than 1 cm over the sole in young persons, and greater than 3 cm on the sole of elderly persons. To accurately test for temperature sensation is time consuming and, in our experience, adds little to the bedside examination in uremic patients.

The peripheral nerves are not usually enlarged in the type of neuropathy that is seen in chronic renal failure. The median nerves of the wrists should be routinely percussed to detect the presence or absence of a positive Tinel's sign in carpal tunnel syndrome.

In observing stance and gait, one should look particularly for a steppage gait with distal weakness and a sensory ataxia (worse with the eyes closed), in which there is significant positional sensory loss. Have the patient walk on heels or toes to detect early weakness of distal lower limb muscles, and rise from the squatting position to detect such weakness proximally.

To test for postural hypotension, the blood pressure should be taken after the patient has been lying flat for at least five minutes. Observe the pulse rate at that time. Have the patient stand, and monitor the blood pressure and heart rate for at least a minute while the patient is still standing. A significant postural hypotension is present if there is a drop in the systolic pressure of 30 mm Hg or more. The heart rate should increase by a factor of at least 1.04, and an abnormal response is one in which there is no change or a decrease (Ewing and Clark, 1987). The presence or absence of sweating should be crudely assessed by inspection and palpation of the skin surfaces proximally and distally. Sweating in the axilla is mediated by apocrine glands, which are stimulated by circulating catecholamines and, hence, are not affected by neuropathy.

Electromyography and Nerve Conduction Studies

These studies are invaluable in identifying and quantifying peripheral nerve dysfunction. They are also useful in following the course of uremic polyneuropathy during the various stages of renal failure. There is strong correlation between the results of such studies and nerve biopsy (Dyck et al., 1984). Compressive neuropathy, such as carpal tunnel syndrome, ulnar neuropathy at the elbow, or peroneal neuropathy at the fibular head can be readily diagnosed. Electrophysiological studies are also useful in cases of myopathy, mainly to rule out neurogenic atrophy as a cause of wasting and weakness of muscle. Repetitive nerve stimulation tests will usually document a defect in neuromuscular transmission due to antibiotic drugs.

While these tests are somewhat uncomfortable, sedatives or analgesic drugs are rarely required. A well-trained and sensitive electromyographic technician will usually ensure a reasonably content patient who will be willing to return for repeat studies. Needle electromyography is the most uncomfortable part of the examination, and it is usually only indicated when there is evidence of moderate or severe muscle or nerve disease (see Neurophysiological Studies, Chapter 5A, for a further discussion of the principles of nerve conduction study in assessing polyneuropathy).

Nerve and Muscle Biopsy

A nerve biopsy (Dyck et al., 1984) will be required in uremic patients only under exceptional circumstances. If after all investigations have been completed, there is still doubt as to the etiology of a polyneuropathy, this procedure will be of benefit. It will supply information as to the type of nerve fiber alterations, for example, whether the neuropathy is of a mainly demyelinating or axonal type, but more importantly, it will usually give information as to whether the neuropathy is due to an underlying vasculitis or amyloidosis. Vasculitis is, of course, specifically treatable by steroids. However, to detect this disorder in tissue sections, it is usually necessary to take a whole-nerve biopsy and one that includes overlying skin, subcutaneous tissue, and adjacent muscle. The sural nerve at the calf may therefore be the best site. The patient will, of course, have sensory loss within the sural nerve distribution afterwards.

If the nature of a primary myopathy is in question, either the biceps or quadriceps muscles are usually most satisfactory for the pathologist (Engel, 1986). A muscle should be chosen that has a moderate degree of weakness and has not been previously needled by therapeutic injections or needle electromyography.

The biopsy, either nerve or muscle, should always be performed by a surgeon who is thoroughly familiar with, and hopefully experienced in, the procedure. Of equal importance is that the pathologist, who must be experienced in examining the tissue, should be notified in advance of the nature of the problem and be prepared to accept the tissue at the time of biopsy for appropriate studies.

References

Dyck PJ, Karnes J, Lais A, et al. Pathologic alterations of the peripheral nervous system of human. In: Dyck PJ, Thomas PK, Lambert EH, Bunge R, eds. Peripheral neuropathy. Vol 1, 2nd ed. Philadelphia: WB Saunders, 1984:760–778.

Engel AG. The muscle biopsy. In: Engel AG, Banker BQ, eds. Myology—basic and clinical. Vol 1. New York: McGraw-Hill, 1986:833–843.

Ewing JD, Clarke BF. Diabetic autonomic neuropathy: a clinical viewpoint. In: Dyck PJ, Thomas PK, Asbury AK, Winegrad AI, Porte D, eds. Diabetic neuropathy. Philadelphia: WB Saunders, 1987:67.

Folstein MF, Folstein SE, McHugh PR. "Mini-Mental State." A practical guide for grading the cognitive state of patients for the clinician. J Psychiatr Res 1975;12:189–198.

Jeannett B, Teasdale G. Management of head injuries. Philadelphia: FA Davis, 1981:77–93.

Kertesz A. Aphasia and Related Disorders. New York: Grune & Stratton, 1979.

Mayo Clinic. Clinical Examinations in Neurology. 5th ed. Philadelphia: Saunders, 1981.

Strub RL, Black FW. The mental status examination in neurology. Philadelphia: FA Davis, 1985.

PART TWO
Neurological Effects of Renal Disease

Chapter 4
Uremic Encephalopathy

Contents

Acronyms

ARF   acute renal failure
BUN   blood urea nitrogen
CAPD   chronic ambulatory peritoneal
       dialysis
CNS   central nervous system
CNV   contingent negative variation
CRF   chronic renal failure
CSF   cerebrospinal fluid
EEG   electroencephalogram
ERP   event-related potential
FM   frequency modulation
FSH   follicle stimulating hormone
LH   luteinizing hormone
LHRH   luteinizing hormone releasing
       hormone
PREP   pattern reversal evoked potential
REM   rapid eye movement
SWS   slow-wave sleep

A

Encephalopathy of Acute Renal Failure

There are few, if any, specific symptoms or signs of central nervous system (CNS) dysfunction in acute uremia that differentiate that condition from other metabolic or toxic encephalopathies (Plum and Posner, 1980). However, the clinician faced with the combination of encephalopathy with hyperventilation (with metabolic acidosis) and myoclonus or seizures should strongly suspect uremia. The acuteness and severity of the encephalopathy reflect the acuteness of the renal failure. The more rapidly the uremic state develops, the less perturbed the measured biochemical abnormalities have to be to produce altered brain function.

Brain dysfunction occurs early in uremic encephalopathy and serves as a sensitive index of acute uremia (Locke et al., 1961). It is necessary to clearly differentiate acute uremic encephalopathy from those systemic conditions that can, on their own, affect both brain and kidneys. Those diseases are dealt with separately in Chapter 6B. In this chapter, we shall refer to CNS manifestations of acute uremia itself.

Clinical Features

Mental Status Changes

Early changes include lethargy and irritable behavior. Disorientation and confusion are the next to occur, also fairly early. Lucid periods are interspersed with periods of abnormal behavior; this fluctuation may also apply to more profound mental status changes (Locke et al., 1961).

Problems with attention and concentration are reflected in difficulty counting backwards and performing calculations and in memory impairment (Locke et al., 1961). Those patients who recover from acute uremia are often amnestic for the acute illness (Locke et al., 1961). Speech may be abnormal, with inappropriate inclusion of parts of words or phrases overheard from other conversations, reflecting distractability. Disorientation is a common accompaniment of acute uremia, as it is for other metabolic encephalopathies (Plum and Posner, 1980). Disorientation for place is as likely to occur as disorientation for time; this feature is sometimes helpful in differentiating metabolic from degenerative CNS diseases, since in the latter time orientation is affected well before place orientation. Rarely, patients may even be disoriented for self, e.g., a married woman might give her maiden name or a patient may only be able to give his or her first name (Locke et al., 1961).

Patients are typically subdued and obtunded to various degrees, but agitation, delirium with hallucinations as part of toxic psychosis, mania with restlessness, and sleep disturbance with insomnia can occur. The more florid behavioral changes may precede stupor or coma and are more likely when the uremia develops very acutely (Plum and Posner, 1980). Catatonia has also been described (Wilson, 1940). Some patients may show other alterations in behavior such as personality change with profanity, depression, or periods of euphoria. Locke et al. (1961) described some acutely uremic patients with anxiety about imminent death.

The level of consciousness can thus be affected along a continuous spectrum from mild clouding, through delirium, to stupor and coma, often with considerable fluctuation. Gowers (1888) pointed out that in uremia deep coma is rare unless the patient is *in extremis.*

Cranial Nerve Abnormalities

Amaurosis with acute uremia has been described in the older literature (Bright, 1836). Usually pupillary reaction is preserved, suggesting that the blindness may be cortical rather than due to problems of the anterior visual pathway. Blindness has not been noted in the more recent series of Locke et al. (1961), and we have not encountered it in acute uremia. It is possible that at least some cases of blindness in acute uremia may have been produced by hypertensive encephalopathy (see Differential Diagnosis, below).

Dysarthria is common, but is not likely due to peripheral cranial nerve neuropathies. It may be related to the encephalopathy, but local oral problems such as dry mucous membranes, aphthous stomatitis, and problems with oral hygiene, may contribute (Locke et al., 1961). Nystagmus was reported by these researchers, but this may have been produced by medication. Other cranial neuropathies have not been reported as complications of acute uremia: extraocular movement problems, pupillary abnormalities, facial sensory loss, weakness, deafness, and lower cranial neuropathies are not features of acute uremia itself. Some of these may be seen in associated conditions, e.g., ophthalmoplegia in Wernicke's encephalopathy.

Seizures

Cerebral seizures secondary to acute uremia are usually generalized convulsions. They typ-ically occur in the anuric or oliguric phase and are often multiple. Occasionally, focal seizures, even with a Jacksonian march (Bionet, 1885), have been noted. These may occur without a structural lesion in the brain at postmortem examination (Raymond, 1885). Generalized convulsions were found in three of 13 acutely uremic patients in the series of Locke et al. (1961). In two, there were early features, and in one patient they occurred just before death. Focal seizures, including adversive movements, were found in two others.

Motor Abnormalities

Most uremic patients feel weak and may show weakness and unsteadiness in movements. Tremor, myoclonus, and asterixis are common in acute uremia and vary in parallel with the mental status (Locke et al., 1961). The myoclonus is typically multifocal, as it is in other metabolic encephalopathies; however, in uremia the myoclonus is more striking. It can be so active that the muscles appear to fasciculate (Plum and Posner, 1980). Action myoclonus, myoclonic movements brought out by voluntary movements, has been reported (Chadwick and French, 1979). Tetany is common. Focal signs such as hemiparesis or reflex asymmetries are not uncommon, are typically transient, resolve with dialysis, and may switch from side to side during the course of the illness. If the morbidity becomes prolonged, wasting from disuse may occur. Locke et al. (1961) found the wasting to be earliest and most marked in the vastus medialis muscle. Such wasting and weakness is most marked in proximal muscles. Tenderness in the affected muscles is common (Locke et al., 1961).

Differential Diagnosis

The condition that is hardest to differentiate from acute uremic encephalopathy is hypertensive encephalopathy. The latter condition may be accompanied by impaired consciousness, fluctuating focal neurological signs, seizures, and renal impairment. Hypertensive encephalopathy is typically accompanied by papilledema and arterial spasm in the optic fundi. Papilledema is not a feature of renal diseases unless complications such as raised intracranial pressure or malignant hypertension supervene. Hypertensive encephalopathy more typically causes focal neurological signs such as aphasia and more rapid fluctuation of those signs than does acute uremia. Another feature more commonly found in hypertensive than in acute uremic encephalopathy is significantly elevated cerebrospinal fluid (CSF) protein concentration. Although renal impairment may occur as a complication of malignant hypertension, it is usually not as striking as that found in acute uremia with encephalopathy. (Hypertensive encephalopathy is discussed in greater detail in Chapter 6.)

Other conditions that could cause encephalopathy and systemic acidosis include certain exogenous toxins, such as methanol, ethylene glycol, formaldehyde, salicylates, and paraldehyde, as well as systemic disorders such as diabetic ketoacidosis, anoxia, circulatory failure, or sepsis with lactic acidosis. The clinical features and commonly available laboratory tests can easily make the distinctions (Plum and Posner, 1980). Each condition requires its own specific treatment (Plum and Posner, 1980).

Penicillin intoxication, either in the context of large doses administered to patients with renal impairment or excessive doses administered to patients with normal renal function, can produce a picture of mental obtundation, myoclonus, and frequent multifocal or generalized convulsive seizures. The mechanism of penicillin-induced seizures and myoclonus is uncertain. It has been shown that penicillin can block inhibitory synapses, and this could be epileptogenic. There may be other effects, e.g., on chloride conductance (Schwartzkroin, 1983).

Penicillin in high doses may be nephrotoxic, which can further compound the problem. It is important to consider the possibility of penicillin intoxication in any patient who develops myoclonus or seizures while receiving large doses of penicillin, especially if renal impairment is present. CSF penicillin levels can be helpful in confirming the diagnosis. Treatment includes stopping the penicillin, symptomatic treatment of the seizures, and an early attempt to reduce the body burden of penicillin. Seizures in this situation can be very difficult to treat. Patients often have refractory, generalized convulsive status epilepticus that requires unconventional measures such as anesthetic barbiturates (Young et al., 1980).

In children, lead intoxication enters the differential diagnosis (Barltrop, 1968). (Adults rarely develop encephalopathy; neuropathy is more common in adults than in children.) Although the accumulation of lead is slow, lead encephalopathy usually presents acutely. Children with lead encephalopathy, especially those under the age of 2 years, most often acquire their intoxication by ingesting lead-based exterior house paint, which apparently has a pleasant, sweet taste. They present with irritability or delirium, convulsions, and coma. Papilledema is commonly present. The raised intracranial pressure may cause splitting of the sutures, which can be seen on skull radiograph. Cerebrospinal fluid shows raised pressure, an excess of protein, normal glucose, and a variable pleocytosis: no white cells or an increase in either mononuclear or polymorphonuclear leukocytes. The encephalopathy is due not to lead acting directly on neurons or glia, but on the cerebral vasculature, causing cerebral edema.

Systemic clues to lead intoxication include a dark line of lead sulfide near the teeth in the gingivae, the presence of a "lead line" in the diaphyseal part of long bones on radiography, and anemia with basophilic stippling of the red blood cells. The kidney is often affected, as lead is toxic to proximal convoluted tubule cells. The glomeruli may also be affected. Typically, there is aminoaciduria, glucosuria, and hyperuricemia, which may even cause gout. Lead can be found as intranuclear inclusions in proximal convoluted tubule epithelium on renal biopsy. The diagnosis can be supported by finding an elevated serum lead level, but this is not reliable, as the blood is cleared of lead fairly rapidly. Increased lead in the urine, especially after a dose of edetate (Versenate), is very helpful. Increased urinary excretion of coproporphyrin III is also helpful diagnostically.

Treatment (Coffin et al., 1966) includes lowering intracranial pressure with steroids and mannitol, controlling seizures with antiepileptic drugs, and the combined use of dimercaprol and sodium calcium edetate once adequate urinary flow is established. Removal from exposure is essential. Common residua include mental subnormality and recurring epileptic seizures. Optic atrophy has also been reported.

Neurophysiological Features

Electroencephalographic (EEG) findings in uremia are dealt with in depth in Chapter 4B. In acute uremia, clinical EEG studies have been less extensive than for chronic renal failure. Furthermore, some of the earlier papers may have included patients who had extrarenal conditions (sepsis, malignant hypertension, disseminated intravascular coagulation, or exogenous toxins) or superimposed fluid and electrolyte disturbances that could themselves affect the brain. EEG abnormalities reflect the level of consciousness, which is often more abnormal in acute uremia than in chronically uremic patients on a regular dialysis program or being closely followed while receiving conservative therapy. The EEG patterns in acute uremia are not sufficiently distinctive to reliably differentiate this condition from other acute metabolic encephalopathies.

In acute uremia, there is a wide spectrum of EEG abnormalities, reflecting the severity of the encephalopathy (Romano and Engel, 1944; Lossky-Nekhorocheff et al., 1959; Locke et al., 1961; Jacob et al., 1965). These do not consistently correlate with the serum urea level (Cadilhac and Ribstein, 1961). The EEG is quite sensitive in acute uremia. Some neurologically normal individuals may show mild but definite abnormalities, which later resolve with improvement in renal status (Cadilhac and Ribstein, 1961). Most often, there are abnormalities, especially in infants and children (Cadilhac and Ribstein, 1961; Jacob et al., 1965). Abnormalities are diffuse, not focal, and consist primarily of slowing of background

rhythms, especially the occipital rhythm (Romano and Engel, 1944; Lossky-Nekhorocheff et al., 1959; Cadilhac and Ribstein, 1961; Jacob et al., 1965).

Bursts of high-voltage slow waves are common, especially if the acute renal failure is severe (Cadilhac and Ribstein, 1961; Jacob et al., 1965), and may be more prominent in either the anterior or posterior head (Lossky-Nekhorocheff, 1959). In children, these high-voltage slow waves are little affected by sensory stimulation (Cadilhac and Ribstein, 1961).

Epileptiform activity (spikes, sharp waves, or spike-and-wave complexes) occurred spontaneously in 25 percent of children with acute uremia in the series of Chaptal et al. (1954). This has not been noted in adults; spontaneous epileptiform activity is not a common feature of acute uremic encephalopathy.

In contrast to the EEG in chronic renal failure (see Chapter 4B), in acute uremia, abnormal responses to intermittent light flashes (photic stimulation) are not a feature (Jacob et al., 1965).

Improvement in the EEG can be expected with dialysis therapy (Kiley and Hines, 1965) or with resolution of the nephrosis (Cadilhac and Ribstein, 1961).

Pathology, Pathophysiology, and Treatment

The pathology and pathophysiology of the encephalopathies of acute and chronic renal failure are similar. The features are discussed in Chapter 4B.

With modern dialysis techniques, acute uremic encephalopathy is readily reversible. After dialysis is begun, there is a variable time lag of hours to two or more days for full recovery in obtunded patients (Schreiner, 1959). Management of convulsions is discussed in Chapter 4B. Appropriate management of the underlying condition (e.g., sepsis, vasculitis, obstructive uropathy) is essential. In some cases the renal impairment itself may be at least partly reversible. General supportive measures are discussed in standard textbooks of internal medicine.

References

Barltrop D. Lead poisoning in childhood. Postgrad Med 1968;44:537–548.

Bionet E. De l'hémiplegie urémique. Rev Med Fr 1885;12:1008.

Bright R. Cases and observations illustrative of renal disease accompanied with the secretion of albuminous urine. Guys Hosp Rep 1836;1:356–357.

Cadilhac J, Ribstein M. The EEG in metabolic disorders. World Neurol 1961;2:296–308.

Chadwick D, French AT. Uraemic myoclonus: an example of reticular reflex myoclonus? J Neurol Neurosurg Psychiatry 1979;42:52–55.

Chaptal J, Passouant P, Puech P. Sur la forme hypertensive des glomerulonéphrites de l'enfant. Arch Fr Pediatr 1954;11:192.

Coffin R, Phillips JL, Stadles EI, Spector S. Treatment of lead encephalopathy in children. J Pediatr 1966;69:198–206.

Gowers WR. A manual of diseases of the nervous system. Philadelphia: P Blakiston, 1888:535–536.

Jacob JC, Gloor P, Elwan OH, et al. Electroencephalographic changes in chronic renal failure. Neurology 1965;15:419–429.

Kiley J, Hines O. Electroencephalographic evaluation of uremia. Arch Intern Med 1965;116:67–73.

Locke S, Merrill JP, Tyler HR. Neurologic complications of acute uremia. Arch Intern Med 1961;108:519–530.

Lossky-Nekhorocheff I, Lerique-Koechlin A, Funck-Brentano JL, Delprat M. L'EEG dans les anuries aiguës hyperazotémiques. Rev Neurol 1959;100:317.

Plum F, Posner JB. The diagnosis of stupor and coma. 3rd ed. Philadelphia: FA Davis, 1980:117–303.

Raymond G. Sur la pathogénie de certains accidents paralytiques observés chez des vieillards: leurs rapports probables avec l'urémie. Rev Med Fr 1885;5:705–708.

Romano J, Engel G. Delirium I. Electroencephalographic data. Arch Neurol Psychiatry 1944;51:356–377.

Schreiner GE. Mental and personality changes in the uremic syndrome. Med Ann DC 1959;28:316–323.

Schwartzkroin PA. Local circuit considerations and intrinsic neuronal properties involved in hyperexcitability and cell synchronization. In: Jasper HH, Van Gelder NM, eds. Basic mechanisms of neuronal excitability. New York: Alan R. Liss, 1983:75–108.

Wilson SAK. Neurology. London: Edward Arnold, 1940:1097.

Young GB, Blume WT, Bolton CF, Warren KG. Anesthetic barbiturates in refractory status epilepticus. Can J Neurol Sci 1980;7:291–292.

B

Encephalopathy of Chronic Renal Failure

Clinical Aspects of Chronic Renal Failure

The brain is the most eloquent spokesperson of the body in uremia. Symptoms and signs of brain dysfunction usually appear before those due to dysfunction in other organ systems, apart from those of the urinary system itself. The severity of uremia as a systemic illness is closely reflected by the clinical CNS features and EEG findings. Further, changes in brain function constitute a sensitive and responsive measure of the success of treatment of renal failure.

The signs and symptoms of chronic renal failure (CRF) do not differ in kind from those seen in acute renal failure (ARF). In ARF they are more acute in onset, more fulminant, and can occur at lower blood urea nitrogen (BUN) or serum creatinine levels. This may reflect the capacity of the brain to adapt more readily to slowly developing than to acute systemic biochemical abnormalities. Furthermore, modern treatment, notably dialysis, has markedly reduced the incidence of some CNS complications, such as coma and seizures. Both ARF and CRF share many clinical features with other metabolic or diffuse brain diseases (Plum and Posner, 1980).

The various alterations in CNS function in uremia will be considered separately, although it should be recognized that they may occur in combination. We shall concentrate on those CNS complications directly due to the uremic state itself, rather than those symptoms and signs due to concomitant diseases, such as systemic lupus erythematosus, that may have caused both the uremia and the CNS dysfunction. The CNS problems that arise as complications of treatment are considered in Chapters 7, 8, and 9. It should be recognized that some of the CNS complications of uremia may be due, at least in some patients, to hypertension or coagulopathy, which are commonly present. Furthermore, treatment of uremia, particularly dialysis and renal transplantation, has greatly modified the prevalence of many of the uremic CNS complications.

Mental Status Abnormalities

Marked alterations in level of consciousness such as delirium, stupor, and coma are now rarely encountered in CRF, mainly due to the prevalence of effective dialysis programs. Also, the brain tends to adapt to disturbed biochemistry if it occurs gradually. These more profound mental status abnormalities are therefore discussed under acute uremia (see Mental Status Changes, Chapter 4A).

Studies of mental status abnormalities in CRF have been imperfect. It has hardly ever been possible to study individuals before they become uremic. Inferences can be drawn after taking a careful history from relatives and by noting the variability in mental status function, whether changes occur spontaneously or as the result of treatment. Many features are common among patients and presumably relate to the uremic state when there is no other common factor. It is difficult to perform complete neuropsychological testing on uremic patients in view of their fatigability, malaise, and problems in maintaining attention. Therefore, the most careful psychological studies of mental status have been limited and very selective in the functions tested.

Usual Findings

Lethargy, slowness in thinking, and general malaise (Addison, 1868; Tyler, 1968; Tyler, 1970; Glaser, 1960) are so commonly encountered in uremic patients that they seem almost universal, whether the patient is untreated or is on peritoneal or hemodialysis. Successful renal transplantation corrects many of these features. Schreiner (1959) emphasized that underlying many of the mental symptoms was marked fatigability, impaired concentration, and pronounced variability in performance time. He described an engineer who could do difficult calculations by working in 15-minute intervals, but who would be completely ineffective for entire days.

Personality changes include apathy, flatness of affect, irritability, and depression. The latter may be reactive, due to awareness of disease or reluctance to assume a dependent role (Tyler, 1970). Occasionally, patients may fluctuate between depression and euphoria (Schreiner, 1959). Patients may become petulant and poorly cooperative, or they may become preoccupied and compulsive in behavior. Others show accentuation of premorbid personality traits. Some patients develop odd tics and mannerisms such as kicking movements of the legs, picking at bedclothes, or doodling. Restlessness is common; sometimes it is due to peripheral nervous system disease as part of the restless leg syndrome. Some patients develop claustrophobia intermittently (Schreiner, 1959). At times they may have paranoid ideation, frank delusions, hallucina-

tions, and delirium (folie Brightique). The last mentioned are features of more acute renal failure, advanced, untreated chronic uremia, underlying causes of both the renal failure and cerebral dysfunction (e.g., systemic lupus), complications such as sepsis, or the effects of therapy (e.g., glucocorticoids). Catatonia has been noted by some authors (Wilson, 1941; Schreiner, 1959). In fact, Wilson (1941) stated that when catatonia appears after the age of 41 years, one should look for uremia. We have not encountered catatonia in patients on dialysis; presumably it is a feature of acute or advanced chronic uremia.

Heilman et al. (1975) studied 24 conservatively managed uremic patients and 12 controls using a psychological battery. Those tests that revealed the greatest difference between uremic patients and controls ($p < .01$) were the early and delayed memory test and trail-making, part B. Interestingly, early and delayed memory function were equally defective; there was no fall-off from the initially impaired value. The authors suggested that the problem, therefore, does not lie so much in the memory storage system of the brain, but in the attention that allows initial registration of information. Other less marked differences between uremics and controls ($p < .05$) were in digit retention and trail-making, part A.

The psychological defects seen in uremics were similar to those found in subjects tested after anesthesia (Parkhouse et al., 1960), which is thought to affect the ascending reticular activating system responsible for arousal (Moruzzi and Magoun, 1949). Arousal, in turn, has been proposed as one of the two components of attention, the other being selection (Meldman, 1970). We shall see a recurring theme that in uremic encephalopathy the brainstem reticular formation is a principal site of involvement.

Peritoneal Dialysis

Most psychological studies have been done on a group basis using small numbers of patients (17 to 26) and comparable numbers of control subjects. Such patients were not in a state of severe uremic encephalopathy, or they would not have been testable. A preliminary study by Kenny et al. (1981) on patients on chronic ambulatory peritoneal dialysis (CAPD) showed that uremic patients yielded scores that were below population norms on tests of speed of psychomotor response, ability to sustain concentration, and general efficiency of memory processes.

Kenny later (1983) conducted a more extensive study using a battery of neuropsychological tests (trail-making, parts A and B [Reitan, 1958], digit-symbol and digit-span tests from the Wechsler Adult Intelligence Scale, the grooved pegboard and finger-tapping tests for dominant and nondominant hands, the Benton visual retention test, and the Minnesota perceptodiagnostic test). Tests were assigned equal value and totaled to give an impairment index between 0.0 and 1.0; the higher the number, the more impaired the patient. Before starting the dialysis program, 45 percent of patients scored in the normal-borderline range, but after six months of dialysis, this percentage rose to 60 percent and after two years, the percentage rose to 70 percent. This study was flawed, however, in that dropouts and transplanted patients were not included in the analysis, and there were not adequate controls in the study. The investigator did show that when patients were stratified into high-index (initially high impairment scores) and low-index (low impairment scores) groups, the high-index group had 43 percent with unfavorable outcome (having to come off CAPD for reasons other than transplantation) compared to 17 percent in the low-index group. Further, the mortality rate in the high-index group was 17 percent compared to 5 percent in the low-index group. Older patients tended to predominate in the high-index group.

Hemodialysis

McDaniel (1971) studied 17 patients on maintenance hemodialysis, 10 patients after renal transplantation, and an age-matched control group of 32 healthy volunteers. Subjects were required to press lighted buttons to match a color or form stimulus, with the problem changing without warning from color to form

or vice versa. Posttransplant patients and controls did not differ, but patients on hemodialysis made significantly more errors than these groups, even though their response time was normal. Those with higher serum creatinine and potassium levels were the more impaired. The normal response time suggests that the problem lay with higher-order processing than just visual-motor integration. The test has similarities to the Wisconsin card-sorting test, which has been used to assess dorsolateral frontal lobe function (Stuss and Benson, 1986). This test also is sensitive to diffuse brain dysfunction. The patients tested showed greater than normal percentage improvement in retest trials, suggesting that other factors, such as problems with attention, could have played a major role in their impairment.

Teschan et al. (1975, 1977) used the continuous memory, choice reaction time, and answer recognition–mental arithmetic tests, along with the power spectral EEG analysis in assessing uremic patients. These tests would be expected to be sensitive to alterations in attention. The results showed that impairment in all these measures occurred in uremia, improved with dialysis, and improved further with renal transplantation. Teschan et al. (1981) studied 19 patients on chronic intermittent hemodialysis for two years or more and found no deterioration in performance of these same psychological tests. Sometimes there was a dissociation of the cognitive function and quantitative EEG: with the D4 Kiil dialyzer, the slow wave–associated power on EEG increased while the cognitive functions improved.

Brancaccio et al. (1981), using a battery of psychological tests, found no differences between 10 undialysed uremic patients and 10 uremics on hemodialysis for more than 8 years. The authors argue that hemodialysis itself does not cause deterioration in mental functioning. Jackson et al. (1987) also found no significant difference in IQs between two groups of patients on hemodialysis: one on dialysis for more than 5 years (long-term group) and the other for less than 5 years (short-term group). However, there was a statistically significant negative correlation between the cumulative oral aluminum intake and performance on cognitive tests in the long-term group, but not in the short-term group. This was a small study that should be repeated. However, it does raise concerns about long-term aluminum exposure in CRF patients.

Although mean IQ values of patients on chronic hemodialysis do not differ from normal population values, some patients do show impairment in some performance tasks, namely digit symbol, block design, and picture arrangement (English et al., 1978). This could produce some difficulty in acquiring new information or new skills in performance of complex duties. The pathophysiology of this observed impairment has yet to be clarified. Further correlations with the accumulated aluminum burden and long-term effects of potential neurotoxins (see Chapter 2) are needed.

Renal Transplantation

Preliminary work of Teschan et al. (1975, 1977) suggests that the cognitive and EEG functions are restored by renal transplantation. This seems likely to be true, providing posttransplant complications, including vascular disease and effects of treatment such as immunosuppression, do not occur (see Chapter 8).

Experimental Work

Impairment in performance time, attention, and learning have also been demonstrated in uremic animal models. Murphy and Sharp (1964) studied the *Macaca mulatta* using an avoidance behavioral paradigm. The monkeys were trained to push a lever to avoid getting a shock following a conditioning stimulus. The experimental situation was then made more complex by introducing a compulsory time window within which the monkey had to respond; i.e., they were shocked if they responded too early or too late. The animals were then made uremic by either performing a ureteric ligation or by reinfusion of filtered urine into the bloodstream. Another group was given an intravenous infusion of urea. After these procedures, animals showed a sig-

nificant worsening in their performance of the task of responding within the time window. This task was clearly more than simple conditioning, but must have relied considerably on vigilance and attention to the task. In addition, the animals showed profound disturbances in serum electrolyte concentrations and osmolality, in addition to elevations of plasma urea nitrogen concentrations. Teschan (1985) showed that uremic rats took longer to learn and remember a maze, although their locomotion was normal.

Convulsions

Cerebral seizures are occasionally encountered in CRF. They are probably less common now than in the past. This may be due to the lower frequency and better treatment of complications such as hypertensive encephalopathy and serious water and electrolyte disturbances, as well as more effective and prompt treatment with dialysis (Mahoney and Arieff, 1982; Raskin and Fishman, 1976).

Cerebral seizures must be differentiated from metabolic and toxic myoclonus. This is often possible on a clinical basis. Generalized convulsive or clonic movements are typically rhythmic, bilaterally synchronous, and predominant proximally. Focal clonic epileptic movements may consist of either rhythmic focal twitching in epilepsia partialis continua, a systematic "march" from one region to a contiguous region of the motor homunculus, or secondary generalization with bisynchronous clonic movements. Uremic myoclonus is usually multifocal, a nonpatterned twitching of groups of muscles of the face and extremities. Intention myoclonus, similar to that described after hypoxic damage to the brain, has also been described in uremia (see Myoclonus, below). Intention or action myoclonus consists of the jerking of an extremity during movement, initiation of movement, or even the intention to move. The EEG usually shows epileptiform activity in association with epileptic myoclonus, and features of a metabolic encephalopathy (see Routine Electroencephalography, below) in metabolic (multifocal or intention) myoclonus.

When cerebral seizures occur in CRF, either they are due to very advanced renal failure accompanied by stupor or coma (Glaser, 1974), or they are often a preterminal event (Raskin and Fishman, 1974). They may be provoked by a rapid change in blood pH or sudden electrolyte changes, such as an increased potassium to calcium ratio or hyponatremia (Tyler, 1968). Seizures also commonly accompany dialytic encephalopathy, dialysis dysequilibrium syndrome, cyclosporine therapy, penicillin intoxication, central nervous system infections, and neoplasms, as well as sepsis. These are discussed separately.

Seizures are usually, but not invariably, generalized convulsions. Focal motor seizures do occur without necessarily implicating a single structural lesion. Focal seizures may be a manifestation of metabolic brain disease (Plum and Posner, 1980), but their localization should vary from one attack to another. Stereotyped focal seizures should raise the possibility of a focal cerebral lesion. It is wise to always look for a structural lesion with the first focal seizure in a uremic patient, in any case.

Prophylaxis against further seizures in CRF may be necessary, especially if they are not due to a readily correctable complication, such as water intoxication. Phenytoin has been the most popular drug, although its kinetics and protein binding are altered in uremia. This is discussed, along with altered handling of other antiepileptic drugs, in Chapter 9.

Phenobarbital is largely cleared through the kidney, so requirements are expectedly less than in nonuremic patients. The drug can be used and is effective in prevention of uremic seizures (Merrill and Hampers, 1971), but its dose is difficult to adjust and patients with uremia may be sensitive to the sedative effects of the drug. Valproic acid, like phenytoin, shows reduced plasma protein binding in uremia, with a higher free fraction that goes even higher during hemodialysis (Bruni et al., 1980).

Status epilepticus is uncommon in CRF. Its management is similar to that of status epilepticus due to other causes (Raskin and Fishman, 1976; Treiman, 1983).

Headaches, Sleep Disturbances, Speech Problems, Hormonal and Vegetative Functions

Headaches are common in uremia. They tend to be generalized and mild and may be nearly constant or recurrent (Schreiner, 1959; Glaser, 1960). Their mechanism is uncertain; there is no clear relationship with meningeal signs or hypertension. Daytime drowsiness is common in uremia. Nighttime sleep is affected by insomnia, disorganized sleep staging, and frequent wakening. The response to hypnotic drugs taken at night is sometimes paradoxical. Speech in uremic patients is commonly mildly dysarthric. Less commonly, aphasic errors occur (Glaser, 1960). Aphasia in a patient with uremia raises the differential diagnosis of a lesion affecting the speech areas in the dominant hemisphere or dialytic encephalopathy.

Patients with CRF typically become anorexic; this may progress to nausea and vomiting if the degree of uremia worsens (Mahoney and Arieff, 1982).

Sexual interests decline; men lose potency and may develop gynecomastia, testicular atrophy, and hypospermatogenesis, while women become oligomenorrheic and infertile. There is increasing evidence that such changes are organic in nature and directly related to the severity of the uremic state. Follicle stimulating hormone (FSH) increases after renal transplantation (Lim and Fang, 1975), providing indirect evidence of hypothalamic-pituitary suppression in uremia. Hyperprolactinemia is common in uremia and may relate to reduced hypothalamic dopaminergic tone (Handelsman, 1985). Further evidence of hypothalamic dysfunction in gonadotropin regulation includes loss of positive estrogen feedback; absence of spontaneous, pulsatile elevations of luteinizing hormone (LH) and temporal asynchrony of LH and estrogen surges; and normal responses of FSH secretion to gonadotropin releasing hormone administration (Handelsman, 1985). These features are present before dialysis therapy but are not corrected by it. Renal transplantation can restore gonadal function in men and women to normal (Handelsman, 1985; Bonomini et al., 1985). There is evidence that in some patients the gonadal dysfunction may be due to zinc deficiency (Mahajan et al., 1982).

Handelsman et al. (1985) confirmed hypothalamic dysfunction in gonadotropin regulation in the uremic rat model by demonstrating lack of luteinizing hormone releasing hormone (LHRH), yet normal pituitary response of LH and FSH to *in vivo* LHRH administration. Further, there was a lack of LH responsiveness to naloxone administration.

There appears to be defective hypothalamic regulation of thyroid hormone function in uremia. There is a lowering of circulating total and free thyroid hormone levels without an increase in reverse triiodothyronine and thyroid stimulating hormone. Although serum cortisol levels, including their diurnal fluctuations, are normal in uremia, suppression of cortisol secretion by dexamethasone is defective, and responses to metyrapone and insulin-induced hypoglycemia are subnormal (Handelsman, 1985). It is not certain whether defective thyroid hormone regulation accounts for the hypothermia seen in the occasional patient with uremia (Glaser, 1960) or whether such patients have defective hypothalamic temperature regulation.

From the above evidence of disturbed hypothalamic endocrine regulation and temperature control and from the evidence of disturbed sleep organization discussed later (see Sleep EEG), it can be inferred that the hypothalamus, like the brainstem reticular formation, is a brain region susceptible to uremic poisoning.

Hormonal status after successful renal transplantation has been thoroughly reviewed by Bonomini et al. (1985). Sexual abnormalities with reduced testosterone production, even after gonadotropic stimulation, were found in five of 42 patients. Growth retardation was observed in four of six children after transplantation but did not appear to be related to decreased levels of growth hormone. Hyperparathyroidism was found to persist after transplantation in six of 71 patients. Erythropoietin production improves, along with hemoglobin concentration in the blood, with good graft function. There can even be an overproduction, with erythrocytosis. Some hormonal changes are related to corticosteroid administration: hyperinsulinism, 1,25-dihydroxyvitamin D_3 deficiency, vasoactive hormone imbalance, and somatomedin inhibition.

Focal Signs and Symptoms in Chronic Renal Failure

Aphasia, apraxia, monoparesis, and hemiparesis occasionally occur in CRF as transient phenomena (Glaser, 1974). Like focal seizures, these signs can be manifestations of metabolic brain disease, in which case they are transient or fluctuating; hemiparesis can even switch sides (Lee et al., 1984; Plum and Posner, 1980). The signs may resolve following further dialysis therapy. As in other metabolic encephalopathies, the pupillary and vestibulo-ocular reflexes are spared, even if the patient is comatose (Plum and Posner, 1980). In most cases appropriate screening should be carried out to exclude a structural lesion, such as a subdural hematoma, which can cause fluctuating signs. Ataxia has also been noted in uremia by some authors (Mahoney and Arieff, 1982), but it is also an early sign of dialytic encephalopathy in children (Foley et al., 1981), as well as part of the established syndrome in adults.

Amaurosis has been associated with uremia for many years (Bright, 1836; Gowers, 1895). It occurred in 0.5 percent of 750 patients with renal failure in the series of Tyler and Tyler (1981). Most often, it is sudden in onset and associated with hypertensive retinopathy, signs of encephalopathy, and intermittent convulsions (Gowers, 1895). Recovery usually occurs within three weeks (Tyler and Tyler, 1981). Occasionally, it is very brief, lasting minutes to hours. Sometimes it is incomplete, consisting of hemianopsia. Pupillary reflexes are usually preserved, indicating that the blindness is cortical rather than ocular (Gowers, 1895). Lennon et al. (1971) found this usually to be the case, but noted that retinal detachment was present in one of their five cases. Others have confirmed retinal detachment in uremia, with fluid overload, hyponatremia, severe hypertension, and retinopathy as common features (Lapco et al., 1965; Buchanan and Ellis, 1964). The retinal detachment and visual defects are usually reversible (Lapco et al., 1965; Steiness, 1968), although macular scarring may persist (Ellis and Fonken, 1965). The cause of the cortical blindness has never been fully determined. It, too, is reversible, but occasional visual-field defects such as a homonymous hemianopia may persist, suggesting that cerebral infarction in the territory of a posterior cerebral artery (or possibly the anterior choroidal artery or a branch of a middle cerebral artery, depending on associated features) may have occurred (Lennon et al., 1971). Ischemia may, therefore, be the main cause, possibly due to severe arterial spasm in malignant hypertension. Tyler (1968) has proposed that cerebral edema is the main factor; this could cause herniation of the brain with compression of the posterior cerebral arteries. The problem needs to be studied using modern technology such as computer tomography and magnetic resonance imaging; however, the complication may be less common now with better control of hypertension, fluid and electrolyte balances, and uremia itself.

More complex, higher-order visual disturbances, such as visual agnosia, are also not uncommon in uremia (Tyler and Tyler, 1981). They likely reflect dysfunction of visual association areas. These deficits may have a course similar to that of classical amaurosis.

Deafness, vertigo, and nystagmus have been reported in uremia (Locke et al., 1961). When carefully studied, deafness and tinnitus are uncommon and are usually related to factors other than the uremia itself (Hutchinson and Klodd, 1982). These include the use of ototoxic drugs; hyponatremia (Yassin et al., 1970), unassociated conditions such as otosclerosis, and syndromes including as features deafness and renal failure (Alport syndrome; dominant urticaria, amyloidosis, nephritis, and hearing loss; and recessive renal, genital, and middle-ear abnormalities) (Lanski, 1982). There are individual case reports of deafness associated with severe uremia that resolves with improvement

in renal failure. The deafness appears to be due to cochlear dysfunction combined with slowing of central conduction (Lucien and Jacob, 1987). Similarly, there is no good evidence for vestibular function abnormality in uremia, other than an increase in caloric response in association with hyponatremia (Yassin et al., 1970).

Transient facial palsy has also been noted in renal failure (Locke et al., 1961). It is probably rare, and its mechanism is obscure. Individual oculomotor nerve palsies are also rare and may recover. Their basis may be small infarctions in the peripheral part of the nerve, similar to that seen in hypertensive individuals (Rucker, 1966).

Diffuse Motor Phenomena

General motor phenomena in uremia include tremor, myoclonus, asterixis, altered tone, reflex changes, and the adoption of certain postures. Tremor and some reflex changes are seen in mild encephalopathy, while the other phenomena are usually seen in the context of more marked clouding of consciousness, stupor, or coma.

Tremor

A coarse, somewhat irregular postural action tremor, noted when the patient extends his limbs and supports them against gravity or reaches for an object, is a more sensitive index of uremic encephalopathy than the other motor phenomena (Leavitt and Tyler, 1964). It appears before asterixis and becomes more marked as the encephalopathy progresses (Raskin and Fishman, 1974). Numerous other conditions can cause a postural action tremor including benign essential tremor, anxiety, hyperthyroidism, drug or alcohol withdrawal, as well as drugs (e.g., lithium, valproic acid, xanthines). It has been debated whether the tremor, especially benign essential tremor, arises from a central or a peripheral mechanism. This is still unsettled. Because the tremor is so closely related to encephalopathy in uremia, it likely arises from a central mechanism.

Myoclonus

Myoclonus usually occurs in a multifocal fashion in uremia, as it does in other metabolic encephalopathies (Plum and Posner, 1980), but it may be bisynchronous (Stark, 1981). Patients usually, but not invariably, show obvious encephalopathic features. Myoclonus seems disproportionately common in uremia and it may even dominate the clinical picture (Chadwick and French, 1979). The twitches may involve a single muscle, a small group of muscles, or even part of a muscle and can be difficult to differentiate from fasiculations, irregular firing of single motor units associated with disease of the lower motor neuron (Tyler, 1968). They can involve proximal as well as distal limb musculature. Involvement of the face and tongue occurs late and is usually associated with severe encephalopathy and a poor prognosis (Tyler, 1968). Myoclonic movements appear spontaneously, but are often stimulus sensitive, provoked by a variety of sensory stimuli. They can also become activated or markedly increased by voluntary movements (Chadwick and French, 1979; Stark, 1981), simulating the intention myoclonus described by Lance and Adams (1963) after anoxic encephalopathy.

Chadwick and French (1979) argue that uremic myoclonus is an example of reticular-reflex myoclonus (Chadwick et al., 1977), features of which include: (1) the myoclonus frequently involves proximal limb and truncal muscles; (2) the myoclonic response to peripheral proprioceptive stimuli involves not only the distal muscles of the limb to which the stimulus is applied but also proximal muscles of the same limb and often muscles of other limbs as well; (3) the associated EEG spike-and-wave activity shows a variable relationship to the muscle twitch associated with the myoclonus; (4) cortical sensory responses to the stimulation of peripheral nerves are not enlarged; (5) during a generalized myoclonic jerk, the brainstem motor nuclei are activated in an ascending manner, e.g., the facial before the trigeminal motor nuclei; (6) the myoclonus is alleviated rapidly by serotonin precursors or clonazepam. This has not been thoroughly studied in intact humans, but criteria 1 through 3 and 5 have been shown to apply in uremic patients studied by Chadwick and French (1979) and by Stark (1981).

An experimental model for uremic myoclonus was developed in the cat by Zuckerman and Glaser (1972) and in the rat by Muscatt et al. (1986). The model was not perfect for uremia, as it involved the infusion of only urea in invert sugar or distilled water. In the cat, asynchronous muscle twitches first appeared in the facial musculature. These then increased in amplitude, became synchronous, and merged with generalized myoclonic jerks. In the rat, there was an initial period of ataxia and shaking before myoclonus appeared. In both animal models, the myoclonus was stimulus sensitive. If the infusion continued, synchronous clonic jerks persisted until the animal died in status epilepticus. Depth electrode studies in both species showed that the muscle jerks were preceded by discharges in the caudal brainstem, particularly the nucleus gigantocellularis and the nucleus reticularis caudalis, and in the cerebellum. As the infusion continued, the epileptiform activity became more active locally, then spread rostrally up the brainstem, and eventually involved the cerebral cortex. The spikes in the bulbar reticular formation were unaffected by sectioning the rostral brainstem but were markedly reduced when the upper spinal cord was sectioned or when the animal was paralyzed with tubocurarine. This implied that the bulbar reticular activation was not dependent on descending influences from higher centers but was greatly augmented by sensory input (from muscle spindle receptors). Further stimulation of a peripheral nerve in the rat produced an ascending spinal withdrawal reflex followed by a descending discharge from the medullary reticular formation, which produced the myoclonic jerk. Myoclonus in the rat abated with clonazepam but not with valproic acid, thus giving support for this model as an example of reticular-reflex myoclonus (Muscatt et al., 1986).

Chung and Van Woert (1986) found that tritium-labeled strychnine, which binds to glycine receptors, showed decreased binding in the medulla of rats infused with urea. Glycine, a putative inhibitory neurotransmitter in the brainstem, was not decreased in concentration in the medulla. Urea may inhibit glycine binding at the receptor site in a manner similar to strychnine, or it may alter the allosteric structure of the glycine receptor protein to decrease its binding activity.

Although the above information suggests a prominent role for the brainstem reticular formation in some of the excitatory phenomena in uremia, it should be recognized that the cortex is also affected, in view of the epileptiform activity (including the photoparoxysmal response) to be discussed later (see Routine Electroencephalography). Uremia may be somewhat analogous to the penicillin model of epilepsy of Gloor (Gloor and Testa, 1974), in which diffuse cortical excitability can be activated by input from the ascending reticular formation.

Asterixis

Asterixis was first described by Adams and Foley (1953) in cases of hepatic coma. It has since been recognized to accompany many metabolic encephalopathies (Plum and Posner, 1980), as well as structural lesions in the midbrain reticular formation (Bril et al., 1979). It also can be seen contralateral to a cerebral lesion (Plum and Posner, 1980). It is most easily demonstrated by having the patient bend the wrists back and extend the fingers. There is at first an irregular oscillation of the fingers followed by a sudden flapping downward movement of the hands at the wrists (Leavitt and Tyler, 1964). The flap is typically bilateral and asynchronous; it can be seen in any body part held against gravity. The asterixis may be so severe that the axial musculature participates. Cases of asterixis mimicking drop attacks, consisting of unpredictable falls unaccompanied by loss of consciousness, have been reported (Massey et al., 1988).

Asterixis comes from the Greek word *sterigma,* which means support. Thus, asterixis means without support. This describes the pathophysiology well, as the phenomenon is associated with brief electrical silence of the

muscles supporting a body part (Tyler, 1968). The mechanisms may be a loss of postural control mediated in the reticular formation or the extension of the ascending reticular activating system to the cortical level.

Other Motor Phenomena

Other motor phenomena include alterations in tone, the appearance of primitive reflexes, and the assumption of certain postures. Paratonic rigidity, or gegenhalten, is a resistance to passive movement that is present throughout the range of movement, but unlike true rigidity, it disappears when the limb is moved very slowly (Plum and Posner, 1980). It is a sign of diffuse forebrain dysfunction. The grasp reflex is seen in lesions of the contralateral supplementary motor region (Travis, 1955) but also in diffuse disturbances in cortical function. Rooting and snouting reflexes also are seen in bifrontal or diffuse cerebral dysfunction. All of these signs can be seen in uremia and other metabolic encephalopathies. Unlike sedative-induced coma, the tone in uremic obtundation is increased (Raskin and Fishman, 1976). Decorticate postures (arms flexed and legs extended) are more common than decerebrate postures (all limbs extended).

Uremic Meningitis

Meningeal signs, cerebrospinal fluid (CSF) pleocytosis, and biochemical abnormalities in the CSF indicative of altered blood-CSF barrier function have been described in uremia, mainly in the older literature. Madonick et al. (1950) tested 30 uremic patients for Kernig's sign and nuchal rigidity. Nine had both, and one had only Kernig's sign. Six of these had pleocytosis and four did not. Pleocytosis of greater than 10 cells/mm^3 was found in the CSF in 16 of 62 consecutive uremic patients in the series of Madonick et al. (1950) but in only three of 56 uremic patients in the series of Merritt and Fremont-Smith (1938). The highest count was 250 cells/mm^3. The cells were lymphocytes, although in some earlier individual case reports, a granulocytic pleocytosis was replaced in a few days by a lymphocytic one (cited by Madonick et al., 1950). In these cases, it is not clear what other factors, such as infection or brain infarction, may have been present in addition to the uremia.

Fishman (1980) points out that when the CSF white count exceeds 50 cells/mm³, other processes apart from uremia, especially stroke or opportunistic infections, should be considered.

Elevated CSF pressure is reported in older individual case reports, but, as Fishman (1980) states, it is difficult to know how often this was due to congestive heart failure with increased central venous pressure. Schreiner and Maher (1961) found CSF protein levels of greater than 60 mg/dL in 30 of 52 uremic patients; in 11 it was greater than 100 mg/dL. Urea concentration in the CSF is normally slightly less than that in the serum (Fishman, 1980). The CSF to serum urea ratio is unchanged except with dialysis, in which case the serum concentration falls faster than that of the CSF. Urea concentration in the CSF had no relation to the pleocytosis. Uremic twitching is more likely with elevation of CSF phosphate concentration to greater than 3.8 mg/dL (Freeman et al., 1962), although such myoclonus can occur without elevation of CSF phosphate (Harrison et al., 1936).

A curious case of hypertrophic, granulomatous pachymeningitis in a patient on chronic hemodialysis was reported by Feringa and Weatherbee (1975). The condition caused blindness by constricting the optic nerves. No cause was found, although the patient had inflammatory pulmonary nodules. Since other cases have not been reported, it is difficult to attribute the condition to uremia alone.

Electrophysiology of Chronic Renal Failure

Routine Electroencephalography

As a test of *function*, the EEG shows changes that reflect the severity of uremic encephalopathy. The fundamental reduction in frequency of EEG waves shows a direct relationship with altered cerebral function, but qualitative changes are also common and give further insight into the disturbance in brain function. The latter include bursts of slow waves, triphasic waves, epileptiform activity, altered response to stimulation, and aberrations in sleep patterns.

In mild renal failure, the EEG may be normal or show low-voltage, fast activity (Tyler, 1965). In a study by Hughes (1980) of 23 patients with CRF, 130 of 362 recordings (36 percent) were abnormal, yet 16 patients (70 percent) had at least one abnormal recording. Hughes's study underlines the sensitivity of multiple recordings in detecting EEG abnormalities (a point made earlier by Pro and Wells [1977]), possibly because of fluctuations in the degree of encephalopathy. As might be expected, with disturbance of the conscious level, the EEG loses its faster frequencies and shows slower rhythms. The frequency decreases in proportion to the degree of encephalopathy, and the amplitude may increase, in the form of bursts of slower rhythmic waves. In the case of delirium, however, in which the patient shows agitation, confusion, and impaired attention, the EEG may show the low-voltage, fast pattern (Pro and Wells, 1977), a pattern most electroencephalographers consider normal or essentially normal.

The occipital rhythm often slows on serial EEGs, even though it may not always fall outside the normal alpha range of 8 to 13 Hz. Most authors cite poor regulation of the occipital rhythm and background in general as the most common and earliest abnormality in CRF (Tyler, 1986; Jacob et al., 1965; Klinger, 1954; Cadilhac and Ribstein, 1961). This is borne out with the quantitative studies described below, although in these, the posterior regions of the head were often selectively examined.

Intermittent bursts of low-voltage, rhythmic 3- to 6-Hz (theta) waves in the frontal regions were the most common abnormality encountered by Hughes (1980), being present in nearly 75 percent of the abnormal records. An example from our own records is shown in Figure 4.1, in which the frontal theta activity extends to the midtemporal and central regions.

Paroxysmal, bilateral, medium high voltage

PROJECTED THETA

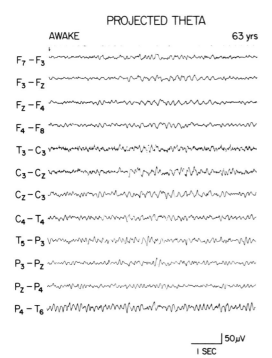

Figure 4.1. A 63-year-old man with chronic renal failure. Intermittent 4- to 5-Hz low-voltage waves are accentuated in the anterior head. (F = frontal, C = central or Rolandic, T = temporal, and P = parietal electrode sites. Odd numbers are left, even numbers are right, and Z are midline or sagittal electrodes.)

PROJECTED DELTA AND ATTENUATION

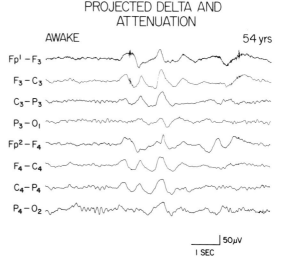

Figure 4.2. A 54-year-old man with chronic renal failure. Intermittent, bisynchronous, rhythmic, frontally predominant delta (< 3-Hz) waves occur, coincident with a reduction in normal rhythms. The burst of delta waves is followed by generalized attenuation of voltage for about two seconds. (Electrode sites as in Figure 4.1; O_1 = left occipital and O_2 = right occipital.)

delta (3-Hz) waves occurred in all 14 CRF patients in the series by Jacob et al. (1965). These are usually frontally predominant, and may represent a variant or extension of the above rhythm described by Hughes (1980). Tyler (1965) pointed out that such projected rhythms are usually, but not invariably, bisynchronous (Figure 4.2). Focal asymmetries or slow waves may occur in CRF, but they are not consistently in the same location; if they are, a focal, structural brain lesion is likely (Tyler, 1965). (See Figure 7.7.)

EEG abnormalities suggestive of dysfunction of the ascending reticular activating system were studied by Jacob et al. (1965). A paradoxical response to eye opening, in which the occipital alpha rhythm becomes more prominent with eye opening rather than with eyes closed (suggestive of impaired alertness), was found in six of 14 patients. Five of the 14 adult patients also showed bursts of synchron-

ous, frontally predominant, rhythmic delta activity on arousal from sleep, rather than the abrupt transition to alpha rhythm seen in normal arousal (Figure 4.3).

Spontaneous epileptiform activity occurs in a minority of regularly hemodialyzed patients with CRF. Tyler (1965) and Hughes (1980) found epileptiform activity in the form of generalized spikes or spike-waves, mainly in

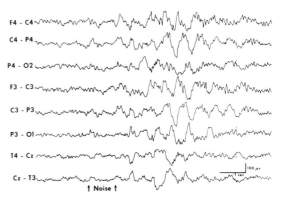

Figure 4.3. Abnormal arousal response to an auditory stimulus in a patient with chronic renal failure. (Reprinted with permission from Jacob et al., 1965.)

advanced uremia. Hughes (1980) noted epileptiform activity in two of his 23 CRF patients and in 18 of 362 records (five percent), in the form of bisynchronous 6-Hz or a mixture of 3- and 6-Hz spike-and-wave forms. They were infrequent: only one patient had more than an average of one every 10 seconds. Jacob et al. (1965) noted that bursts of bisynchronous slow waves occasionally evolved into an irregular spike-and-wave pattern (see Figure 4.4).

Mises et al. (1968) reported that patients with epileptiform activity had hypocalcemia or disturbances in water metabolism, although other authors have not noted any specific correlation with any single biochemical abnormality. Zynso (1970) found that paroxysmal dysrhythmias correlated with the presence of clinical seizures, that they abated with improved dialysis therapy, but that they recurred when the patient was terminally ill. Hughes (1980) found that when paroxysmal activity was present, an elevation of BUN was the most common biochemical accompaniment (found in seven of the 11 cases with epileptiform activity), followed closely by increased serum creatinine (five cases).

Triphasic waves are found in a minority of patients with renal failure; they are always associated with impairment of conscious level. They are bilaterally synchronous complexes with an initial spikelike negative component and a prominent positive wave, followed by a more variable negative component (Figure 4.5).

Typical triphasic waves with frontal predominance, frontal-occipital lag time, and in groups or runs with slowed or suppressed background activity (Figure 4.6) were thought to be specific for hepatic encephalopathy (Bickford and Butt, 1955; Silverman, 1962; Reiher, 1970). However, a recent study by Karnaze and Bickford (1984) showed that triphasic waves also occur in azotemia (10 of their 50 cases). We have seldom seen them in CRF if the patients are hemodialyzed thrice weekly, unless a complication such as sepsis or occasionally dialytic encephalopathy (see Chapter 7A) causes decompensation. The associated conscious level ranges from mild somnolence, through stupor or delirium, to coma.

Sleep Electroencephalography

Prolonged polygraphic recordings have revealed profound sleep alterations in uremia (Passouant et al., 1970; Zynszo, 1970; Reichenmiller et al., 1971). Total duration of

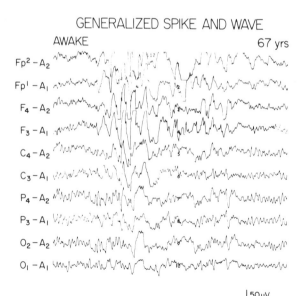

GENERALIZED SPIKE AND WAVE
AWAKE   67 yrs

Fp2 – A2
Fp1 – A1
F4 – A2
F3 – A1
C4 – A2
C3 – A1
P4 – A2
P3 – A1
O2 – A2
O1 – A1

50 μV
I SEC

Figure 4.4. A 67-year-old woman with chronic renal failure. A spontaneous burst of 3-Hz waves with spikes lasts just less than two seconds.

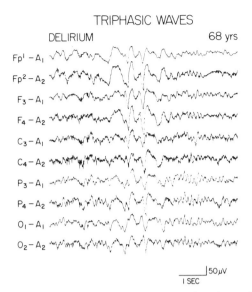

TRIPHASIC WAVES
DELIRIUM   68 yrs

Fp¹ – A₁

Fp² – A₂

F₃ – A₁

F₄ – A₂

C₃ – A₁

C₄ – A₂

P₃ – A₁

P₄ – A₂

O₁ – A₁

O₂ – A₂

⎪50μV
I SEC

Figure 4.5. A 68-year-old woman with chronic renal failure during a transient delirium of uncertain etiology. She was drowsy during the burst of triphasic waves. They were not present at times when the patient was awake and agitated.

nighttime sleep is reduced, and frequent wakening occurs. Sleep cycles are irregular and poorly defined, especially in the first half of the night's sleep. One sometimes sees rapid eye movement (REM) onset sleep, similar to that described in narcolepsy (Dement et al., 1966). REM may also intrude into deeper stages of slow-wave sleep (SWS). Myoclonus in both REM and SWS is increased, except in deep SWS (Passouant et al., 1970). Apneic periods in the middle of SWS, as well as a

periodic pattern of respirations similar to that seen in Pickwickian syndrome, have been described (Reichenmiller et al., 1971). Hemodialysis can lengthen the nighttime sleep, reduce the frequency of wakening, and improve the organization of stages, but total REM sleep remains shorter than normal, and the increase in myoclonus in sleep persists (Passouant et al., 1970). Passouant et al. (1970) also showed a rough correlation of the degree of sleep disturbance with the serum urea level. The pathophysiology of the sleep disturbance and the presumed biochemical alterations in neurotransmitters have not been adequately explored.

Kimmel et al. (1989) examined sleep apnea in patients with CRF. Nineteen men plus seven from their dialysis population of 166 patients were studied with polysomnography (EEG tracings in which respirations, eye movements and concentrations of capillary oxygen and carbon dioxide tension are simultaneously recorded). These patients were partly selected on the basis of symptoms: 22 gave histories suggestive of sleep apnea; the four who did not served as controls. Sixteen of the 22 symptomatic patients, including three women, had sleep apnea, usually of the obstructive type. This study had design flaws because of the selectivity and inadequate controls, but it does raise the possibility that a significant portion of patients with CRF have sleep apnea syndrome. A better study is needed to assess the prevalence of the problem. This is potentially very important as sleep apnea, by producing

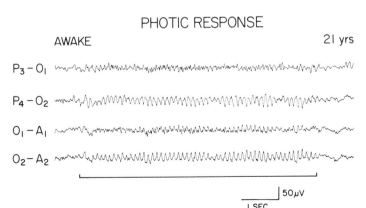

PHOTIC RESPONSE
AWAKE   21 yrs

P₃ – O₁

P₄ – O₂

O₁ – A₁

O₂ – A₂

⎪50μV
I SEC

Figure 4.6. A 21-year-old man with chronic renal failure. The long line at the bottom represents the time a bright light was flashed at nine times per second. Note that the right occipital response (P₄–O₂ and O₂–A₂) is at the same frequency as the flash, while the left occipital region (P₃–O₁ and O₁–A₁) has a higher harmonic. Such prominent responses can be found in healthy individuals but have a higher prevalence in uremic patients.

hypersomnolence in the daytime, could contribute to the disability suffered by patients with CRF. Symptomatic treatments are available to control the sleep apnea and to alleviate the daytime hypersomnolence.

Photic Stimulation

Photic stimulation may elicit a number of possible responses in CRF. An exaggerated photic driving response, in which a medium-voltage occipital rhythm follows the fundamental flash frequency or a harmonic of it at higher-than-usual amplitude or voltage, is common (see Figure 4.6) (Klinger, 1954; Tyler, 1965; Gastaut et al., 1968). Klinger (1954) found the photic driving response to be greatest at 10 flashes per second, with the amplitude of the occipital response sometimes achieving 100 μV. The latency of the response is 30 to 40 ms (Klinger, 1954). The response on bipolar derivation is sometimes biphasic, with a small positive wave followed by a larger negative wave (Klinger, 1954). Interestingly, in one patient with "uremic amaurosis" in which pupillary responses were preserved (cortical blindness), the photic driving response was present, but with a voltage of only 40 μV. With recovery of vision, the amplitude of the photic response increased significantly (Klinger, 1954).

The photomyogenic (formerly photomyoclonic) response was found in three of 14 patients with CRF by Jacob et al. (1965). The phenomenon consists of muscle twitches, especially in the face, that closely follow each flash. The amplitude of the twitch typically augments during the flash train and stops abruptly when the flash train terminates. The photoparoxysmal (formerly photoconvulsive) response is characterized by the appearance of epileptiform activity during the flash train. This is usually most prominent in the frontocentral regions, but spiking in response to the flash can also be seen in the occipital regions (Figure 4.7). Jacob et al. (1965) showed that in CRF a photoparoxysmal response has a high association with recurrent spontaneous seizures. Photic stimulation may trigger generalized

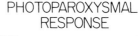

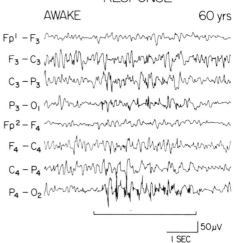

Figure 4.7. A 60-year-old woman with chronic renal failure. During a train of flashes delivered at 12 times per second (long horizontal line), a burst of irregular spike-and-wave forms and individual spikes occurs from the posterior head, higher on the right (P_4–O_2).

tonic-clonic seizures in CRF; these may arise from either the photomyogenic or photoparoxysmal response (Gastaut et al., 1968).

It seems reasonable that all the above responses to photic stimulation reflect enhanced neuronal excitability in CRF, in a spectrum ranging from the increased amplitude of photic driving response to generalized convulsive seizures. The photomyogenic response is thought to be due to subcortical excitation, possibly at the level of the brainstem reticular formation (Naquet and Meldrum, 1980). The photoparoxysmal response, when seen maximally in the frontocentral regions, is now thought to arise, at least in part, from a decrease in stimulation from the ascending reticular activating system. Increased synchronization occurs with repetitive stimulation; this can be blocked by reticular activation (Naquet and Meldrum, 1980). The myoclonus that can occur as a result of the photoparoxysmal response probably is due to spread of the cortical excitation to the reticular formation in the lower brainstem (Naquet and Meldrum, 1980).

Quantitative Electroencephalography

Quantifying the EEG allows for more objective comparison of both intra- and inter-individual recordings. Because of limitations such as the loss and oversimplification of data, quantitative methods have not been widely utilized. Progress is being made in this area. Standardized yet sensitive quantitative EEG analysis is achieving a more prominent role in research, investigation, and management of patients with CRF.

General Comments

The goal of spectral analysis is to reduce the subjectivity of EEG reading and to provide a standardized, quantitative assessment of brain function. While this has been accomplished to some degree, there are a number of problems. By the nature of the mathematical treatment of the EEG signal, some information is lost: transients such as epileptiform potentials and triphasic waves are "absorbed" in the analysis and not detected; suppression, possibly the most significant EEG change, is deemphasized or not specified. Unwanted artifacts contaminate the analysis. A major concern has been the dependence of the EEG spectrum on state—can drowsiness or altered vigilance be separated from an encephalopathic picture? Furthermore, the EEG shows considerable inherent variability, creating potential problems in comparing short epochs of EEG analysis. Some reassurance on the latter point was given by Gasser et al. (1985), who analyzed 20-second epochs recorded 10 months apart on a group of school children. The authors found that the topography of the frequency bands was very consistent. There was more variability in the frequencies themselves. Delta and beta rhythms showed considerable variability, but alpha rhythms showed good reliability.

Event-related potential testing has to focus on specific parameters. These can be fairly reliably performed for shorter-latency subcortical responses and for responses in the primary sensory cortical areas. However, relations between higher cortical functions and later cortical responses are not simple and may be more variable than subcortical and primary sensory cortical responses.

Further quantitative work may be fruitful, but this should be coupled with further research into the physiological mechanisms responsible for the various EEG signals we record.

Manual Counting Methods

The first quantitative technique applied to the EEG in uremic patients was developed by Engel et al. (1944). A frequency spectrum was developed for 300 consecutive seconds of the EEG tracing by counting the number of waves in each second and then tabulating the results. The frequencies from one to 12 were rounded off to the nearest whole number, with higher frequencies grouped as fast activity. The technique ignored voltage and epileptiform activity and underemphasized other transient phenomena, such as projected rhythms. Despite these shortcomings, these pioneering efforts provided a clinically useful method of quantifying the severity of the systemic effects of renal failure. The selection of frequency as the measured parameter was a wise choice, as frequency changes are probably the most physiologically important variable of neuronal function (Gerard, 1936).

Romano et al. (1944) applied their quantitative method to the study of delirium due to various causes. The method was resurrected and applied to the study of uremia by Kiley and Hines in 1965. These authors found that if each of the seconds counted contained fewer than eight waves, the immediate prognosis was poor; death was usually imminent unless dialysis was commenced. They then used the quantitative EEG as a major guide to the initiation of dialysis therapy. They showed that as the patient improved, the EEG frequencies shifted to higher values. In a follow-up of the application of this technique, Kiley et al. (1976b) showed that most patients with CRF had a higher than normal percentage of slower frequencies, and that this percentage was reduced by increasing dialysis frequency from two to three times per week. Renal transplantation can further improve the frequency spectrum. This simple quantitative method can detect significant EEG changes which may not be obvious on visually read records (Di Paolo et al., 1982).

Goldstein et al. (1980) used the method of Engel et al. (1944) in their study of 20 uremic patients on chronic hemodialysis. They showed a strong correlation between the degree of EEG slowing (percentage of seconds showing seven waves) in individual EEGs and N-terminal parathyroid hormone levels. They also found that the suppression of parathyroid hormone levels by administration of 1,25-dihyroxyvitamin D_3 was associated with an improvement in the quantitative EEG. The same EEG technique was used in a study of chronic uremia in the dog model by Akmal et al. (1984). The percent of seconds with less than seven waves was significantly lower in those animals that underwent thyroparathyroidectomy before five-sixths nephrectomy than in animals with intact parathyroid glands. The abnormal EEGs also correlated with the brain calcium level. The authors argued that it was not the elevation in brain calcium alone that produced the EEG abnormality, as the brain calcium levels were still elevated in the thyroparathyroidectomized animals with normal EEGs. They concluded that the EEG abnormality may be due to the parathyroid hormone itself or to a combination of parathyroid hormone and elevated calcium levels.

Manual period analysis (Sulg, 1969) is a more refined manual counting method in which, over a 30-second segment of EEG, the duration of each wave is noted. A graph is then constructed based on the number (activity) of the individual wavelengths; this is easily converted into a frequency spectrum. Using Sulg's method, Hagstrom (1971) determined activity times for the various frequency classes and also derived certain parameters that emphasized the amount of each frequency class. He found a significant correlation between the weighted EEG parameters and serum creatinine, nonprotein nitrogen, serum urea, and serum phosphate concentrations. Adjusting for creatinine concentration, the serum phosphate correlation was still valid. There was not, however, a significant EEG correlation with serum electrolyte values or hemoglobin concentration.

Automated Analysis

An automated method of counting various frequencies using a computer of average transients to determine the reciprocals of (time) distances between baseline crossovers can be used to plot a frequency spectrum (Kiley et al., 1976b). Other quantitative methods consider the frequency but also give a measure of the voltage or square of the voltage (power) for each frequency band. The EEG can be recorded on frequency modulation (FM) tape or computer disk and later analyzed (off-line) by various techniques. On-line analysis by computer is now also feasible.

In sonic analysis, the FM tape is played back at 100 times normal speed through sweep-type filters. Voltage or power versus frequency can be plotted. A simpler system is Ollf's analysis, in which the input of each EEG channel goes through two different filters. The first filters out all frequencies below 1 Hz and above 6 Hz, while the second allows 1- to 25-Hz frequencies through. The output of each filter is measured on a voltmeter. The percentage of the EEG signal occupied by the 1- to 6-Hz band is then calculated from the integrated voltage from the 1- to 6-Hz filter divided by that from the 1- to 25-Hz filter, multiplied by 100.

In a study by Kiley et al. (1976a), these techniques were found to be as useful as the power spectral analysis described in the following paragraph. The above methods were equally effective in determining the mean frequency for most records. The manual counting methods probably underestimate the dominant frequencies when the latter are under 5 Hz. Automated analyses that consider power (voltage squared) overemphasize low-frequency waves when they make up more than 50 percent, and underemphasize them when they account for less than 10 percent, of the trace.

Power spectral analysis has been the most popular method of automated analysis of EEG rhythms. This method uses fast Fourier algorithms to construct a plot of power versus frequency. These plots can be shown for representative epochs for each channel (Figure 4.8), or the sequential epochs for a given channel can be stacked on one another to form a

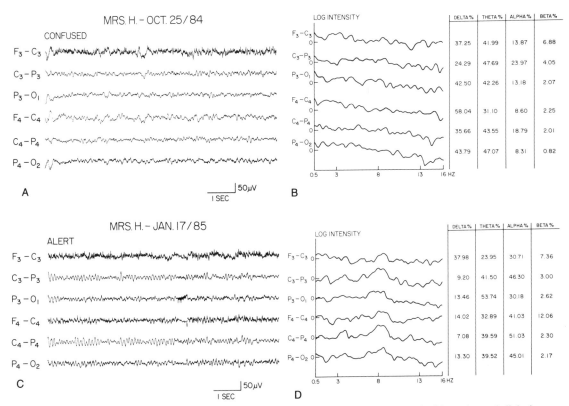

Figure 4.8. (A) The EEG of a 65-year-old woman with chronic renal failure treated with peritoneal dialysis. In October, 1984, she was confused. The tracing shows diffuse slowing in the theta (3- to 7-Hz) and delta (< 3-Hz) ranges. (B) The power spectral analysis (see text) of the same EEG trace. (C) and (D) The patient's EEG and power spectral analysis three months later. Her encephalopathy cleared and the EEG frequencies improved with an increased frequency of dialysis.

compressed spectral array (Bickford et al., 1971) (Figure 4.9).

The compressed spectral array allows easier recognition of artifact contamination and easier visualization of the quantity of lower frequencies compared with time-averaged autocorrelation and subsequent Fourier analysis (Bourne et al., 1975). Autoregressive analysis has some advantages over the Fourier transformation if sudden or subtle changes in EEG frequency occur, in that short (e.g., 1-second) segments are separately analyzed. In routine use, however, there is no real advantage of one method over the other (Jansen et al., 1981). Both methods rely on reproducible results when the same individual is retested under identical physiological conditions. Gasser et al. (1985) showed that the alpha rhythm shows good reliability, and that 20 seconds of recording effectively reduces the natural vari-

ability inherent in the EEG and reduces the effects of artifacts to a minor role.

The group at Vanderbilt University has extensively used power spectral analysis, using an ipsilateral parietal-occipital derivation, in following patients with CRF. They have shown the technique to be sensitive to frequency and adequacy of dialysis (Bourne and Teschan, 1983). An index of slow-wave frequency power constructed as the percent power of the 3- to 7-Hz band over that of the 3- to 13-Hz band, was found to be a convenient way of representing the relative amount of low frequencies present. Bowling and Bourne (1978) subsequently found that if the record were of low voltage, low-frequency artifacts could cause significant contamination. This was overcome by the use of discriminant analysis (Bowling and Bourne, 1978): "weights" were attached to 34 frequency values based on a reference

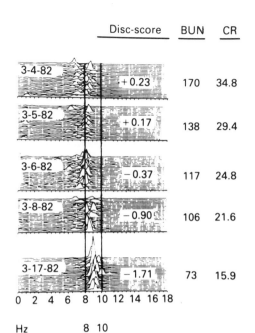

Figure 4.9. Serial compressed spectral array preparations in a patient with chronic renal failure. Following the initiation of dialysis therapy on March 4, 1982, there is a progressive improvement in the EEG frequency spectrum and discriminant score (Disc-score). The latter represents a mathematical weighting of the relative amount of lower-frequency activity. The improvement is commensurate with a reduction in blood urea nitrogen (BUN) and serum creatinine (CR) levels. (Reprinted with permission from Bourne et al., 1983.)

population of normal, mildly azotemic, and markedly azotemic subjects.

An objective assessment of which quantitative EEG parameters correlated best with predialysis azotemia, frequency of dialysis, and the effects of renal transplantation was made by Chotas et al. (1979). Those measures showing the highest correlation with the severity of uremia included average mean frequency, mean frequency of the averaged spectrum, average mean peak, and maximum 1-Hz and 2-Hz bands. An automated program (syntactical analysis) (Giese et al., 1979) notes these parameters and, using a standard covariance matrix, compares channels and sequential one-second periods of time. This program correctly identified drowsiness and artifact and classified the degree of encephalopathy in over 80 percent of records.

A more highly abstracted form of spectral analysis of EEG is "Hjørth's EEG descriptors" (Hjørth, 1970). These are time domain measures of the following: activity (power), mobility (central or peak frequency), and complexity (frequency spread). The descriptors are based on a physical model for EEG signals that obeys certain principles (Hjørth, 1973). The technique uses autocorrelation in a more comprehensive manner than do other methods.

Event-Related Potentials

Event-related potentials (ERPs) are EEG signals occurring at a reproducible interval after a well-defined event, usually a brief sensory stimulus. Some types of ERPs can be identified by superimposition of traces, but usually computer averaging techniques are used to more reliably identify the signal related to the particular event. Those that have been studied in CRF include visual, auditory, and somatosensory responses. A special category of ERPs, long-latency responses, are beginning to be studied as well.

Visual-Evoked Responses

Several studies have shown prolongation of the latency of the cortical visual-evoked response to diffuse flash in CRF (Hyman and Kooi, 1969; Hamel et al., 1978; Lewis et al., 1978; Di Paolo et al., 1982; Rossini et al., 1981). A series of waves are produced with this test; some studies examined latencies of all the major waves, some selected certain waves, and others examined the time difference between individual waves (interpeak latencies). All studies concur in showing prolongation of the measured parameter in CRF, with improvement following the commencement of dialysis or after renal transplantation. Furthermore, there is a modest but significant correlation with BUN and serum creatinine (Hamel et al., 1978; Lewis et al., 1978; Rossini et al., 1981) and with the continuous memory test, which depends largely on attention (Hamel et al., 1978).

Lewis et al. (1978) reported a significant increase in the amplitude or voltage of flash-evoked responses in hemodialysed patients compared to controls. Hyman and Kooi (1969) noted a tendency for this to occur, but statistical significance was not achieved. In the larger series of Hamel et al. (1978) and Rossini et al. (1981) no increase in mean amplitude of flash-evoked response was found in uremic compared to control subjects.

It is of interest that the power spectrum of the EEG (see Automated Analysis, above) is affected promptly when dialysis or transplant is instituted, while the effects on the flash-evoked response take longer to stabilize to new values (Hamel et al., 1978).

Pattern reversal evoked potentials (PREPs) are elicited using a checkerboard pattern on a television screen. They show much less inter- and intraindividual variability than do flash-evoked responses (Jeffreys, 1977). They may also test the visual system in a more physiologically relevant manner than the flash: Hubel and Wiesel (1977) have shown that neurons in the visual cortex respond to certain specific characteristics of the stimulus, such as the straight lines separating white from black squares.

Using PREPs, Rossini et al. (1981) showed that the major positive peak was unrecognizable or delayed in 37 percent of nondialysed and in 54 percent of dialysed uremic patients. Smaller check sizes (30 minutes of arc) are more effective than large check sizes in demonstrating an abnormality, possibly because small checks more effectively test the macular-calcarine system, which may require a higher level of processing than the luminance channel tested by larger checks. Furthermore, when steady-state responses are measured, noting the fidelity with which the cortical response follows the frequency of the stimulus reversal, uremic patients show a lack of response or a phase shift when higher frequencies of stimulus reversal are used (Rossini et al., 1981). There are no significant amplitude differences between uremic and nonuremic subjects (Rossini et al., 1981). Serum creatinine, BUN, serum parathyroid hormone level and the glomerular filtration rate are statistically correlated with PREP latency when small checks (7.7 and 15 minutes) were used (Rossini et al., 1981).

Auditory-Evoked Potentials

Albertazzi et al. (1985) showed that the short-latency auditory-evoked responses, which are generated in the brainstem within 10 ms of the click stimulus, are normal in uremia unless the patient is severely ill, often with grossly encephalopathic signs and symptoms. Such patients have prolongation of interpeak latencies (I–III, I–V, III–V), as well as an increase in latency of individual waves from the time of the stimulus.

Komsuologm et al. (1985) studied brainstem auditory-evoked potentials in a group of CRF patients on hemodialysis. They found a prolongation in central conduction times for the I–II and III–V intervals *predialysis*. These were reversed by dialysis, but there was an increase in the III–V interval (compared to normals) that was unaffected by dialysis. These findings indicate that the physiological disturbance in uremia acts differently than most drugs or physiological changes in attention and arousal, which do not affect brainstem auditory-evoked potentials.

Knoll et al. (1982) studied the major waves occurring within 80 ms after auditory click stimuli in 43 uremic patients and 32 healthy volunteers (Figure 4.10). The N30 component was used in comparison studies. The authors found that latencies of N30 are significantly prolonged in uremic patients compared to the control subjects. Further, those patients with uremic symptoms have significantly prolonged N30 potentials compared with uremic patients without such symptoms. Also, when patients begin dialytic therapy there is a reduction of N30 latency into the normal range (see Figure 4.10B).

Such auditory-evoked response testing may be a valuable quantitative method of assessing uremic encephalopathy, as the values for healthy individuals and mildly uremic patients are clearly separated from those with uremic symptomatology. The results are quantitative and easily measured. Further, the test is less

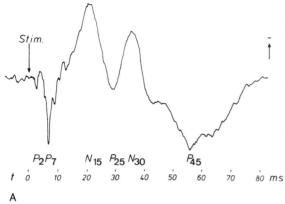

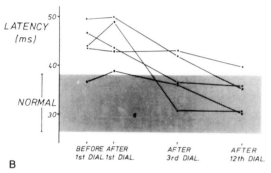

Figure 4.10. (A) Early auditory-evoked response components: 2,048 responses averaged. Stim = stimulus; t = time. Note the N30 peak. (B) Latencies of the N30 component during initiation of regular dialysis treatment (DIAL.) in five patients with chronic renal failure. (Reprinted with permission from Knoll et al., 1982.)

subject to the variability in results that can occur with altered vigilance or drugs than the compressed spectral array or longer-latency ERPs. It may thus provide a sensitive, if not specific, index of uremic encephalopathy.

Somatosensory-Evoked Responses

Somatosensory-evoked responses are produced by electrical stimulation of peripheral nerves, with the various waves produced along the somatosensory pathway up to and including the cerebral cortex. Studies by Lewis et al. (1978), Serra et al. (1979), and Albertazzi et al. (1985) showed that the cortical potential recorded from over the Rolandic region is delayed in uremia. Serra et al. (1979) found that

the delay is largely in the central, rather than in the peripheral, nervous system. This delay is reversed by renal transplantation (Lewis et al., 1978). Because of the crossover of the sensory pathway, the largest initial cortical potential is generated in the contralateral postcentral gyrus. Serra et al. (1979) also found a cortical response ipsilateral to the side of stimulation. The delay between the contralateral and ipsilateral responses was attributed to conduction across the corpus callosum. These authors also found that the transcallosal conduction time was increased in uremia.

The series of Lewis et al. (1978) and Serra et al. (1979) showed that the amplitude of the somatosensory response is increased in uremic patients on dialysis.

Albertazzi et al. (1985) found that central delay with somatosensory responses is more marked with stimulation of the peroneal than of the median nerve. They propose that the CNS is affected in a similar fashion to the peripheral nervous system in uremia, with longer axons being more affected than shorter axons (see Chapter 5 for a discussion of the peripheral nervous system in CRF). Uremia, they suggest, causes a distal axonopathy.

Long-Latency Event-Related Potentials

If a certain stimulus is followed by a second stimulus to which the subject makes a voluntary response, a negative baseline shift in the EEG, the contingent negative variation (CNV), can be recorded (Walter et al., 1964). The area of the CNV following the first stimulus has been called A_1 and that after the second stimulus (when a choice of response is required) is A_2. In a preliminary report by Teschan (1975), the area of A_2 is reduced in uremia.

Other long-latency ERPs (greater than 100 ms after event) have been called endogenous ERPs. They depend more on higher-order signal processing than the earlier components and are not as dependent on the physical features of the stimulus. The P300 is such an ERP, generated approximately 300 ms after the presentation of a novel stimulus or event. The

P300 may even occur when a regularly recurring, stereotyped signal is omitted, the absence of the anticipated signal constituting the novel event (Syndulko et al., 1982).

The P300 has been studied in uremic patients by Cohen et al. (1983). Patients were divided into two groups: the first had mild azotemia with patients only on a low-protein diet; the second had patients who required thrice weekly hemodialysis. Prolongation of P300 was found in 33 percent of the first group and 54 percent of the second group. Within the second group, there was no clear relationship between P300 prolongation and level of BUN, serum parathyroid hormone level, or serum aluminum level, although numbers of patients used for comparison were small.

Pathology of the Central Nervous System

Olsen (1961) performed the classic study on the pathological changes in brains of humans dying with acute and chronic renal failure. Gross and light microscopic findings were reported on 104 patients. Although the study was carefully done, it was, in several aspects, not well controlled. Many of the changes noted were due to complications of uremia, rather than the metabolic effects of uremia itself. The pathogenesis of the other changes are uncertain and so is their significance. The various abnormalities will be discussed in the order Olsen presented them.

Nerve Cell Changes

A variety of changes were noted: simple shrinkage, cellular swelling with intracytoplasmic vacuoles, central chromatolysis, and frank "ischemic cell change" with eosinophilic cytoplasm and nuclear pyknosis. Simple shrinkage is somewhat controversial; it may be a fixation artifact. Although these various changes were described in both acute and chronic renal failure, all such changes result from a recent insult. Since "ischemic cell change" and cellular swelling with intracytoplasmic vacuoles are progressive changes in

anoxic-ischemic neuronal damage (Brown and Brierley, 1968), it seems likely that they arise by such a mechanism operating shortly before death. Neuronal death may occur from a number of causes, possibly all acting through a common pathway with calcium influx into the neuronal cytoplasm (Farber, 1981). Central chromatolysis has been described after axonal injury and in pellagra (Meyer, 1901), particularly affecting large motor neurons.

Olsen grouped these changes together in noting their occurrence in various brain regions: they were most prominent in the sensory nuclei of the brainstem, followed by the brainstem reticular formation and the large neurons of the cerebral cortex. Despite the uncertain significance of these cellular changes, it is of interest that there is clinical and experimental evidence for dysfunction of the reticular formation in uremia (Jacob et al., 1965; Zuckermann and Glaser, 1972).

Conglutination of the cerebellar granule cells was unusually prominent in Olsen's material. The significance of conglutination of the cerebellum is uncertain; many pathologists regard it as an artifact or due to postmortem autolysis.

Lacunar Infarcts

Small deep infarcts were described particularly in the pons and corpus striatum in association with hypertension and were attributed to arteriosclerosis. This observation was later corroborated by Fisher (1965).

Demyelination

Knutson and Baker (1945) reported several cases of subacute and chronic uremia in which there was focal perivascular, as well as large confluent areas of, demyelination. Perivascular myelin sheaths were swollen and fused with fine vacuolated spaces after five days of uremic illness. The larger areas of demyelination were found in cases of longer duration. Olsen (1961) described demyelination in only eight of his 104 cases. Six had very small foci in one to three of the sampled regions; the other two had foci up to a few millimeters in diameter. There was no attendant inflammation, and the tissue was not frankly infarcted. It is possible that these demyelinative lesions were a complication of hypertensive arteriolar disease and represent early stages of the controversial Binswanger's disease (subcortical arteriosclerotic encephalopathy) (Olszewski, 1962).

Glial Changes

Olsen (1961) noted glial nodules in six of 104 patients. These were mainly in the medullary reticular formation. He postulated that at least some were in response to neuronal death (neuronophagia), noting remnants of a neuron in the center and activation of microglia. Other glial reactions were in response to tissue necrosis. No Alzheimer type II astrocytes, as seen in hepatic encephalopathy, were encountered.

Hemorrhages

Hemorrhages were found in 69 of the 104 cases studied by Olsen (1961). These were usually microscopic, but four patients had large macroscopic hemorrhages involving the brain parenchyma or meninges. There was no significant association with the use of dialysis or anticoagulant drugs. Many patients with larger hemorrhages had complicating factors such as hepatic failure, hypertension, or sepsis.

Inflammatory Changes

Olsen (1961) found inflammation in the form of perivascular infiltrates of mononuclear cells or as microabscesses. The former were the most common. Their occurrence was unassociated with any evidence of infection elsewhere in the body or on history in at least half the cases in which they were noted. Microabscesses were associated with sepsis or bacterial endocarditis; this is supported by the recent study of Jackson et al. (1985). In some cases, fungi such as *Candida* or *Aspergillus* organisms were responsible.

Vascular Changes

These clearly relate to associated conditions such as hypertension, diabetes, or hyperlipidemia. Large-vessel changes in the form of atherosclerosis (sometimes complicated by large brain infarcts) as well as arteriolar damage (which can result in lacunar infarcts or hypertensive hemorrhages) have been reported. When the risk factors are taken into consideration, it is unsettled whether patients with uremia, including those on dialysis have accelerated atherosclerosis (Lundin and Friedman, 1978).

Meningeal Involvement

Although a chemical meningitis occasionally occurs in uremia, Olsen (1961) found little evidence of meningeal inflammation or fibrosis in his pathological series.

Cerebral Edema

Cerebral edema is defined as an increase in water content of the brain. Diffuse cerebral edema is difficult to prove by ordinary anatomical methods; a more reliable method is to measure the percentage of water in the brain. This has been done for humans and experimental animals with uremia (Strobel, 1939; Olsen, 1961), and no significant difference between uremics and controls was noted in any study. Although there is no good evidence for cerebral edema in uremia per se, it should be recognized that cerebral edema may accompany certain complications of uremia such as vascular disease or osmotic dysequilibrium.

References

Adams RD, Foley JM. The neurological disorder associated with liver disease. Res Publ Assoc Res Nerve Ment Dis 1953;32:198–237.

Addison T. A collection of the published writings of the late Thomas Addison. Wilks S, Daldy TM, eds. London: New Sydenham Society, 1868.

Akmal M, Goldstein DA, Multani S, Massry SG. Role of uremia, brain calcium and parathyroid hormone on changes in electroencephalogram in chronic renal failure. Am J Physiol 1984; (Renal, Fluid Electrolyte Physiol 16):F575–F579.

Albertazzi A, Di Paolo B, Capelli C, Del Rosso G. Evoked responses in uremia. Contrib Nephrol 1985;45:60–68.

Bickford RG, Butt HR. Hepatic coma: the electroencephalopathic pattern. J Clin Invest 1955;34:790–799.

Bickford RG, Fleming JI, Billinger TW. Compression of EEG spectra by isometric power spectral plots. Electroencephalogr Clin Neurophysiol 1971;31:632.

Bonomini V, Campieri C, Feletti C, et al. Hormonal abnormalities in renal transplantation. Contr Nephrol 1985;70–77.

Bourne JR, Miezin FM, Ward JW, Teschan PE. Computer quantification of electroencephalographic data recorded from renal patients. Comput Biomed Res 1975;8:461–473.

Bourne JR, Teschan PE. Computer methods, uremic encephalopathy and adequacy of dialysis. Kidney Int 1983;24:496–506.

Bowling PS, Bourne JR. Discriminant analysis of electroencephalograms recorded from renal patients. IEEE Trans Biomed Eng 1978;25:12–17.

Brancaccio D, Damasso R, Spinnler H, et al. Neuropsychological performances of patients dialysed for more than 10 years. In: Giordano C, Friedman EI, eds. Uremia—pathobiology of patients treated for 10 years or more. Milan: Wichtig Editore, 1981:126–129.

Bright R. Cases and observations illustrative of renal disease accompanied by the secretion of albuminous urine. Guys Hosp Rep 1836;1:338–400.

Bril V, Sharpe JA, Ashby P. Midbrain asterixis. Ann Neurol 1979;6:362–364.

Brown AW, Brierley JB. The nature, distribution and earliest stages of anoxic-ischemic nerve cell damage in the rat brain as defined by the optical microscope. Br J Exp Pathol 1968;49:87–106.

Bruni J, Wang JL, Marbury TC, et al. Protein binding of valproic acid in uremic patients. Neurology 1980;30:1233–1236.

Buchanan WS, Ellis PE. Retinal separation in chronic glomerulonephritis. Arch Ophthalmol 1964;71:182–186.

Cadilhac J, Ribstein M. The EEG in metabolic disorders. World Neurol 1961;2:296–308.

Chadwick D, French AT. Uremic myoclonus: an example of reticular reflex myoclonus. J Neurol Neurosurg Psychiatry 1979;42:52–55.

Chadwick D, Hallett M, Harris R, et al. Clinical, biochemical and physiologic factors distinguishing myoclonus responsive to 5-hydroxytryptophan, tryptophan plus a monoamine oxidase inhibitor, and clonazepam. Brain 1977;100:455–487.

Chotas HG, Bourne JR, Teschan PE. Heuristic techniques in the quantification of the electroencephalogram in renal failure. Comput Biomed Res 1979;12:299–312.

Chung E, Van Woert MH. Urea myoclonus: possible involvement of glycine. In: Fahn S, Marsden CD, Van Woert MH. Advances in neurology: myoclonus 1986;43:565–568.

Cohen SN, Syndulko K, Rever B, et al. Visual evoked potentials and long latency event-related potentials in chronic renal failure. Neurology (Cleve) 1983;33:1219–1222.

Dement W, Rechtschaffen A, Gulevich G. The nature of the narcoleptic sleep attack. Neurology (Minneap) 1966;16:18–33.

Di Paolo B, Cappelli P, Spisni C, et al. New electrophysiological assessments for the early diagnosis of encephalopathy and peripheral neuropathy in chronic renal failure. Int J Tissue Reac 1982;4:301–307.

Ellis PT, Fonken HA. Retinopathies of chronic glomerulonephritis. Arch Ophthalmol 1965;75:36–41.

Engel GL, Romano J, Ferris EB Jr, et al. A simple method of determining frequency spectrums in the electroencephalogram. Arch Neurol Psychiatry 1944;51:134–146.

English A, Savage RD, Britton PG, et al. Intellectual impairment in chronic renal failure. Br Med J 1978;1:888–889.

Farber JL. The role of calcium in cell death. Life Sci 1981;29:1289–1299.

Feringa ER, Weatherbee L. Hypertrophic granulomatous pachymeningitis causing progressive blindness in a chronic dialysis patient. J Neurol Neurosurg Psychiatry 1975;38:1170–1176.

Fisher CM. Lacunes: small, deep cerebral infarcts. Neurology 1965;15:774–784.

Fishman RA. Cerebrospinal fluid in diseases of the nervous system. Philadelphia: WB Saunders, 1980:303–304.

Foley CM, Polinsky MS, Gruskin AB, et al. Encephalopathy in infants and children with chronic renal disease. Arch Neurol 1981;38:656–658.

Freeman RB, Sheff MF, Maher JF, et al. The blood-cerebrospinal fluid barrier in uremia. Ann Intern Med 1962;56:233–240.

Gasser T, Bacher P, Steinberg H. Test re-test reliability of spectral parameters of the EEG. Electroencephalogr Clin Neurophysiol 1985;60:312–319.

Gastaut H, Papy JJ, Toga M, et al. The epilepsy of renal insufficiency and incidental epileptic attacks during extrarenal detoxification. Electroencephalogr Clin Neurophysiol 1968;25:92.

Gerard RW. Factors influencing brain potentials. Trans Am Neurol Assoc 1936;62:55–60.

Giese DA, Bourne JR, Ward JW. Syntactic analysis of the electroencephalogram. IEEE Trans Systems Man Cybernet 1979;9:429–435.

Glaser GH. Metabolic encephalopathy in hepatic, renal and pulmonary disorders. Postgrad Med 1960;27:611–619.

Glaser GH. Brain dysfunction in uremia. In: Plum F, ed. Brain dysfunction in metabolic disorders. New York: Raven Press, 1974:173–199.

Gloor P, Testa G. Generalized penicillin epilepsy in the cat: effects of intracarotid and intravertebral pentylenetetrazol and amobarbital injections. Electroencephalogr Clin Neurophysiol 1974;36:499–515.

Goldstein DA, Feinstein EI, Chiu LA, et al. The relationship between the abnormalities in the electroencephalogram and blood levels of parathyroid hormone in dialysis patients. J Clin Endocrinol Metab 1980;51:130–134.

Gowers WR. Lectures on the diagnosis of diseases of the brain. London: Churchill, 1895:114.

Hagstrom K-E. EEG frequency content related to chemical blood parameters in chronic uraemia. Scand J Urol Nephrol 1971;(5) Suppl 7:1–56.

Hamel B, Bourne JR, Ward JW, Teschan PE. Visually evoked cortical potentials in renal failure: transient potentials. Electroencephalogr Clin Neurophysiol 1978;44:606–616.

Handelsman DJ. Hypothalamic-pituitary gonadal dysfunction in renal failure, dialysis and renal transplantation. Endocr Rev 1985;6:151–182.

Handelsman DJ, Spaliviero JA, Turtle JR. Hypothalamic-pituitary function in experimental uremic hypogonadism. Endocrinology 1985;117:1984–1995.

Harrison TR, Mason MF, Resnik H. Observations on the mechanism of muscular twitchings in uremia. J Clin Invest 1936;15:463–464.

Heilman KM, Moyer RS, Melendez F, et al. A memory defect in uremic encephalopathy. J Neurol Sci 1975;26:245–249.

Hjørth B. EEG analysis based on time domain properties. Electroencephalogr Clin Neurophysiol 1970;29:306–310.

Hjørth B. The physical significance of time domain analysis. Electroencephalogr Clin Neurophysiol 1973;34:321–325.

Hubel DH, Wiesel TN. Functional architecture of macaque monkey visual cortex. Proc R Soc Lond [Biol] 1977;198:1–59.

Hughes JR. Correlations between EEG and chemical changes in uremia. Electroencephalogr Clin Neurophysiol 1980;48:583–594.

Hutchinson JC, Klodd DA. Electrophysiologic analysis of auditory, vestibular and brainstem dysfunction in chronic renal failure. Laryngoscope 1982;92:833–843.

Hyman PR, Kooi KA. Visual evoked cortical responses in renal insufficiency. Univ Mich Med Center J 1969;35:177–179.

Jackson AC, Gilbert JJ, Young GB, Bolton CF. The encephalopathy of sepsis. Can J Neurol Sci 1985;12:303–307.

Jackson M, Warrington EK, Roe GJ, Baker LRI. Cognitive function in hemodialysis patients. Clin Nephrol 1987;27:26–30.

Jacob JC, Gloor P, Elwan OH, et al. Electroencephalographic changes in chronic renal failure. Neurology 1965;15:419–429.

Jansen BH, Bourne JR, Ward JW. Autoregressive estimation of short segment spectra for computerized EEG analysis. IEEE Trans Biomed Eng 1981;28:630–638.

Jeffreys DA. The physiological significance of pattern visual evoked responses. In: Desmedt JE, ed. Visual evoked potentials in man. Oxford: Clarendon Press, 1977:134–167.

Karnaze DS, Bickford RG. Triphasic waves: a reappraisal of their significance. Electroencephalogr Clin Neurophysiol 1984;57:193–198.

Kenny FT. Neurotoxicity, cognitive function and the outcome of CAPD. Peritoneal Dialysis Bull 1983;(3) Suppl 3:S43–S47.

Kenny FT, Oreopoulos DG. Neuropsychological studies of CAPD: preliminary findings. Peritoneal Dialysis Bull 1981;1:129–133.

Kiley J, Hines O. Electroencephalographic evaluation of uremia. Arch Intern Med 1965;116:67–73.

Kiley JE, Pratt KL, Gisser DG, Schaffer CA. Techniques of EEG frequency analysis for evaluation of uremic encephalopathy. Clin Nephrol 1976a;5:279–285.

Kiley JE, Woodruff MW, Pratt KL. Evaluation of encephalopathy by EEG frequency analysis in chronic dialysis patients. Clin Nephrol 1976b;5:279–285.

Kimel PL, Miller G, Mendelson WB. Sleep apnea syndrome in chronic renal disease. Am J Med 1989;86:308–314.

Klinger M. EEG observations in uremia. Electroencephalogr Clin Neurophysiol 1954;6:519.

Knoll O, Harbort U, Schulte K, Zimpel F. Quantitative survey of uremic brain dysfunction by auditory evoked potentials. In: Courjon J, Mauguiere F, Revol M, eds. Clinical applications of evoked potentials in neurology. New York: Raven Press, 1982:227–232.

Knutson J, Baker AB. The central nervous system in uremia. Arch Neurol Psychiatry 1945;54:130–140.

Komsuologm SS, Mehta R, Jones LA, Harding GFA. Brainstem evoked potentials in chronic renal failure and maintenance hemodialysis. Neurology 1985;35:419–423.

Lance JW, Adams RD. The syndrome of intention or action myoclonus as a sequel to hypoxic encephalopathy. Brain 1963;86:111–136.

Lanski LL. Abnormalities of hearing. In: Swaiman KF, Wright FS, eds. The practice of pediatric neurology. St. Louis: CV Mosby, 1982:232–245.

Lapco L, Weller JM, Greene JA Jr. Spontaneously reversible retinal detachment occurring during renal insufficiency. Ann Intern Med 1965;63:760–766.

Leavitt S, Tyler HR. Studies in asterixis. Arch Neurol 1964;10:360–368.

Lee KS, Powell BL, Adams PL. Focal neurological signs associated with hyperkalemia. South Med J 1984;77:792–793.

Lennon PA, Adam WR, Bladin P, et al. Transient blindness associated with chronic renal failure. Aust NZ J Med 1971;4:346–352.

Lewis EG, Dustman RE, Besk EC. Visual and somatosensory evoked potential characteristics of patients undergoing hemodialysis and kidney transplantation. Electroencephalogr Clin Neurophysiol 1978;44:223–231.

Lim VS, Fang VS. Gonadal dysfunction in uremic men. A study of the hypothalamo-pituitary-testicular axis before and after renal transplantation. Am J Med 1975;58:655–662.

Locke S, Merrill JP, Tyler HR. Neurological complications of acute uremia. Arch Intern Med 1961;108:519–530.

Lucien JC, Anteunis MA, Jacob MVM. Hearing loss in a uraemic patient: indications of involvement of the VIIIth nerve. J Laryngol Otol 1987;10:492–496.

Lundin AP, Friedman EA. Vascular consequences of maintenance hemodialysis—an unproven case. Nephron 1978;21:177–180.

Madonick MJ, Berke K, Schiffer I. Pleocytosis and meningeal signs in uremia. Arch Neurol Psychiatry 1950;64:431–436.

Mahajan SK, Abbasi AA, Prasad AS, et al. Effect of oral zinc therapy on gonadal dysfunction in hemodialysis patients: a double-blind study. Ann Intern Med 1982;97:357–361.

Mahoney CA, Arieff AI. Uremic encephalopathies: clinical, biochemical and experimental features. Am J Kidney Dis 1982;2:324–336.

Massey EW, Bowman MH, Rozear MP. Asterixis mimicking drop attacks in chronic renal failure. Neurology 1988;38:663.

McDaniel JW. Metabolic and CNS correlates of cognitive dysfunction with renal failure. Psychophysiology 1971;8:704–713.

Meldman MJ. Diseases of attention and perception. Oxford: Pergamon Press, 1970.

Merrill JP, Hampers CL. Uremia: progress in pathophysiology and treatment. New York: Grune and Stratton, 1971.

Merritt HH, Fremont-Smith F. The cerebrospinal fluid. Philadelphia: WB Saunders, 1938:212.

Meyer A. On parenchymatous systemic degenerations mainly in the central nervous system. Brain 1901;24:47–115.

Mises J, Lerique-Kocchlin A, Rombot B. The electroencephalogram during renal insufficiency. Electroencephalogr Clin Neurophysiol 1968;25:91.

Moruzzi G, Magoun HW. Brainstem reticular formation and activation of the EEG. Electroencephalogr Clin Neurophysiol 1949;1:455–473.

Murphy GP, Sharp JC. Timed behavior in primates during various experimental uremic states. JSR 1964;4:550–553.

Muscatt S, Rothwell J, Obeso J, et al. Urea-induced stimulus-sensitive myoclonus in the rat. In: Fahn S, Marsden C, Van Woert M, eds. Advances in neurology, Vol 43: Myoclonus. New York: Raven Press, 1986:553–563.

Naquet R, Meldrum BS. Myoclonus induced by intermittent light stimulation in the baboon: neurophysiological and neuropharmacological approaches. In: Fahn S, Marsden CD, Van Woert M, eds. Advances in neurology, Vol 43: Myoclonus. New York: Raven Press, 1980:611–628.

Olsen S. The brain in uremia. Acta Psychiatr Neurol Scand 1961;36(Suppl 156):3–129.

Olszewski J. Subcortical atherosclerotic encephalopathy. World Neurol 1962;3:359–375.

Parkhouse J, Henrie JR, Duncan GM, Rome HP. Nitrous oxide analgesia in relation to mental performance. J Pharmacol Exp Ther 1960;128:44–54.

Passouant P, Cadilhac J, Baldy-Moulinier M, Mion C. Etude du sommeil nocturne chez des urémiques chroniques soumis à une épuration extrarénale. Electroencephalogr Clin Neurophysiol 1970;29:441–449.

Plum F, Posner JB. The diagnosis of stupor and coma. 3rd ed. Philadelphia: FA Davis, 1980:177–303.

Pro JR, Wells CE. The use of the electroencephalogram in the diagnosis of delirium. Dis Nerv Syst 1977;38:804–808.

Raskin NH, Fishman RA. Neurologic disorders in renal failure (first of two parts). N Engl J Med 1976;294:143–148.

Reichenmiller HE, Reinhard U, Durr F. Sleep EEG and uremia. Electroencephalogr Clin Neurophysiol 1971;30:263–264.

Reiher J. The electroencephalogram in the investigation of metabolic coma. Electroencephalogr Clin Neurophysiol 1970;28:104P.

Reitan RM. Validity of the trailmaking test as an indicator of organic brain damage. Percept Mot Skills 1958;8:271–276.

Romano J, Engel GI. Delirium I. Electroencephalographic data. Arch Neurol Psychiatry 1944;51:356–377.

Rossini PM, Pirchio M, Treviso M, et al. Checkerboard reversal pattern and flash VEPs in dialysed and non-dialysed subjects. Electroencephalogr Clin Neurophysiol 1981;52:435–444.

Rucker CW. The causes of paralysis of the third, fourth and sixth cranial nerves. Am J Ophthalmol 1966;61:1293–1298.

Schreiner GC, Maher JF. Uremia: biochemistry, pathogenesis and treatment. Springfield, IL: Charles C Thomas, 1961.

Schreiner GE. Mental and personality changes in the uremic syndrome. Med Ann DC 1959;28:316–323.

Serra C, Romano F, D'Angelillo A, et al. Somatosensory cerebral evoked responses in uremic polyneuropathy. Acta Neurol 1979;34:1–14.

Silverman D. Some observations of the EEG in hepatic coma. Electroencephalogr Clin Neurophysiol 1962; 14:53–59.

Stark RJ. Reversible myoclonus with uremia. Br Med J 1981;282:1119–1120.

Steiness IB. Reversible retinal detachment in renal insufficiency. Acta Med Scand 1968;183:225.

Strobel T. Uber den Trockensubtanzgehalt verschiedener Hirnteille. Ztschr f d ges Neurol u Psychiat 1939;166:161.

Stuss DT, Benson DF. The frontal lobes. New York: Raven Press, 1986:209–211.

Sulg IA. Manual period analysis. Acta Neurol Scand 1969;45:431–458.

Syndulko K, Hansch EC, Cohen SN, et al. Long latency event-related potentials in normal aging and dementia. In: Courjon J, Mauguiere F, Revol M, eds. Clinical applications of evoked responses in neurology. New York: Raven Press, 1982;32:279–285.

Teschan PE. Electroencephalographic and other neurophysiological abnormalities in uremia. Kidney International 1975;7:S210–S216.

Teschan PE. Central and peripheral nervous system in uremia: an overview. Clin Nephrol 1985;45:1–8.

Teschan PE, Ginn HE, Bourne JR, et al. Quantitative neurobehavioral responses to renal failure and maintenance hemodialysis. Trans Am Soc Artif Intern Organs 1975;21:488–491.

Teschan PE, Ginn HE, Bourne JR, Ward JW. Neurobehavioral probes for adequacy of dialysis. Trans Am Soc Artif Intern Organs 1977;23:556–560.

Teschan PE, Ginn HE, Bourne JR, et al. Neurobehavior in long-term hemodialyzed patients. In: Giordano C, Friedman EI, eds. Uremia—pathobiology of patients treated for 10 years or more. Milan: Wichtig Editore, 1981;25:117–125.

Travis AM. Neurological deficiencies following supplementary motor area lesions in *Macaca mulatta*. Brain 1955;78:174–198.

Treiman DM. General principles of treatment: responsive and intractable status epilepticus in adults. In: Delgado-Escueta AV, Wasterlain CG, Treiman DM, Porter RJ, eds. Advances in neurology status epilepticus. New York: Raven Press, 1983;34:377–384.

Tyler HR. Convulsions and EEG changes in uremia. Trans Am Neurol Assoc 1965;90:76–79.

Tyler HR. Neurologic disorders in renal failure. Am J Med 1968;44:734–748.

Tyler HR. Neurologic disorders seen in the uremic patient. Arch Intern Med 1970;126:781–786.

Tyler HR, Tyler KL. Neurologic complications. In: Eknoyan G, Knochel JP, eds. The systemic complications of renal failure. Orlando, FL: Grune & Stratton, 1981;12:311–330.

Walter WG, Cooper R, Aldridge VJ, et al. Contingent negative variation: an electric sign of sensori-motor association and expectancy in the human brain. Nature (Lond) 1964;203:380–384.

Wilson SAK. In: N Bruce (ed), Neurology, Vol. 2. Baltimore: Williams & Wilkins, 1940:1047.

Yassin A, Badry A, Fatt-hi A. The relationship between electrolyte balance and cochlear disturbance in cases of renal failure. J Laryngol 1970;84:429–435.

Zuckermann EC, Glaser GH. Urea-induced myoclonic seizures: an experimental study of the site of action and mechanism. Arch Neurol 1972;27:14–28.

Zynso EA. The EEG in uremia. Electroencephalogr Clin Neurophysiol 1970;29:212–213.

Chapter 5
Uremic Neuropathy

Contents

Acronyms

ATPase   adenosine triphosphatase
CAP   compound action potential
CAPD   continuous ambulatory peritoneal
    dialysis

A

Uremic Polyneuropathy

Despite the beneficial effects of hemodialysis and successful renal transplantation, uremic polyneuropathy remains a significant factor in the ongoing morbidity of patients in chronic renal failure. It should be regarded as a sign of the degree of renal failure, or the lack of control of such failure by hemodialysis, and hence is a prime indication for renal transplantation. Uremic neuropathy must be distinguished from other types of neuropathy that may occur in renal failure patients, such as diabetic neuropathy. For these and many other reasons, those who are responsible for caring for these patients should have a thorough knowledge of uremic polyneuropathy.

In a series of articles published between 1970 and 1978, Nielsen (1967;1971a; 1971b; 1973a; 1973b; 1973c; 1973d; 1974a; 1974b; 1974c; 1974d; 1974e; 1978; Nielsen and Winkel, 1971) recorded remarkably detailed and wide-ranging observations on uremic polyneuropathy. Even though severe uremic neuropathy is much less common now, many of Nielsen's observations are still relevant. A number of centers in the world have remained active in the investigation of uremic polyneuropathy, and this chapter will attempt to bring together these various observations and opinions.

Clinical Features

Clinical assessment is often difficult, no matter how severe the neuropathy, perhaps explain-ing why the neuromuscular complications of uremia escaped detection for so many years. The encephalopathy of chronic uremia may make elicitation of the clinical features of neuropathy difficult. Reduction of deep tendon reflexes may be the only reliable clinical sign of neuromuscular disease. Electrophysiological abnormalities are the earliest and most objective method of demonstrating the presence and type of neuromuscular disease. Nonetheless, worthwhile clinical signs may still be elicited that provide important information on the type and severity of the neuromuscular disease.

There is little evidence, if any, of uremic polyneuropathy on clinical examination in acute renal failure. Locke et al. (1961) studied 13 such cases and noted only variable degrees of muscle wasting and weakness, somewhat depressed deep tendon reflexes, and normal sensation. But, as emphasized, there are great difficulties in examining such patients. None have apparently been studied by electrophysiological techniques. Using such techniques in an animal experimental model of acute uremia, Brismar and Tegner (1984) have shown electrophysiological evidence of neuropathy.

When renal disease develops insidiously, mental symptoms are less marked, and a worthwhile clinical assessment can often be made. Asbury et al. (1963) have given the best description, made from observations on the four patients that were the subject of this classic paper. All were young males whose primary renal diseases were of different types, and none had been treated by hemodialysis. Thus, the neuropathy seemed entirely due to the renal failure.

> In each of our patients, pain, numbness and tingling of the toes and feet were the initial symptoms. In the early stages, the feet were sensitive to light touch and pressure. As these symptoms progressed over a period of weeks, weakness of the feet and atrophy of the leg muscles became evident. The feet and legs were always affected first, and more severely than the hands and arms. The trunk and face were spared, as were the structures innervated by the lower sacral segments. A sensory loss affecting all of the modalities, more or less equally, was demonstrable over the feet and legs, and to a lesser extent the hands. The upper borders of sensory impairment were indefinite with the zones of altered sensation shading into normal areas. The tendon reflexes were abolished. There had been no abrupt worsening of renal function just prior to or at the time of onset of the polyneuropathy, although in case 4 the uremia was steadily worsening at the time of onset.

Since then, the clinical features have been documented by a number of investigators, who have reported an incidence ranging from 10 percent to 83 percent (Table 5.1). The most comprehensive study was by Nielsen (1971) of 109 patients, most in advanced stages of renal failure, the creatinine clearances varying from 0 to 80 mL/min, with a median of 8 mL/min. This was a particularly valuable study because none of these patients had received hemodialysis, eliminating an important confounding factor.

The incidence of the various symptoms and signs is noted in Table 5.2. Those symptoms with the highest incidence—restless legs, cramps, and paresthesias—are nonspecific and not necessarily due to polyneuropathy. They may be related to transient disturbances of peripheral sensory receptors induced by fluctuation in water and electrolyte balance or in the as-yet-unknown uremic toxins. Muscle cramps involve various muscle groups and occur mainly at night. The restless leg syndrome may be particularly distressing (Callaghan, 1966). It occurs prior to or during a regular hemodialysis procedure, but otherwise is typical of the syndrome originally described by Eckbom (1960). (In patients not in renal failure, it is usually associated with mental depres-

sion, various types of peripheral neuropathy, or rarely, a familial tendency.) In the evening or when attempting to sleep at night, there is an extremely uncomfortable, often indescribable sensation in the legs that can only be relieved by movement of the legs. At times, this may reach bizarre proportions, such that the patient literally dishevels not only her or his bed but the entire bedroom with restless activities. Diazepam often provides symptomatic relief, as does increasing the frequency and duration of the hemodialysis treatments.

Transient numbness, tingling, itching, and pricking, often in the distal extremities, are also nonspecific symptoms of the uremic syndrome that may not necessarily be related to uremic neuropathy.

Persistent, severe pain or a burning sensation in the feet, "the burning foot syndrome," now is an uncommon manifestation of uremic neuropathy due to uremic toxins (Asbury, 1984). It is a well-known symptom of neuropathy due to thiamine deficiency. This vitamin, being water soluble, is easily removed during hemodialysis. Thus, when hemodialysis was first begun, it was commonly reported. However, with the regular administration of thiamine and other vitamins during terminal renal failure, particularly during regular hemodialysis, this syndrome is now rarely encountered.

The earliest concrete clinical evidence of uremic polyneuropathy is loss of vibration sense in the toes and reduction of deep tendon reflexes, beginning with the ankle jerks. Jennekens et al. (1971) noted that such signs developed only when the creatinine clearance was 5 mL/min or less and were more likely to be present in more advanced stages of renal failure. While there is some correlation between the incidence of clinical signs of polyneuropathy and the severity of the nerve conduction velocity changes, it is not a close one (Nielsen, 1973b). The possible reasons for this discrepancy are discussed under Pathophysiology, below.

Thus, clinical signs of uremic polyneuropathy are unlikely to be present in acute renal failure and do not appear until the more advanced stages of chronic renal failure. Inexplicably, the neuropathy is more common in

Table 5.1. The Incidence and Course of Uremic Polyneuropathy during Regular Hemodialysis

Year	Location	Investigator	No. of Patients	Type of Hemodialysis	Clinical Signs		Electrophysiological Signs	
					Incidence (%)	Course	Incidence (%)	Course
Part I. Studies of Adults								
1965	London, England	Konotey-Ahulu et al., 1965	20	Kiil, 14 hr, 2/wk	75	Improved	75	Improved
1967	Seattle, United States	Jebsen et al., 1967	20	Kiil	45	2 stabilized, 3 improved, 4 worsened	?	10 stabilized, 10 improved
1968	Germany	Dobblestein et al., 1968	12	Kolff twin-coil, 7 hr, 2/wk	30	All worsened	100	All worsened
1969	London, England	Curtis et al., 1969	32	Kiil dialyzer, 14 hr, 2/wk	20	Improved	63	8/15 improved, 3/15 worsened
1971	Holland	Jennekens et al., 1971	20	Kiil dialyzer, 2/wk	60	Improved	70	?
1974	Copenhagen, Denmark	Nielsen, 1974a	16	Kiil, 10 hr, 2/wk	51	Improved, 2 worsened	97	Stabilized, 1 improved
1975	Rochester, United States	Dyck et al., 1975a	20	Cordis-Dow, 8 hr, 3/wk	10	No follow-up	59	No follow-up
1978	France	Cadilhac et al., 1978	213	?	62	?	85	Stable, 7% improved, 3 worsened
1981	Boston, United States	Ackil et al., 1981b	18	?, 3/wk	83	No follow-up	87	No follow-up
Part II. Studies of Children								
1975	Toronto, Canada	Arbus et al., 1986	20	8 hr, 2/wk	?	?	57	Stable
1981	Boston, United States	Ackil et al., 1981a	17	3/wk	29	?	59	?
Part III. Studies by Bolton et al.								
1970	Saskatchewan, Canada	Bolton et al., 1970	30	Kolff twin-coil, 6 hr, 2/wk	53	3 stabilized, 9 worsened	77	11 stabilized, 12 worsened
1976	London, Canada	Bolton et al., 1976	18	Hospital, Gambro 17, 2/wk, 15 m²·hr	33	4 stabilized, 2 worsened	89	14 stabilized, 2 worsened
1976	London, Canada	Bolton et al., 1976	12	Home, Gambro 17, 3/wk, 18 m²·hr	17	2 worsened	83	10 stabilized, 2 worsened

Table 5.2. Clinical Neurological Findings in 109 Patients with Chronic Renal Failure

Finding	No. of Patients (%)
Symptoms	84 (77)
Motor	76 (70)
Restless legs	43
Cramps	55
Muscular weakness	10
Sensory	44 (40)
Paresthesia	34
Dysesthesia	20
Pain	6
Burning feet	7
Signs	56 (51)
Paresis	15 (14)
Muscular atrophies	13 (13)
Abnormal reflexes	31 (28)
Achilles	30
Patellar	23
Biceps	7
Impaired vibratory perception	42 (38)
Pulp, big toe	37
Medial malleolus	34
Pulp, thumb	10
Hypesthesia	17 (16)

Source: Reprinted with permission from Nielsen (1971b).

males than in females, but is not more frequent in the elderly than in younger patients when the degree of renal failure is taken into account (Nielsen, 1973b). In the occasional patient, a very severe polyneuropathy will develop in which there is severe weakness and wasting of muscles and impaired sensation in all four limbs. In modern times, dialysis, either hemodialysis or peritoneal dialysis, has been instituted early enough in the course of renal failure that severe cases are now rarely observed (Bolton, 1980b).

An important variant is a rapidly progressive, predominantly motor polyneuropathy (McGonigle et al., 1985). It is most likely to occur in the early stages of hemodialysis, usually in association with, to quote Tenckhoff and colleagues (1965), "critical illness—a catabolic state with septicemia, pneumonia or other forms of infection and rapid muscle wasting." These authors noted that improvement in neuropathy occurred with more frequent and longer dialysis times. Such cases were subsequently noted by Dobblestein et al. (1968),

Thomas et al. (1971), and Lynch et al. (1971). The patient reported by Willett (1964) likely had coincidental Guillain-Barré syndrome. In the report by McGonigle et al. (1985), two patients improved following transplantation and a third patient, after treatment by a charcoal hemoperfusion type of hemodialysis. However, McGonigle et al. noted that nerve conduction studies remained grossly impaired. Recent studies by Bolton et al. (1984;1986) have shown that a polyneuropathy, at times severe, develops in association with critical illness, a syndrome of sepsis and multiple organ failure. However, the renal failure in this situation may be only mild. The mechanism appears to be the same one that causes dysfunction of all organs in this syndrome, and the neuropathy will improve once the sepsis comes under control. One must speculate, therefore, that these early cases of accelerated, predominantly motor polyneuropathy, all of which occurred in terminal renal failure but also in association with sepsis, may have been due as much to the sepsis as to the renal failure. Thus, the lessening incidence of severe uremic polyneuropathy in recent years may not simply be due to improved methods of hemodialysis, but may be due to the lower incidence of, or better treatment of, sepsis. In particular, the use of arteriovenous fistulas for access, rather than various types of shunts that were remarkably prone to septic complications, may be a chief reason for this change.

The cerebrospinal fluid protein may be normal or elevated in uremia per se, but Jennekens et al. (1971) showed that it was more likely to be elevated in association with polyneuropathy, particularly more severe types. The level might reach 200 mg/dL (Figure 5.1). The cell counts were not increased. Jennekens et al. (1971) suggested that a breakdown in the blood-brain barrier might account for the elevated protein and at the same time play a role in the development of the polyneuropathy.

Autonomic Neuropathy in Uremia

There has been debate as to whether autonomic dysfunction occurs in uremia. For ex-

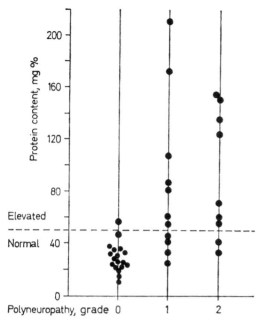

Figure 5.1. Protein content of the cerebrospinal fluid in 40 patients with chronic and severe renal insufficiency. Note the increasing concentration of protein in patients with more severe uremic polyneuropathy. (Reprinted with permission from Jennekens et al., 1971.)

ample, Mathias et al. (1983) found through extensive physiological testing that the evidence for autonomic neuropathy was unconvincing and was unlikely to account for hemodialysis-induced hypotension in the majority of patients with chronic renal failure. Wehle et al. (1983), using a technique of carotid sinus stimulation by neck suction in nine patients, was also unconvinced of an abnormality.

However, Solders et al. (1985) have not only extensively reviewed the literature on the subject but have performed comprehensive testing on 44 uremic patients. They note that various investigators have found abnormalities in uremic patients in the Valsalva test and the tilt test, both of which evaluate parasympathetic and sympathetic nerves. Tests of the sympathetic nervous system that have been used in uremic patients include the forced handgrip test, the cold pressure test, the mental stress test, and the sweat test, and the results have been abnormal. Solders et al. (1985) investigated only the parasympathetic nervous system, and their findings largely con-

firmed several other reports in the literature. The normal variation in the RR interval of the electrocardiogram tended to be abolished (Figure 5.2), this abnormality being more marked in relationship to the severity of the renal failure. A single hemodialysis treatment had no effect on the RR variation. The abnormality was more marked in those patients who had abnormal lowering of the amplitude of the sensory compound action potential of the sural nerve, suggesting that the axonal degenelation of peripheral nerves affects both the somatic and autonomic nerves. Thus, Dyck et al. (1971) noted a degeneration of nonmyelinated as well as myelinated fibers in nerve biopsies in patients who had uremic polyneuropathy. Signs of autonomic dysfunction are more marked in the elderly.

Despite the more recent, well-documented evidence for autonomic neuropathy in uremia,

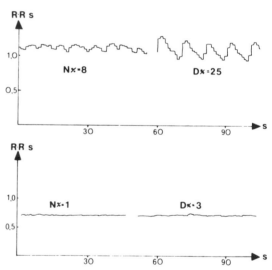

Figure 5.2. Abnormality in the cholinergic autonomic nervous system in chronic renal failure. (Top) Electrocardiographic RR variation in a patient in advanced renal failure. At this time, the RR variation was normal in the resting state and after deep breathing (N% and D% refer to the percentage variation with normal breathing and with deep breathing). (Bottom) The same patient developed more marked renal insufficiency, which required intermittent hemodialysis. The RR interval is now abnormal, with very little variation either at rest or with deep breathing, indicating cholinergic autonomic insufficiency. (Reprinted with permission from Solders et al., 1985.)

in an earlier study (Bolton, 1980) found that few patients exhibited overt symptoms or signs of severe autonomic insufficiency at any time during the course of chronic renal failure, i.e., orthostatic hypotension, impotence, or bowel or bladder disturbance. However, in the ill uremic patient, orthostatic hypotension could be erroneously attributed to volume depletion or antihypertensive drugs, impotence to a variety of other causes, bladder problems to decreased urine volumes from renal failure, and bowel problems and constipation to aluminum-containing antacids. Thus, the incidence and type of autonomic disturbance is very difficult to assess in the uremic patient on a purely clinical basis.

Neurophysiological Studies

In 1963, just three years after regular hemodialysis had been instituted in several centers throughout the world, Chaumont et al. in France reported reduced nerve conduction velocities in uremic patients. This was subsequently confirmed by Versaki et al. (1964) in the United States and by Preswick and Jeremy (1964) in Australia. Of particular importance was the observation that the abnormality often occurred when patients had no clinical signs of neuropathy. This discovery initiated many studies and the application of new physiological techniques. The effect of renal failure on these various electrophysiological tests is discussed in this chapter.

Standard Nerve Conduction and Electromyographic Studies

In uremia, both motor and sensory conduction velocities are reduced (Nielsen, 1973a), distal latencies being prolonged to a similar degree. Conduction velocity has remained as one of the best measures of peripheral nerve function. It changes during the various stages of renal failure, largely reflecting its severity (Figure 5.3) (Bolton, 1980b). Amplitudes of muscle and sensory compound action potentials (CAPs) are considerably reduced, the re-

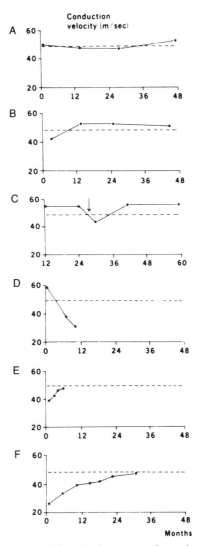

Figure 5.3. Variations in the course of uremic neuropathy in individual patients as reflected in median motor conduction velocity (.... = 2 standard deviations below mean control value). Other nerves tested showed similar results. (A) Stable course in a 54-year-old man on three times weekly home dialysis. (B) Improvement in uremic neuropathy in a 55-year-old man on three times weekly home dialysis. (C) Transient worsening of uremic neuropathy in a 48-year-old woman during intercurrent illness (→: hysterectomy, septicemia and uremic encephalopathy). (D) Rapidly progressing neuropathy in a 21-year-old man on twice weekly hemodialysis with a Kolff twin-coil unit. (E) Rapid recovery after successful renal transplantation in a 43-year-old man with only a subclinical neuropathy. (F) Gradual recovery after successful renal transplantation in a 21-year-old man with severe, quadriplegic neuropathy. (Reprinted with permission from Bolton et al., 1980.)

duction being due partly to a dispersion of the action potential as a result of disproportionate slowing of conduction in some nerve fibers. The main reason for the reduction, however, is axonal degeneration and loss of conduction in affected fibers (Bolton, 1976) and denervation of muscle (Figure 5.4). Of the various nerve conduction measurements, reduction of the amplitude of both muscle and sensory nerve CAPs is the most marked (Ackil et al., 1981b). Needle electromyography shows abnormalities only when the neuropathy has become moderate or severe. At this time, positive sharp waves and fibrillation potentials appear mainly in distal muscles, and the number of motor

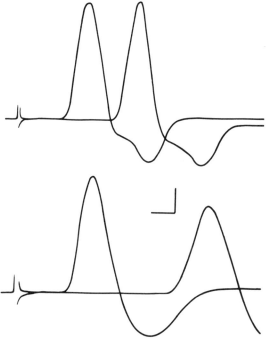

Figure 5.4. Median nerve conduction study in a 21-year-old man with a rapidly progressive uremic polyneuropathy (see Fig 5.3D). The first study (upper tracing), a normal result, was performed after one month of hemodialysis with a Kolff twin-coil unit. The second study (lower tracing), an abnormal result, was performed after 10 months of hemodialysis. Thenar muscle compound action potentials from wrist and elbow stimulation are shown. Conduction velocity fell from 57 to 29 m/s. The CAP became dispersed, consistent with demyelination secondary to an underlying primary axonal degeneration. (Calibration: vertical, 2 mV; horizontal, 2 ms.)

unit potentials on voluntary recruitment becomes moderately decreased in number (Bolton, 1980b; Bolton et al., 1971). The sural nerve, a purely sensory nerve, is possibly the site of the earliest abnormality (Ackil et al., 1981b; D'Amour et al., 1984). In general, the degree of slowing of nerve conduction in proximal segments is at least equal to, or perhaps more marked than, in distal segments (Nielsen, 1973b; Chokroverty, 1982). Moreover, van der Most van Spijck et al. (1973) demonstrated that there was slowing in conduction in small as well as large myelinated fibers. The excitation threshold to peripheral nerve stimulation is increased in comparison to controls (Wright and McQuillen, 1973), but the variability in this test is too great to make it of any clinical value.

In Nielsen's comprehensive studies of 56 patients with chronic renal failure who were not yet receiving regular hemodialysis (1973b), he demonstrated that nerve conduction was significantly slowed once the 24-hour creatinine clearance fell below 10 mL/min for a 1.73-m^2 membrane area. In fact, there was a linear relationship between reduced peroneal nerve conduction velocity and creatinine clearance (Figure 5.5) (Nielsen, 1973b). Slowing of nerve conduction was more marked in males than females, but age was not a factor when the degree of renal failure was taken into account. There was a relatively poor correlation between the prevalence of clinical signs and abnormalities of nerve conduction, the latter often being present when clinical signs were absent.

Arbus et al. (1986) found that peroneal conduction velocities were abnormal in about 60 percent of children in chronic renal failure. However, more recent studies by Ackil et al. (1981a) and Alderson et al. (1985) indicate that standard nerve conduction abnormalities are less frequent in children than in adults, approximately 20 percent versus 60 percent, respectively. On the other hand, Ackil et al. (1981a) showed that if sural nerve conduction is measured, as well as H-reflex and F-responses (late responses), approximately 60 percent of children will show abnormalities. In children, as well as in adults, nerve con-

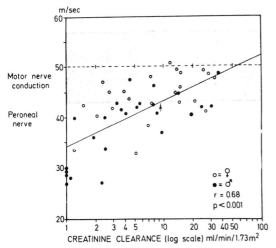

Figure 5.5. Fall in conduction as kidney function declined in 56 patients prior to institution of hemodialysis. The arrow indicates when 50 percent of patients will show abnormal values. The conduction velocities tended to be lower in males than females (*p* <0.01). (Reprinted with permission from Nielsen, 1973b.)

1.7°C for the hand, and 29.5 ± 1.1°C for the foot. The second method, which Bolton uses for research studies, is to measure the temperature and then apply a correction factor. This factor in abnormal (i.e., uremic) nerve (Bolton, 1981) is so small for compound muscle and sensory action potential amplitudes that correction for differences in temperature need not be done. However, correction factors are substantial in uremic nerve for conduction velocity and F-wave measurement: +1.5 m/s/°C (Bolton, 1981), and for the F-response latency: −1.5 m/s/°C (Bolton et al., 1982).

Sex is an important factor only when considering antidromic sensory conduction studies in the upper limb, where the amplitude of the sensory CAP in females is higher than that in males (Bolton and Carter, 1980). Age is a factor for both conduction velocity and action potential amplitude measurement, these values decreasing with advancing age (Ludin and Tackmann, 1981). These correction factors should be calculated for the individual laboratory.

In doing serial nerve conduction studies in the same patient to determine the effect of treatment, i.e., hemodialysis or transplantation, it is important to know the repeatability of the test. This was first examined by Kominami et al. (1971) for motor nerve conduction velocity in healthy and uremic patients. We repeated these studies and found similar results but extended them to include measurements of action potential amplitudes (Table 5.3). It can be seen that if one takes into account 95 percent confidence limits, conduction velocity may vary as much as 10 m/s, and CAP amplitudes by as much as 5 mV for muscle CAP amplitudes and 18 μV for sensory CAP amplitudes. The variation is likely to be greater in uremic than control patients, perhaps because the axon membrane is somewhat more unstable in uremic patients. Thus, in assessing the effect of any form of treatment on uremic polyneuropathy, nerve conduction studies should be performed in a reasonably large group of patients and, in individual patients, should be repeated a number of times to be certain that any trend is genuine.

duction values tend to stabilize during chronic hemodialysis but consistently improve after successful renal transplantation (Alderson et al., 1985).

Thus, Bolton has found nerve conduction measurements to be of great value in assessing peripheral nerve function in chronic renal failure. There is little discomfort when the procedures are performed by experienced technicians. Needle electromyography is somewhat more uncomfortable, but it need only be performed in more severe neuropathies and need not be repeated in most cases.

Each laboratory should establish its own control values. However, it should be recognized when interpreting such values that there are a number of important variables. Maynard and Stolov (1972) and Ludin and Tackmann (1981) have discussed the experimental error in conduction velocity measurements. CAP amplitude is also affected by these variables (Bolton, 1981). Temperature is the most important factor. It can be handled in two ways. At the time of nerve conduction testing, the limbs can be warmed to a mean physiological level, which Bolton has found to be 31.8 ±

Table 5.3. Repeatability of Nerve Conduction Measurements (Median Nerve)*

	Mean	SD	Coefficient of Variation (%)
Motor conduction velocity (ms)			
Normal	62.5	3.7	5.9
Uremic	48.1	3.6	7.4
Compound thenar muscle action potential amplitude (mV)			
Normal	12.6	1.7	13.2
Uremic	7.8	1.2	17.4
Compound digital nerve action potential amplitude (μV)			
Normal	45.8	7.8	18.0
Uremic	19.1	3.2	19.5

*Repeated four times at 3-month intervals in six persons on chronic hemodialysis and in six healthy subjects.
Source: Bolton CF and Carter K, unpublished data.

Studies of the Motor Unit

The number of motor units in the extensor digitorum brevis muscle of the foot of 30 patients on chronic hemodialysis was estimated by Hansen and Ballantyne (1978) using a computer technique. They found that the total number of units in the muscle was reduced to approximately one-third the normal value.

Thiele and Stålberg (1975) and Konishi et al. (1982) studied uremic patients by the technique of single fiber electromyography. By placing a very fine recording needle electrode within the belly of the muscle, it is possible, using this technique, to calculate the density of muscle fibers within each unit and also to detect variation in the interval at which two fibers within a unit fire. The former gives evidence on the amount of collateral reinnervation of muscle, and the latter, on impairment of neural transmission due to demyelination. It was the final conclusion of these investigators that in uremia the fiber density was normal, suggesting a failure of reinnervation. However, there was an abnormality in the variation in the interval between the firing of two single fibers, so-called jitter, likely related to peripheral demyelination. Thus, these investigations point to significant peripheral demyelination and failure of collateral reinnervation, both presumably secondary to axonal degeneration.

Somatosensory Evoked Potential Studies

In this technique (Brown, 1984), a peripheral nerve, such as a median nerve, is stimulated submaximally as many as 1,000 or 2,000 times, and the resulting propagated sensory impulse is recorded with surface electrodes at various places along the peripheral nerve and its central connections: the spinal cord, brainstem, and cerebral hemispheres. Computer averaging allows detection of the very low voltage action potentials. The technique is moderately time consuming and tedious but causes relatively little discomfort to the patient. In fact, patients are encouraged to relax and they often go to sleep.

There is general agreement (Serra et al., 1979; Ganji and Mahajan, 1983; Lewis et al., 1978; Obeso et al., 1979; Rossini et al., 1983; Vaziri et al., 1981) that conduction is slowed along both the peripheral segment and the central segments of primary sensory neurons, but only through the spinal cord, not higher in the brainstem or cerebral hemispheres. The only exception to this was the observation by Serra et al. (1979) that transcallosal conduction time was increased. Lewis et al. (1978) and Serra et al. (1979) reported that the amplitude of the evoked potentials recorded over the cerebral hemispheres was abnormally increased in comparison to controls, suggesting excessive synchronization of the traveling impulse.

Late Response Measurements

The development of H-reflex and F-wave studies have made it possible to study conduction in the proximal, as well as the distal, segments of peripheral nerves. The H-reflex (Kimura, 1983b) is simply an electrophysiological elucidation of the deep tendon reflex by electrical stimulation of group 1A afferent fibers. The tibial nerve is stimulated at the knee, and the resulting muscle response is recorded from the soleus muscle. The latency represents conduction along sensory fibers to the spinal cord, through central connections to the anterior horn cells, and then down the motor nerves to activate the muscle fibers. Thus, slowing of conduction, or abolition of the impulse, can occur through dysfunction at any site along the pathway. Relatively weak stimuli are required to elicit the response, so there is very little discomfort to the patient. Moreover, the technique is highly reproducible. Unfortunately, it is only the tibial nerve that regularly gives the response on stimulation; all other nerves in the body, at least in adults, are usually unresponsive.

The F-wave (Kimura, 1983a) is recorded by stimulating a peripheral nerve with much stronger currents. The resulting action potential is transmitted antidromically up the axon, turns around near the anterior horn cell, and in a small proportion of the motor fibers passes down the same axon orthodromically to reactivate the muscle fibers. With each stimulus, which is usually repeated 10 to 15 times, the number of motor units responding and accounting for the F-wave is only one or two, and the latencies of these units will vary somewhat, depending on the conduction velocity of the alpha motor neurons involved. Here, also, dysfunction could occur from a lesion located anywhere along the motor unit, from the anterior horn cell to the muscle fiber membrane. While the technique is somewhat more uncomfortable than the H-reflex method, the F-wave technique can be successfully applied to virtually all peripheral nerves. Thus, it is much more commonly utilized than the H-reflex, which can usually only be elicited in the tibial nerve.

Several studies (Ackil et al., 1981b; Guihneuc and Ginet, 1973; Panayiotopoulous and Scarpalezos, 1977; Panayiotopoulous and Laxos, 1980) have shown that the F-wave latency is abnormally prolonged in up to 86 percent of patients in chronic renal failure. The latency has been shown to shorten towards normal in some patients during the course of hemodialysis and in all patients following successful renal transplantation. The H-reflex response is abnormal in an equally high percentage of patients and may be abnormal in approximately 20 percent of the patients who have normal nerve conduction studies (Ackil et al., 1981b).

Quantitative Testing of Sensation

Disordered sensation is the first of the various symptoms and signs to develop in uremic polyneuropathy. A method to detect it that is both sensitive and subject to quantitation would be advantageous. Nielsen (1972) used a bioesthesiometer (Chagrin Falls, Ohio), which is a hand-held device that can be applied to the skin and transmits vibrations at a frequency of 10 Hz. The patient reports a level at which vibration is first detected—the vibratory threshold. The stimulus strength is expressed as the square of the voltage of electrical energies applied to the vibrator. The effect of the viscoelastic resistance of the skin on the amplitude of the vibrations is an important variable (Nielsen, 1975).

Male uremic patients are significantly more affected than female patients, particularly the elderly. Vibratory perception deteriorates significantly with advancing renal failure, the deterioration being most marked in the lower limbs. The earliest change occurs in the pulp of the great toe. In normal males, Nielsen (1972) found that the threshold was 2.00 ± 0.37 in controls ($n = 27$), and 2.50 ± 0.60 in uremic patients ($n = 49$). He concluded that the test had high specificity but low sensitivity. However, it provided a quantitative measure that was readily applicable to bedside examination.

Lowitzsch et al. (1981) utilized this technique in studying 18 patients immediately before and immediately after a single hemo-dialysis procedure. They noted that there was only slight improvement in vibratory perception thresholds, and the improvement was not statistically significant. However, they found that there was significant improvement in sural nerve conduction velocities, in the duration but not the amplitude of the sural nerve CAP, and in the refractory period, which returned to normal.

Read et al. (1982) studied 92 patients at various stages of chronic renal failure. They found vibratory perception impaired in uremic patients prior to the beginning of hemodialysis. These patients had no clinical evidence of peripheral neuropathy, but vibratory perception tended to deteriorate during the first years of dialysis, after which it remained relatively constant. It returned towards normal within one week of successful kidney transplantation. It seemed unrelated to the type of dialyzer, acetylator status, average serum creatinine values, or serum aluminum levels.

At the Karolinska Hospital, Stockholm, Sweden, vibratory perception thresholds and other physiological tests were performed on 81 patients with chronic renal failure (Tegner and Lindholm, 1985). A hand-held vibrator was used in which an accelerometer recorded the movement of the stimulator head. Neuropathy was found in 83 percent of patients. The most common abnormalities were reduced nerve conduction velocities, increased vibratory perception thresholds, loss of deep tendon reflexes, and impaired temperature sensibility. A special method was used to measure thermal sensation, and these investigators found that the incidence of abnormality was much higher than had been previously reported. In a further study, they found that during treatment with low-protein diets, vibratory threshold in uremic patients correlated better with clinical grading of the neuropathy than did conduction velocities or distal motor latencies, but during hemodialysis the situation was the reverse. Of the various tests, they found the vibratory perception threshold recorded on the foot to be the best. Finally, it was demonstrated that in healthy individuals vibratory sensation decreases with a rise in temperature. The same

phenomenon occurs in uremic patients but not in diabetic patients, leading Tegner (1985) to suggest that diabetic neuropathy is predominantly demyelinating, as opposed to uremic neuropathy, and with warming the refractory period of the distal sensory nerves is decreased.

As discussed by Dyck et al. (1984), new knowledge has been gained about the physiology of peripheral sensation and particularly about sophisticated methods of testing it. As these methods become more refined and less demanding and time consuming, they may be used routinely in clinical investigations and provide a more sensitive means of detecting early polyneuropathy than current methods.

Pathophysiology

While there is still no generally accepted theory as to the precise cause of uremic polyneuropathy, nor of the chief mechanism by which it occurs, the subject has been studied by many investigators using a variety of techniques. Important information has been obtained from electrophysiology, pathology, measurements of various nutrients in the blood to detect deficiency syndromes, measurements of abnormal product accumulation in blood that might be toxic, and finally, studies of the vascular supply to peripheral nerves. The subject has been comprehensively reviewed by Nielsen (1978) and by Savazzi et al. (1982).

Physiological Changes

Disturbances in physiology are widespread throughout the peripheral nervous system. Conduction velocity along motor and sensory fibers of both large and small myelinated fibers is slowed, both proximally and distally. The degree of slowing is greater than one would expect from the fallout of larger, faster-conducting myelinated fibers and is consistent with significant segmental demyelination (Bolton, 1976; Bolton et al., 1971). The presence of underlying demyelination is also indicated by the relative preservation of the amplitude of the CAPs and the fact that the action potentials are somewhat dispersed (Figure 5.4). However, particularly in more advanced neuropathy, needle electromyography shows a reduction in the number of motor unit potentials and the presence of fibrillation potentials and positive sharp waves, indicating clear-cut denervation of muscle. This indicates that axonal degeneration is occurring, in addition to demyelination. These electrophysiological abnormalities are more marked in the lower limbs than in the upper limbs, and on needle electromyography the more distal muscles are affected (Bolton, 1976; Bolton et al., 1971). This predominant involvement of more distal nerve segments suggests a dying-back polyneuropathy. Thus, the segmental demyelination could conceivably be secondary to a primary axonal degeneration (Dyck et al., 1971).

However, there have been other studies that have suggested early, widespread changes of a purely functional nature, all suggesting fundamental defects at the cell membrane level. The excitation threshold to electrical stimulation is considerably elevated, even when nerve conduction velocities are normal (Bolton, 1980b; Wright and McQuillen, 1973). The refractory period, both absolute and relative, is increased for sensory fibers (Lowitzsch et al., 1979; Tackmann et al., 1974) but apparently not for motor fibers (Delbeke et al., 1978). The refractory period results suggest a lowering of the "safety factor" for the axonal membrane at the nodes of Ranvier.

Uremic nerves respond abnormally to changes in temperature. In the nonuremic individual, with reduced limb temperature, conduction velocity slows and both the amplitude and the duration of CAPs increase (Bolton et al., 1982). In uremia, conduction velocity falls more rapidly, but there is a less rapid rise in amplitude and increase in the duration (Bolton et al., 1982). This also suggests an axonal membrane defect, possibly involving sodium channels (Chiu et al., 1979).

Studies on the effects of ischemia of peripheral nerves also favor a basic membrane abnormality. The observed phenomena have been called "resistance to ischemia." As opposed to healthy nerves, when uremic nerves are rendered ischemic, vibratory perception is retained longer and sensory CAPs can be recorded for a longer period of time. Castaigne et al. (1972) showed that this abnormality was increased the day after dialysis, when blood volume was low, but the phenomenon could be almost completely reversed when the low blood volume was corrected with infusion of a macromolecular plasma expander. These results could be explained by a decreased extracellular potassium concentration due to increased permeability of the cation binding barrier substance in the nodal gap (Seneviratne and Peiris, 1970) or by expansion and then retraction of the endoneurial space (Jakobsen, 1978).

Nielsen has advanced the theory that the fundamental membrane defect in uremia may be a toxin that inhibits the ouabain-sensitive, sodium-potassium-activated adenosine triphosphatase (ATPase) enzyme, resulting in a reduced flux, and increased intracellular sodium concentration, and a resulting decrease in the transmembrane potential difference (Nielsen, 1973a; 1974b; 1978). Several investigations of membrane function at various sites in uremia have supported this argument. There is a reduction of the muscle membrane potential (Bolte et al., 1963; Cunningham et al., 1971), and there have been abnormalities of sodium transport in erythrocyte membranes (Welt et al., 1964), crab muscle fibers (Bittar, 1967), frog skin (Bourgoignie et al., 1971), cells in uremic rats, and leukocytes from uremic patients (Edmondson et al., 1975). The sodium-potassium ATPase activity improves dramatically and the intracellular sodium concentration appropriately decreases after successful renal transplantation (Cole and Maletz, 1975; Cole et al., 1978).

Tegner and Brismar (1984) studied the peripheral nerves of rats that were rendered acutely uremic. They observed that conduction velocity decreased and the refractory period did not change, but that in potential recordings and potential clamp of isolated myelinated fibers, there was a decrease in excitability, related to a decrease in the specific sodium permeability of the nodal membrane. It was their opinion that this explained a decreased nerve conduction velocity. They believe that some of the changes could be caused by elevated intracellular calcium or an intracellular accumulation of cation metabolites.

Pathology

In the original classic report by Asbury et al. (1963), pathological examination at autopsy revealed both segmental demyelination and axonal degeneration in peripheral nerves, which was more marked distally. In the spinal cord, there was evidence of chromatolysis of anterior horn cells, indicating primary axonal damage. However, in particularly severe uremic polyneuropathy, there may be demyelination more proximally at the level of the lumbosacral nerve roots (Bolton and Rozdilsky, unpublished data, 1971). Teased fiber studies reveal paranodal demyelination, segmental demyelination, axonal degeneration, and segmental remyelination (Figure 5.6). Quantitative studies show that there is reduction of large and small myelinated, as well as unmyelinated, fibers (Dyck et al., 1971). However, none of the pathological observations to date, including electron microscopic studies, have shown any changes that appear specific for uremic polyneuropathy. Said et al. (1983) studied 10 uremic patients who had single nerve biopsies at various stages of renal failure: at the beginning of dialysis treatment, during the course of regular hemodialysis, or during continuous ambulatory peritoneal dialysis. A variety of pathological changes were demonstrated, including acute axonal neuropathy, axonal neuropathy with secondary segmental demyelination, and a predominantly demyelinating neuropathy. All patterns were associated with distal degeneration of nerve fibers.

Some early pathological studies suggested that the primary defect was at the level of the Schwann cell. These conclusions arose from teased fiber studies (Dinn and Crane, 1970) and light and electron microscopy and biochemical analysis by gas-liquid chromatography of whole peripheral nerves (Appenzeller et al., 1971). However, Dyck et al. (1971) and Thomas et al. (1971), from comprehensive pathological studies, indicated that the seg-

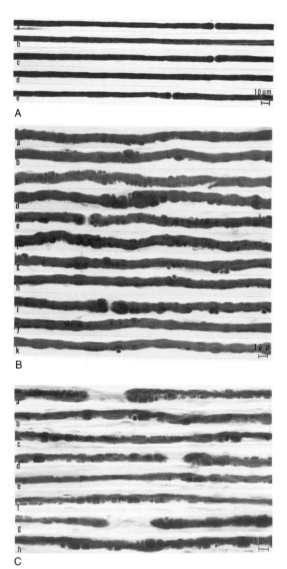

Figure 5.6. (A) Teased fiber preparation from a normal sural nerve. The myelin sheath interrupted by nodes of Ranvier appears black. Letters indicate consecutive segments of the same nerve fiber. (B) Teased fiber preparation of sural nerve in a patient who had moderately severe uremic polyneuropathy. This particular fiber showed only irregularity of the myelin sheath, a variation of normal. (C) Early stages of demyelination. (D) The stage of segmental demyelination. (E) An advanced stage of demyelination. Linear rows of myelin ovoids are seen. (F) Numerous areas of segmental demyelination along the length of a single nerve fiber. This and all the other changes in this patient represent demyelination secondary to an underlying primary axonal degeneration. (All, original magnification ×380.) (Reprinted with permission from Dyck et al., 1971.)

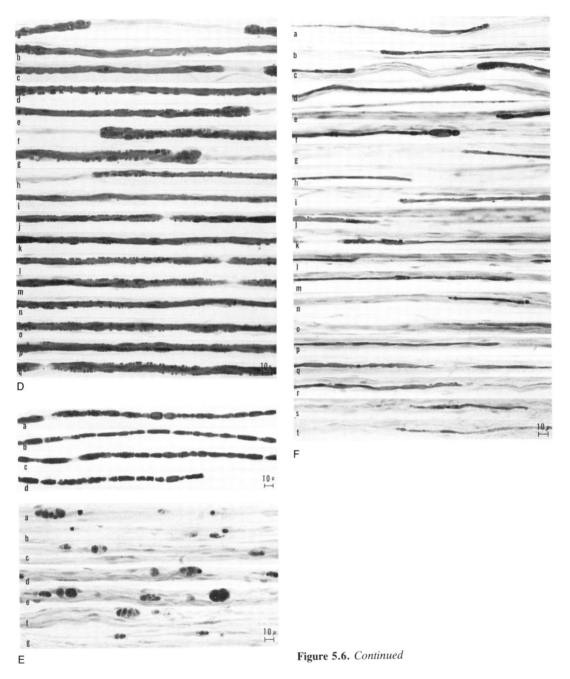

Figure 5.6. *Continued*

mental demyelination was secondary to a primary axonal degeneration. The ratio of the circumference of axis cylinders to the number of myelin lamellae was decreased in distal nerve fibers, compared with proximal axons, suggesting axonal shrinkage. Segmental demyelination tended to occur only on certain fibers, completely sparing others, suggesting that de-

myelination was secondary to axonal disease. Finally, these authors confirmed Asbury's original observation that demyelination and axonal degeneration were much more severe distally.

Thus, the pathological evidence strongly suggests that if there is a primary axonal degeneration, any segmental demyelination or remyelination that is present is secondary to the underlying axonal disease. The axonal disease is most pronounced distally, suggesting a dying-back phenomenon, possibly due to dysfunction at the level of the nerve cell body.

Deficiency Syndromes

Deficiency of B vitamins, which are water soluble and would tend to be washed out by dialysis procedures, were initially considered to be a cause of uremic polyneuropathy (Tyler, 1968). This may, indeed, have been an important cause, since the burning foot syndrome was commonly observed at that time, but it is now rarely seen. Nonetheless, the administration of large amounts of vitamins, including B vitamins, seemed to have little overall effect on the incidence of uremic neuropathy or on its progression (Asbury et al., 1963; Tenckhoff et al., 1965). Even after vitamin administration had been tried, one of the B vitamins, thiamine, remained a primary candidate. Measurements of erythrocyte transketolase activity, which is depressed in thiamine-deficient states, was found to be depressed in uremic patients, even though they were receiving oral thiamine. The transketolase activity returned towards normal following dialysis (Egan and Wells, 1979; Lonergan et al., 1970). However, Koppell et al. (1972) found transketolase activity was increased in uremic patients, suggesting that thiamine deficiency was not a factor in uremic polyneuropathy.

Yatzidis et al. (1981) reported decreased levels of biotin in uremic patients undergoing chronic hemodialysis. Treatment with biotin resulted in improvement in both uremic encephalopathy and polyneuropathy. However, this is a preliminary report and further observations are needed.

A series of studies of magnesium metabolism in uremia (Fleming et al., 1972; Hollinrake et al., 1970; Posen and Kaye, 1967; Stewart et al., 1967) provides no convincing evidence that either an excess or a deficiency of this electrolyte bears any relationship to polyneuropathy.

Protein malnutrition may occur as a result of accelerated breakdown of muscle protein or through dietary restriction. Considerable muscle atrophy may occur on this basis, although polyneuropathy could conceivably be a significant cause of this atrophy. Further proteins are lost through both hemodialysis and peritoneal dialysis. However, whether protein depletion per se is a cause of polyneuropathy is still purely speculative. As noted earlier, it is more likely that a severe catabolic state is more commonly associated with surgery and infection during chronic hemodialysis and this, in itself critical, illness (Bolton et al., 1984; 1986) may be the chief reason for polyneuropathy developing at this time in uremic patients.

Circulating Toxins

A comprehensive discussion of this is given in Chapter 2. The present discussion will focus on those toxins that are most likely to affect peripheral nerves.

It has been known for many years that methyl guanidine and phenols accumulate in uremic plasma but there is no evidence that they account for polyneuropathy (Savazzi et al., 1982). A more significant role has been proposed for *myo*-inositol, a growth factor important in the metabolism of the myelin sheath. It is abnormally elevated in uremia. When *myo*-inositol was administered to rats, reduced nerve conduction velocities were noted (Clements et al., 1973; DeJesus et al., 1974). However, Reznek et al. (1977) were unable to show a relationship between nerve conduction velocities and the level of blood *myo*-inositol in patients.

Urea and creatinine, being of relatively low molecular weight, have been considered the main uremic toxins for years, and there is good evidence that they play an important role in the toxicity of acute uremia (see Chapter 2). However, there is no good evidence that they are responsible for uremic polyneuropathy. Levels of these two substances could not be related to the incidence or severity of neuropathy in conservatively managed patients studied by Nielsen (1971b). However, there was a strong relationship between the incidence of neuropathy and the degree of renal failure, as measured by the creatinine clearance (Figure 5.5).

The most widely accepted hypothesis for uremic neuropathy is that molecules of medium molecular weight are toxic to the peripheral nerves. This theory was originally proposed by Babb et al. (1971) following the now apparently erroneous claim that the incidence of polyneuropathy was lower in patients who were receiving peritoneal dialysis than in those receiving hemodialysis. Presumably, the peritoneal membrane was more porous to substances in the middle-molecule range—500 to 500,000 daltons molecular weight. This theory spawned an exhausting number of studies, all designed to develop hemodialysis techniques that would selectively clear middle molecules, followed by attempts to determine whether such procedures, in fact, lessened the incidence of the various toxic uremic syndromes, including polyneuropathy. The subject has been comprehensively reviewed by Bergstrom and Furst (1983) and by Savazzi et al. (1982). A number of basic investigations strongly implicate the toxic effect of middle molecules on the nervous system. These molecules, specifically B_{4-2}, impair the function of the frog sural nerve *in vitro* (Bergstrom and Furst, 1983; Man et al., 1980) and cause a reduction in motor nerve conduction velocity in uremic rats (Boudet et al., 1980). They also cause degeneration of nerve fibers but not of nerve cells through inhibition of glucose phosphate dehydrogenase and pyruvate kinase enzymes in chick embryo cultures of spinal dorsal root ganglion (Kumegawa et al., 1980). Such toxicity has been shown in similar basic studies for a variety of other body systems (Bergstrom and Furst, 1983).

However, many of the studies on patients have given disappointingly conflicting results. Further studies with patients using a variety of dialysis techniques; peritoneal dialysis; varying dialysis flow rates, membrane size, and type of membrane; cellulose acetate membranes; cellophane membranes; hemofiltration techniques; and hemoperfusion over activated charcoal have failed to give a clear-cut answer (Savazzi et al., 1982). In the study by Lindsay et al. (1983) using a careful crossover-design protocol, platelet and peripheral nerve function were measured in relationship to a conventional hemodialyzer and to one that

combined hemodialysis and hemoperfusion so as to improve the clearance of middle molecular weight substances. The study suggested that these substances were toxic to platelets but not to peripheral nerve.

However, there are a number of studies which still strongly support the middle-molecule theory. These have been led by the Necker group in Paris. They used a membrane highly permeable to middle molecules (the polyacrylonitrile membrane) and measured these molecules in the plasma and dialysate. Six patients with severe neuropathy improved when, in particular, the b4-2 fraction of middle molecules was removed (Lindsay et al., 1983; Man et al., 1973; 1974). Botella et al. (1980) found that crude middle-molecule accumulation caused reduced motor nerve conduction velocity in uremic patients.

Asaba et al. (1983), at the Karolinska Institute, Sweden, have shown that the 7C fraction of the middle molecule seemed to be particularly toxic to peripheral nerve in patients. Such patients had a high incidence of acute infections which, as already noted, are particularly deleterious to peripheral nerve in patients who are uremic. Finally, middle molecules of uremia inhibit the formation of microtubules in the axons of tissue cultures of nerve cells (Braguer et al., 1983).

Higher molecular weight compounds, particularly hormones, are known to accumulate abnormally in uremia—insulin, growth hormone, glucagon, prolactin, gastrin, and corticotropin (Bergstrom and Furst, 1983). Parathyroid hormone has been most strongly implicated in nervous system damage, where it is thought to be an important cause of uremic encephalopathy and other uremic complications. The hormone was purported to cause impaired peripheral nerve function (Massry and Goldstein, 1979; Goldstein et al., 1978). However, Schaeffer et al. (1980) failed to show any correlation between serum parathyroid hormone and nerve conduction velocity in patients on regular hemodialysis.

Vascular Mechanisms

In various pathological studies to date, no clear-cut lesion of the vascular supply to the peripheral nerves, the vasa nervorum, has been demonstrated. However, Bundschu (1977) and Savazzi et al. (1980) have shown thickening of the basal membrane in capillaries and arterioles, along with calcium deposits in the microcirculation of muscle in uremic patients. Moreover, Gilchrest et al. (1980) have shown a microangiopathy of the skin of patients, which did not improve during dialysis but did improve following successful renal transplantation. The histological changes consisted of endothelial cell activation and/or necrosis, basement membrane zone thickening, and reduplication of the basal lamina, involving both venules and arterioles. Thus, the vascular supply to peripheral nerve clearly needs further investigation—in particular, studies of the microenvironment of the peripheral nerve similar to those by Low et al. (1987) at the Mayo Clinic, which have shed so much light on diabetic polyneuropathy. As described in Chapter 5B, uremic nerves seem particularly susceptible to damage from ischemia induced by arteriovenous shunts or fistulae.

Treatment and Prevention

Hemodialysis

In 1963, within three years of the Seattle group's first demonstration that chronic hemodialysis was feasible (see Chapter 1), Chaumont et al. (1963) demonstrated that nerve conduction velocities were often reduced in uremia. It then became obvious that electrophysiological tests could provide an objective and quantitative assessment of peripheral nerve function. As already noted, a remarkable number of tests, most of them electrophysiological, have since been devised in an attempt to accomplish this objective. In particular, it had been hoped that these tests would provide one method of assessing the adequacy of the various types of dialysis. Unfortunately, the results have been controversial, the discussion centering around two main problems. Initially, it was assumed that electrophysiological measurements, notably nerve conduction velocity, were much more precise than they actually are. When the variability was realized, opinion

shifted too far in the opposite direction, and many centers have now entirely discarded this method of patient assessment. The second problem has been that even when nerve conduction studies are properly evaluated, they have borne a poor relationship, so it seemed, to the course of the neuropathies assessed by symptoms and signs or by other methods of measuring uremic toxicity. Thus, it was the recommendation in a recent review (Jennekens and Kemmelems-Schinkel, 1983) that nerve conduction studies are of little value in assessing patients during chronic hemodialysis.

This section critically reexamines the entire subject. While there is little doubt that chronic hemodialysis halts the progression of uremic polyneuropathy and that modern methods are associated with an extremely low incidence of moderate or severe polyneuropathy, electrophysiological tests still disclose an incidence of approximately 60 percent (Bolton, 1980a) (Table 5.1) in patients receiving chronic hemodialysis. There would seem little doubt, therefore, that this complication remains a significant contributing factor to the morbidity associated with this group of patients. Thus, it is our view that objective methods of measuring peripheral nerve function should continue to be regularly utilized in patients receiving chronic hemodialysis, and such methods should be taken into account in evaluating a dialysis method that claims to be an improvement. Nerve conduction measurements have been strongly correlated with underlying pathological changes (Dyck et al., 1971; 1975a) and are, in our opinion, still the best method of peripheral nerve assessment.

Uremic Neuropathy during Regular Hemodialysis

In 1962, Hegstrom and colleagues in Seattle observed uremic polyneuropathy in four patients who were receiving regular hemodialysis. One patient had a severe polyneuropathy. These investigators were initially concerned that the hemodialysis procedure itself was responsible for the polyneuropathy, but they then noted that the neuropathy seemed to improve when the number of hours per week on dialysis was increased. At the same time, Asbury and colleagues (1963) reported their classic observations on four patients who suffered from uremic neuropathy, none of these patients having had hemodialysis. Thus, there seemed no doubt that the chronic renal failure, itself, was responsible for the polyneuropathy, not the dialysis procedure.

Greater experience with peripheral neuropathy in relationship to regular hemodialysis was reported by the Seattle group in two classic papers in 1965 and 1967 (Tenckhoff et al., 1965; Jebsen et al., 1967). In the initial report, they described 10 patients on regular hemodialysis, using the Kiil unit. Two of these patients, both septic and critically ill, developed a rapidly progressive, ultimately severe, predominantly motor neuropathy soon after hemodialysis was started. A patient studied by Bolton in 1967 provides an example of the rapidity with which severe polyneuropathy can develop (Figure 5.3D). A further three patients in Seattle had a more slowly progressive polyneuropathy. Intensification of the dialysis schedule caused improvement, but only slowly, over a matter of months.

Jebsen et al. (1967) in Seattle reported 20 patients who had been followed by chronic hemodialysis. They emphasized the electrophysiological results, which stabilized in 10 patients and improved in a further 10 patients. Again, the improvement occurred slowly, over a year or more. The Seattle group emphasized that uremic neuropathy could potentially be prevented by starting hemodialysis earlier in the course of chronic renal failure and by intensifying hemodialysis should evidence of polyneuropathy develop. They also emphasized that nerve conduction values were an important method of detecting the neuropathy in its early stages and following its course. In fact, they stated that a change of more than 3 m/s in the mean of the combined conduction velocity measurements for median, ulnar, and peroneal nerves should be regarded as a significant change. Finally, this group reported, for the first time, that two patients successfully treated by transplantation showed striking improvement in clinical signs and in nerve conduction results. Thus, the main observations

and conclusions in these two papers even now must be regarded of fundamental importance and, as will be seen, have been largely borne out by subsequent studies. The main areas of disagreement have been how sensitive the nerve conduction studies are in monitoring the course of the neuropathy and whether manipulation of the dialysis schedule truly affects the cause of uremic polyneuropathy.

Subsequent experience from various centers throughout the world is summarized in Table 5.1. From this, it can be seen that, in general, patients being treated with coil dialyzing units have had a higher incidence of uremic polyneuropathy and of progressing polyneuropathy. On the other hand, the record with the Kiil unit appears to be much better.

As various refinements in the hemodialysis techniques have taken place over the years, it has been noted that the incidence of uremic polyneuropathy, certainly the clinical symptoms and signs of such a neuropathy, have fallen dramatically. Overt uremic polyneuropathy must now be considered a relatively rare entity (Bolton, 1980a; Funck-Brentano et al., 1968). As will be noted later, alterations in dialysis methods are unlikely to be the only reason. Others to be considered are institution of chronic hemodialysis earlier in the course of renal failure when there is still some residual renal function and more severe peripheral nerve damage has not yet occurred (Figure 5.7), and earlier renal transplantation when uremic "toxicity" cannot be controlled.

A point we made earlier needs reemphasis. Rapidly progressive and ultimately severe polyneuropathy seems to develop in association with critical illness; that is, sepsis and malfunction of other organs of the body, in addition to the kidney. We have noted in the last 10 years that an acute axonal type of polyneuropathy is a specific complication of sepsis and multiple organ failure (Bolton et al., 1984; 1986). Thus, one would anticipate that in a patient with advanced renal failure, any episodes of sepsis or injury such as surgery might be particularly harmful to peripheral nerves. This was noted by Tenckhoff et al. (1965). Williams et al. (1973) observed worsening in polyneuropathy during an epidemic

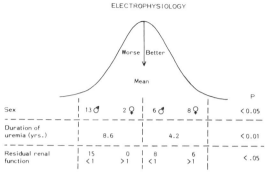

Figure 5.7. Factors influencing peripheral nerve function during chronic hemodialysis. Twenty-nine patients on a thrice weekly home dialysis program in London, Ontario, Canada were tested by nerve electrophysiological methods at yearly intervals for three years. Electrophysiological values remained constant over this period. Based on the results, the patients were classified as having better or worse peripheral nerve function. Those with better function tended to be females, had had uremia a shorter period of time, and had better residual renal function based on creatinine clearance values. (Reprinted with permission from Del Campo et al., 1983.)

of hepatitis in their renal unit. Thus, it is possible that the improvement in polyneuropathy over the years is due not to refinements in the type of dialyzer but to the advent of the Brescia-Cimino fistula, which has dramatically reduced the incidence of recurring sepsis.

Dialysis Schedules

After the first 10 years of experience with regular hemodialysis, there was the general feeling that uremic polyneuropathy was an indication of the adequacy of hemodialysis. It was thought that if signs of polyneuropathy developed during hemodialysis, particularly as detected by changes in nerve conduction results, improving the dialysis would result in improvement in the uremic neuropathy (Konotey-Ahulu et al., 1965; Jebsen et al., 1967; Curtis et al., 1969; Pendras and Erickson, 1966). If one could measure the adequacy of dialysis by various techniques and then adjust the type of dialysis accordingly, theoretically an ideal dialysis method would eventually result. Uremic polyneuropathy was regarded as a major index of the adequacy of dialysis.

However, it has been difficult to prove that optimal hemodialysis regularly improves uremic polyneuropathy (Bolton et al., 1971; 1975). In his study of 14 patients, Nielsen (1974a) observed only a stabilization in nerve conduction studies, although symptoms improved. In a much larger study of 213 patients, Cadilhac et al. (1978) again found mainly a stabilization, a few patients improving or worsening.

Deliberately manipulating the dialysis schedule also seems to have little effect. In 1975, Dyck et al. (1975b) at the Mayo Clinic, using a crossover method halfway through the one-year trial period, found that patients treated with restricted intake of protein and fluid and infrequent dialysis had no worsening of peripheral nerve function, compared to a conventional hemodialysis treatment schedule. However, of all patients initially entered in the study, only five were able to complete it for various reasons. Thus, despite the use of sensitive and comprehensive methods of testing, it is difficult to draw firm conclusions from this study.

In 1977, Lindsay and Bolton (unpublished data) chose six adult patients who had been treated for two years on a Gambro 17 dialyzer, twice weekly for a total of 15 m^2 · hr/wk and switched them while still on hospital dialysis to three times per week, 18 m^2 · hr/wk, using the same type of dialyzer. There were no significant changes in nerve conduction measurements in individual patients or in the mean values of these measurements for the group, when assessed every four months for a year. Six healthy controls were tested at the same time by the same methods. In this study, each patient served as her or his own control.

Bolton and colleagues have also found no convincing differences in incidence or severity while managing patients on either home or hospital dialysis (Bolton et al., 1975; 1976). Some preservation of residual renal function, perhaps induced by starting regular hemodialysis earlier, is associated with less severe uremic polyneuropathy (Figure 5.7) (Funck-Brentano et al., 1968; Del Campo et al., 1983).

A concept that is still in vogue arose from Babb and colleagues (1971). They believed that patients on peritoneal dialysis did not have the same tendency to uremic polyneuropathy as those on hemodialysis. They theorized that the peritoneal membrane was much more permeable to middle-molecule substances than the artificial membrane in dialysis machines. It might also explain the observation that patients being dialyzed by the Kiil machine, in which there would theoretically be a greater clearance of middle molecules, had a lower incidence of uremic neuropathy than those being dialyzed by the Kolff twin-coil machine. Clearance of these middle molecules, or higher molecular weight than urea and creatinine or approximately 500 to 3,000 daltons, could be calculated by multiplying the number of hours of dialysis per week by the surface area of the dialyzing membrane and dividing this by the body weight in kilograms—the so-called square meter–hours per kilogram body weight. This middle-molecule concept was then subject to intensive investigation (Bergstrom and Furst, 1983).

Funck-Brentano et al. (1968) treated four uremic patients with a dialysis machine containing a polyacrylonitrile membrane that had a high clearance for vitamin B_{12}, which is in the same molecular range as the middle molecules. Dramatic improvement in uremic polyneuropathy was claimed by this treatment. However, Lowrie et al. (1976) assessed, among other factors, peripheral nerve function, measuring the ulnar nerve conduction velocity and distal latency in a carefully randomized study. They reported improvement in nerve conduction measurements when small-molecule clearance was increased, and middle-molecule clearance had no effect on the neuropathy. Results in the 1983 study by Lindsay and colleagues also failed to substantiate the middle-molecule theory. In 14 patients with end-stage renal disease who had been established on hemodialysis, treatment was compared with a conventional hemodialyzer and an experimental device that combined hemodialysis and hemoperfusion in such a way that *in vitro* vitamin B_{12} clearances and, hence, middle-molecule clearances, were improved. A crossover design was used, switching between these two techniques every two months. While there was an improvement in the velocity of platelet

aggregation in response to 10 uM adenosine diphosphate and to a standard collagen preparation associated with treatment with the experimental device, there was no demonstrable influence on nerve conduction studies (Figure 5.8). Thus, enhanced middle-molecule clearance seemed to improve platelet, but not peripheral nerve, function. Alternatively, the crossover may have been too often (every two months) to allow sufficient time for measurable changes in peripheral nerve function to have occurred.

However, as noted in the discussion under Pathophysiology above, the arguments for middle molecules as factors in the production of peripheral neuropathy are strong. Asaba et al. (1983), by using the technique of gel chromatography followed by ion exchange gradient lucent chromatography, were able to separate various middle-molecule fractions. Among 65 regularly hemodialyzed patients, six had sig-

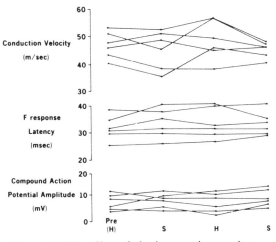

Figure 5.8. The effect of altering uremic retention products on peripheral nerve function. Fourteen patients were studied at two-month intervals in a crossover trial. Treatment with a conventional Cuprophan membrane dialyzer, the Hemoclear (H) (Medical Incorporated, Minneapolis, Minn.) was compared to a Sorbiclear (S) dialyzer (Medical Incorporated) which had better clearance of middle, but not smaller, molecular weight substances. There was no significant change in peripheral nerve function, and the same result occurred when the sequence of treatments was reversed. Thus, there was no evidence for improved peripheral nerve function with enhanced removal of middle molecules. (Reprinted with permission from Lindsay et al., 1983.)

nificantly elevated plasma concentrations of middle molecules, including 7C, 7B, and 7D fractions. These patients had a high incidence of acute infections, which seemed to be associated with elevation of the 7C fraction. Three of these patients developed a progressive peripheral neuropathy.

Finally, Braguer et al. (1983) have shown by *in vitro* methods that tubulin, an intracellular protein that polymerizes microtubules, essential components of the axons of nerve cells, is inhibited by the middle molecules of uremia.

The Effect of Treatment by a Single Hemodialysis Procedure

Studies on this subject have provided somewhat conflicting results. Jebsen et al. in 1967, reported that a single hemodialysis procedure had no effect on peripheral nerve conduction studies. But Solders et al. (1985) reported a rise in the amplitude of the sensory CAP. The most detailed study has been by Lowitzsch et al. (1981). These authors studied several neurophysiological conditions in 18 patients one hour before and two hours after a single hemodialysis procedure. There was an increase in the conduction velocity and the duration of the sensory nerve CAP, but not its amplitude. However, the most striking abnormality was a decrease in the refractory period of the nerve immediately after this procedure. There was no change in vibratory perception or in visual-evoked potentials.

The pattern of changes suggested that there is a decreased resting membrane potential in uremia which is reversible by a single hemodialysis procedure.

Effects of Hemodialysis on Children

There is general agreement that the incidence and severity of uremic polyneuropathy is less in children than in adults during chronic hemodialysis (Alderson et al., 1985). Only five (29 percent) of 17 children had signs or symptoms of peripheral neuropathy, and the neuropathy was mild. The most sensitive electrophysiological sign in detecting neuropathy in these children was the measurement of sural nerve conduction and the late re-sponses—H-reflex and F-response. These were abnormal in 59 percent (10/17) of the children (Ackil et al., 1981a). Arbus et al. (1975) observed that, as in adults, the polyneuropathy failed to improve during chronic hemodialysis.

General Effects of Chronic Hemodialysis

A large number of studies have been performed to assess the dysfunction of the various organ systems that occurs in chronic uremia. Attempts have been made to relate these to the adequacy of hemodialysis. In the main, the results have been conflicting.

Lowrie et al. (1981) studied 151 patients who were divided into four treatment groups: (1) long dialysis time and high serum urea, (2) long dialysis time and low serum urea, (3) short dialysis time and low serum urea, (4) short dialysis time and high serum urea. Over a period of one year, it was found that morbid events, such as anorexia and nausea, pericarditis, pleuritis, and convulsions, were associated with a relatively high blood urea nitrogen. Only two of the patients developed polyneuropathy, one who was receiving a long dialysis treatment time and a high blood urea. Evans et al. (1985) studied the quality of life in 859 patients undergoing either dialysis or transplantation. Seventy-nine percent of the transplant recipients were able to function at near-normal levels, compared to only 47 to 59 percent receiving dialysis (depending on the type).

In these studies, it would have been interesting to measure peripheral nerve function, clinically and electrophysiologically, since one suspects that in the hemodialysis group, those who functioned poorly probably had evidence of peripheral neuropathy in addition to other long-term complications.

Peritoneal Dialysis

There is now at least 10 years' experience with peritoneal dialysis. The subject was recently reviewed by Gokal (1987). In the United Kingdom, this form of treatment is now used twice as often as it was five years ago, accounting for one-third of all dialysis patients. Patients on hemodialysis who are then started on peritoneal dialysis immediately notice an improved sense of well-being, and there is a rise in hemoglobin concentration. Hypertension is easier to control, and there is improvement in renal osteodystrophy. Patients that were previously thought unacceptable for hemodialysis can now be treated by this method. They include patients who are elderly, very small children, and those who suffer from diabetes mellitus or cardiovascular disease. The patient who has just developed end-stage renal failure is now often placed on continuous ambulatory peritoneal dialysis (CAPD) first, if he or she is a good candidate for transplantation.

The main problems are recurring attacks of peritonitis, poor catheter function, and damage to the peritoneal membrane. The infecting organisms are often skin contaminants. A peritonitis rate of at least one episode per 24 patient-months of treatment occurs. However, one-third of all CAPD patients will remain peritonitis-free over several years. Rarely, the peritoneal membrane may develop into a state of sclerosing encapsulating peritonitis that ultimately proves fatal.

Initial observations suggested a low incidence of polyneuropathy (Tenckhoff and Curtis, 1970). It was theorized that the higher permeability of the peritoneal membrane compared to the dialysis membrane would allow more efficient removal of middle molecules. This originally helped form the basis of the m^2/hr or middle-molecule hypothesis (Babb et al., 1971). However, progressive uremic polyneuropathy was subsequently observed during peritoneal dialysis (Kurtz et al., 1983; Lindholm et al., 1982). Tegner and Lindholm (1985a) compared CAPD and hemodialysis in 21 and 22 patients, respectively. Motor nerve conduction and vibration sensation decreased, more in CAPD patients. Paradoxically, clinical testing suggested improvement. A similar paradox was noted by Nielsen (1974b) in relationship to chronic hemodialysis, apparent clinical improvement occurring but only a stabilization in electrophysiological tests. Pierratos et al. (1981) found no significant change in nerve conduction velocities during peritoneal dialysis, perhaps because most of their patients were women, in whom the incidence of polyneuropathy is quite low.

Amair et al. (1982) studied 20 diabetic patients with end-stage renal disease who were treated for 36 months with CAPD. While 15 of the 20 patients (75 percent) had clinical evidence of polyneuropathy before treatment, follow-up for one year revealed no change in the clinical signs or in the nerve conduction velocities of median, ulnar, and peroneal nerves. However, polyneuropathy in diabetic patients may not improve even after successful renal transplantation, suggesting that the neuropathy in these patients may be due to the diabetes mellitus.

Thus, despite the theoretical advantages of CAPD, uremic polyneuropathy seems to behave the same for this procedure as it does for chronic hemodialysis: that is, it mainly stabilizes, worsening or improving in a few patients or with various methods of assessment.

Kidney Transplantation

Kidney transplantation has been the centerpiece of transplant development. The history of the developments is reviewed in Chapter 1. So successful has this procedure been that in the United States it is being performed at an increasingly rapid rate: from 4,697 per year in 1980 to 7,695 per year in 1985, approximately a 10 percent annual increase (Egges, 1988).

The one-year survival of cadaveric transplants has improved, partly due to the use of cyclosporine, from 53 percent in 1977 to 68 percent in 1984. The quality of life is better than with dialysis. Moreover, the procedure is much more cost effective. Thus, there is a great pressure to use this procedure for the management of end-stage renal disease, particularly in patients under 65 years of age.

Early Experience with Kidney Transplantation and Uremic Polyneuropathy

Rapid developments were taking place in both hemodialysis and transplantation procedures in the 1960s, and there was active debate as to which would be the most effective in controlling uremic polyneuropathy. Versaki et al. (1964) stated that nerve conduction studies failed to improve following renal transplantation. But Dinapoli et al. (1966) and Tenckhoff et al. (1965) noted clear-cut improvement in nerve conduction studies and in clinical signs, respectively, in two patients following successful renal transplantation. Jebsen et al. (1967) later expressed some pessimism that even successful renal transplantation could improve severe uremic polyneuropathy. This view was also expressed by Merrill and Hampers (1970). Tyler (1968) stated that uremic polyneuropathy improved following successful renal transplantation.

However, several systematic studies clearly proved the beneficial effects of successful renal transplantation on uremic polyneuropathy. Using both clinical observation and electromyographic techniques, Dobblestein et al. (1968) in Germany and Funck-Brentano et al. (1968) in France reported consistent improvement in the polyneuropathy, even in severe forms, following successful renal transplantation.

In Canada, Bolton and colleagues observed a case of severe uremic polyneuropathy that improved dramatically after successful renal transplantation in March of 1967 (Bolton et al., 1971) (see the case report below). During the next two years, these investigators carried out systematic clinical and electrophysiological studies on uremic patients to observe the polyneuropathy during conservative management prior to the institution of hemodialysis, during the hemodialysis procedure itself, and following successful renal transplantation. There were 14, 30, and 10 patients in the three groups, respectively. In comparing the hemodialysis and transplant groups, it was obvious that conduction velocities were much better in the transplant group. At follow-up, those on chronic hemodialysis either worsened or stayed the same, while those who had successful renal transplantation progressively improved in both clinical and electrophysiological measurements (Bolton et al., 1970; 1971; Bolton, 1976). Nielsen, through careful studies, made similar observations (1974b; 1974c).

Changes in Clinical Signs following Successful Renal Transplantation

After this procedure has been successfully accomplished, renal function rapidly returns to near normal within one month (Figure 5.9). The following case report illustrates polyneuropathy progressing rapidly during chronic hemodialysis to a severe form and then improving dramatically following successful renal transplantation.

A 38 year old salesman was admitted to the hospital in April, 1966, when physical examination and tests showed findings consistent with severe renal failure; the blood urea was 400 mg, and the serum creatinine 18.6 mg per 100 ml. He was treated conservatively by regulation of fluid balance, control of acidosis, protein restriction, androgenic steroids, multivitamin tablets and methyldopa, but was readmitted to the hospital in December, 1966, in end-stage renal failure. The blood urea was 406 mg, and the creatinine 27.6 mg per 100 ml. Twice a week, he was given hemodialysis with the use of the Kolff twin-coil dialyzing unit; the average creatinine was 18.0 mg per 100 ml before and 9.0 mg per 100 ml after dialysis.

One month before chronic dialysis was started, and 4 months before transplantation, he noticed impotence, an unsteady gait and distal paresthesia and weakness in all limbs, particularly the legs. The neuropathy progressed, and one month before transplantation, he was unable to walk without assistance. Neurologic examination at that time revealed moderate reduction in the brachioradialis reflexes, the only abnormal sign in the upper limbs. However, in

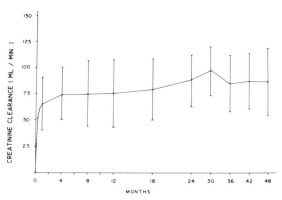

Figure 5.9. Renal function (mean values ± SD) after successful transplantation in 17 patients. Note prompt return to near normal values within one month. This was associated with improvement in symptoms and nerve conduction studies. (Reprinted with permission from Bolton, 1976.)

the lower limbs, muscle weakness was so severe distally that only minimal voluntary movements of the feet and ankles were possible, and intrinsic muscles of the feet were quite wasted. Mild weakness was present proximally. The quadriceps reflexes were reduced, and the Achilles absent. Vibration and position sense were lost at the toes. There was moderate hypesthesia to pain and touch distal to the ankles. Two-point discrimination was 2 mm at the fingertips but absent in the feet. Nerve conduction studies showed abnormalities consistent with polyneuropathy (Figure 5.10). Needle electrode examination disclosed a moderate number of fibrillation potentials and absence of motor-unit potentials (many of which were polyphasic) in the tibialis anterior muscle; the quadriceps muscle was normal.

On March 10, a cadaveric kidney was transplanted into the right iliac fossa (previously, both polycystic kidneys had been excised); 600 R was directed at the site of the grafted kidney. He did well after operation and was initially given prednisone in high dosage but was later maintained on

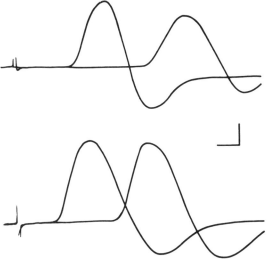

Figure 5.10. Return of nerve conduction to normal after successful renal transplantation. Upper trace: three months before transplantation when the patient had a severe uremic polyneuropathy. Lower trace: 27 months after transplantation when almost complete recovery had occurred. The median nerve was stimulated at the wrist and elbow, and the recording was made from the thenar muscle. Conduction velocity rose from 39 to 55 m/s, and the previously dispersed compound action potential became normal, consistent with segmental remyelination. (See the case report in this chapter.) Calibration: vertical, 2 mV; horizontal, 2 ms. (Redrawn from Bolton et al., 1971, with permission.)

prednisone, 15 mg, azathioprine, 250 mg, and methyldopa, 1 g daily in divided dosage.

One month after transplantation, renal function was in the normal range; the creatinine was 0.8 mg per 100 ml, and the creatinine clearance 80 ml per minute. At that time he began to notice improvement in the numbness and weakness in the feet, but he still had to be fitted with leg braces and clinical and nerve conduction studies were unchanged. Thereafter, improvement of the neuropathy was rapid, however. Impotence disappeared. Two months after transplantation, he was able to discard the leg braces and 3 months later, he returned to work full time as a salesman.

One year after transplantation the deep tendon reflexes were moderately depressed at the knees and absent at the ankles. There was mild weakness of dorsiflexion of the feet, and vibration sense was absent at the toes. Considerable improvement in nerve conduction studies had occurred. Needle electrode study of the right tibialis anterior muscle revealed disappearance of fibrillation potentials and return of motor unit potentials, many of which were polyphasic. He remained well except for the development of mild diabetes mellitus, which was thought to be steroid induced.

Twenty-seven months after transplantation there was only minimal weakness of dorsiflexion of the feet, moderate reduction in ankle jerks and moderate loss of vibration sense at the toes. Nerve conduction studies showed further improvement (Figure 5.10). However, an evoked CAP could still not be obtained from the extensor brevis muscle of the foot; this finding, in addition to the clinical signs, suggested that, whereas recovery from the neuropathy had been considerable, there was likely to be residual evidence of it on a permanent basis. (Reprinted with permission from Bolton et al., 1971.)

The first symptoms to improve, within a few days or weeks, are distal numbness and tingling (Nielsen, 1974b). However, even patients who have had no signs or symptoms of polyneuropathy have a greater feeling of well-being soon after the transplantation, and this coincides with improvement in nerve conduction velocities (Bolton et al., 1971). Moreover, during this early stage, Nielsen noted a dramatic improvement in previously elevated thresholds to vibratory perception (Nielsen, 1974b).

Clinical recovery seems to occur in two phases (Nielsen, 1974b; Dobblestein et al., 1968): initial rapid improvement over days or weeks and then more protracted improvement over months. The rate of improvement is related mainly to the severity of the neuropathy, being more protracted in severe cases (Bolton et al., 1971). Even in these severe cases, walking may be possible within two to three months, and reasonably satisfactory function may eventually occur. Patients will then be able to perform fine movements with their hands, such as buttoning their clothes, writing, etc. In severe neuropathy, a disabling action tremor may develop during the recovery phase, but this will eventually disappear and allow normal function of the hands (Casano, personal communication, 1972).

However, in severe polyneuropathy, residual clinical signs often remain. Ankle jerks may remain absent, and distal muscles may be moderately weak and wasted, particularly in the lower limbs. Despite evidence of impotence and signs of autonomic dysfunction during regular hemodialysis, potency and fertility virtually return to normal (Bolton et al., 1971; Phadke et al., 1970).

Improvement in these various manifestations of polyneuropathy will only occur if the transplanted kidney continues to function successfully for a matter of months. Should acute or chronic rejection occur, not only will uremic polyneuropathy fail to improve, but progressive worsening will likely occur (Dobblestein et al., 1968; Bolton et al., 1971). However, with successful renal transplant, clinical and electrophysiological improvement will prevail for a second time (Bolton, 1976). This observation provides strong evidence that immunosuppressive methods such as irradiation, steroids, and azathioprine, which are used following successful renal transplantation, are not in themselves responsible for the recovery from uremic polyneuropathy. There is little doubt the restoration of near-normal function is responsible for this improvement.

Mononeuropathies, particularly of a compressive nature, of the ulnar nerve at the elbow and the peroneal nerve at the fibular head occasionally occur during terminal renal failure, particularly if the patient is cachectic and bedridden for any length of time.

Successful renal transplantation will restore the function of these individually damaged nerves, as it does the more general polyneuropathy (Bolton, 1976).

Mallamaci et al. (1986) observed that autonomic nervous system function was equally impaired in patients on hemodialysis and peritoneal dialysis but was essentially normal in patients who had successfully received a renal transplant.

Studies of the effects of transplantation on diabetics with end-stage renal disease have been of great interest. Carrillo et al. and Van der Vliet et al. (1987) noted no convincing improvement in the polyneuropathy of such patients after successful renal transplantation. In a careful, well-controlled study, Solders et al. (1987) observed that polyneuropathy not only failed to improve in 15 diabetics who had renal transplantation, but also in a further 13 diabetics who had combined kidney and pancreatic transplantation; a third group of nondiabetic patients evinced complete recovery from "pure" uremic polyneuropathy after renal transplantation alone. Thus, the polyneuropathy in diabetic patients who are in renal failure would seem to be due mainly to the diabetes mellitus, this type of neuropathy being resistant to even combined kidney and pancreatic transplantation.

Kidney transplantation is a successful method of managing end-stage renal disease in children. In Canada, approximately 2 percent of all new patients entering the dialysis transplantation program are children, and of all transplants performed, 9 percent are performed on children (Arbus et al., 1986). Uremic polyneuropathy fails to improve during chronic hemodialysis, but improves regularly after successful renal transplantation, although the recovery phase may be somewhat more protracted than in adults (Alderson et al., 1985).

*Electrophysiological Changes
following Successful Renal
Transplantation*

Chaumont et al. (1963), Funck-Brentano et al. (1968), and Dobblestein et al. (1968) were the first to report that nerve conduction studies consistently improved following successful renal transplantation. Dobblestein et al. emphasized the clinical improvement along with the electrophysiological improvement and indicated that, as with the clinical signs, recovery occurred in two phases. Funck-Brentano et al. indicated, however, that electrophysiological recovery might be incomplete:

> In all 10 cases, tracings definitely showed denervation of a number of motor units despite apparent complete motor recovery. This observation suggests that the healing process occurs only in fibers which are partially functional at the time of transplantation.

These observations were largely substantiated and then expanded by more detailed studies by Bolton (Bolton et al., 1970; 1971; Bolton, 1976) and Nielsen (1974b; 1974c).

Just how early electrophysiological changes begin following the transplant is debatable. Neither Nielsen nor Bolton systematically tested nerve conduction in the days and weeks immediately before and then following the transplant procedure. Bolton, however, did perform nerve conduction studies in nine patients at least once in the two months before and once within two months after transplantation. No significant change was demonstrated in either median or peroneal nerve conduction velocities. However, Ibrahim et al. (1974) and Oh et al. (1978) measured nerve conduction velocity at frequent intervals immediately before and then following transplantation. They noted statistically significant rises in the conduction velocity within a week following the transplantation. This suggested a rapidly reversible metabolic effect on the peripheral nerve. In fact, Oh et al. demonstrated that the rise in conduction velocities coincided with a fall in the previously abnormally elevated levels of *myo*-inositol.

A word of caution should be introduced in interpreting these last results. Ibrahim et al. failed to measure limb temperature. Oh et al. recorded limb temperature and applied a correction factor to their nerve conduction results. However, the correction factor was one based on changes in normal nerve (Ibrahim et al., 1974). Bolton et al. (1982) have demonstrated that in peripheral neuropathy, specifically

uremic neuropathy, the speed of impulse conduction tends to rise more rapidly with increasing limb temperature than in normal nerve. Thus, the results following transplantation may be spurious if limb temperature rose, as it often does postoperatively, and appropriate correction factors were not applied.

There is little doubt that the more definitive rise in conduction velocities that occurs in the weeks following transplantation (Figure 5.3E) (Bolton et al., 1981) parallels the significant clinical recovery and likely represents segmental remyelination. The later, less rapid, more protracted rise in conduction velocities may represent axonal regeneration, a slower process (Nielsen, 1974b; Bolton et al., 1981). However, a rise in the amplitude of muscle and sensory CAPs also occurs. In observing the change in the shape of the action potential when comparing proximal and distal stimulation, Nielsen (1974b) and Bolton et al. (1971) (Figure 5.10) noted that the reversal of dispersed action potentials occurs as a result of segmental remyelination. However, the action potentials do not recover to the same degree as conduction velocities, particularly in more severe neuropathies (Bolton, 1976; Bolton et al., 1971), indicating that recovery may be incomplete as originally suggested by Funck-Brentano et al. (1968). Presumably, axons have been irreversibly damaged. The improvement in speed of nerve conduction occurs in distal segments, as well as more proximal segments, as indicated by the shortening of distal latencies. Needle electromyography shows eventual disappearance of fibrillation potentials and positive sharp waves. The number of motor unit potentials, which was previously decreased, increases towards normal values. The potentials assume a more polyphasic form, an indication of the reinnervation process (Nielsen, 1974b; Bolton et al., 1971).

Should the kidney graft that was initially successful later show evidence of rejection and deteriorating renal function, the polyneuropathy will again appear. This phenomenon was originally noted by Dobblestein et al. (1968). Bolton et al. confirmed this observation by systematic studies in four patients, noting the deterioration of clinical and electrophysiological studies as the first transplant failed, and then noting with a second successful renal transplant the subsequent partial recovery (Bolton, 1976).

Conclusion

Uremic polyneuropathy is a symmetrical impairment of muscle strength and sensation that occurs mainly distally and in the legs. It is not clinically evident in acute renal failure. In chronic renal failure, the earliest sign is abnormal nerve conduction, particularly prolongation of F-responses, decreased sural nerve conduction velocity, and decreased action potential amplitudes. As the degree of renal failure progresses, as measured by the creatinine clearance, conduction velocity gradually falls until end-stage renal failure is reached, when approximately half of such patients will have abnormal nerve conduction. A rapidly progressive, predominantly motor polyneuropathy may rarely occur, particularly when renal failure is further complicated by sepsis or major surgery. Tests of autonomic dysfunction are often abnormal, but overt evidence of such dysfunction is not usually present.

The pathophysiology is complex. Basic physiological testing of peripheral nerve reveals increase in the peripheral nerve excitation threshold, prolongation of the refractory period, decrease in the transmembrane potentials, and dysfunction of sodium channels. There is also a decrease in the resting membrane potential of muscle. Peripheral nerve pathology reveals a combination of axonal degeneration and segmental demyelination, the latter presumably being a secondary effect. However, the precise site and mechanism of the dysfunction is still not known.

A variety of etiologies have been considered. There is no good evidence for a deficiency of B vitamins (particularly thiamine), biotin, magnesium, or certain proteins (i.e., protein malnutrition). There is also no evidence for a toxic effect of substances known to accumulate in the blood during uremia: guanidine, phenols, *myo*-inositol, urea, creatinine, and middle molecules. A number of hormones also accumulate, notably parathyroid hormone, but again, there is no evidence that this causes dysfunction of peripheral nerves. Studies of the peripheral vasculature have revealed several abnormalities of capillaries and arterioles in the skin, but no such abnormalities have yet been reported in peripheral nerves. These, and other methods, should be applied to determine the etiology of this important complication of chronic renal failure.

Uremic polyneuropathy stabilizes during chronic hemodialysis, but manipulating the type, frequency, or duration of this procedure may not alter the course of the polyneuropathy. To prevent this complication, chronic hemodialysis should be started early in the course of chronic renal failure, when there may still be some preservation of residual renal function and more serious polyneuropathy has not yet developed. There is still no convincing evidence that selective removal of middle molecules by dialysis affects the polyneuropathy. Similarly, CAPD appears to have the same effect as hemodialysis on the polyneuropathy. If the patient also has diabetes mellitus, CAPD fails to improve the polyneuropathy.

Successful renal transplantation regularly results in improvement within a matter of weeks for mild cases and months for more severe cases. Should the transplant be rejected, the polyneuropathy may then recur, only to improve again with a second successful transplant. Autonomic function, particularly potency in the male, returns to normal after this procedure. However, if the patient is diabetic, transplantation seems to have little effect on the polyneuropathy, suggesting that the neuropathy may be mainly on the basis of diabetes mellitus. If the patient is a child, the polyneuropathy will improve following transplantation.

The peripheral nervous system should be routinely assessed, at least every 12 months, by clinical methods and nerve conduction studies.

References

Ackil AA, Shahani BT, Young RR. Sural nerve conduction studies and late responses in children undergoing hemodialysis. Arch Phys Med Rehabil 1981a;62:487–491.

Ackil AA, Shahani BT, Young RR, Rubin NE. Late response and sural conduction studies. Usefulness in patients with chronic renal failure. Arch Neurol 1981b;38:482–485.

Alderson K, Seay A, Brewer E, Petajan J. Neuropathies in children with chronic renal failure treated by hemodialysis. Neurology 1985;35 (Suppl): 94.

Amair P, Khanna R, Leibel B, et al. Continuous ambulatory peritoneal dialysis in diabetics with end-stage renal disease. N Engl J Med 1982;306:625–630.

Appenzeller O, Kornfeld M, Macgee J. Neuropathy in chronic renal disease. A microscopic, ultrastructural and biochemical study of sural nerve biopsies. Arch Neurol 1971;24:449–461.

Arbus GS, Barnor HA, Hsu AC, et al. Effect of chronic renal failure, dialysis and transplantation on motor nerve conduction velocity in children. Can Med Assoc J 1975;113:517–520.

Arbus GS, Geary DF, McLorie GA, et al. Pediatric renal transplants: a Canadian perspective. Kidney Int 1986;30:S31–S34.

Asaba H, Alvestrand A, Furst P, Bergstrom J. Clinical implications of uremic middle molecules in regular hemodialysis patients. Clin Nephrol 1983;19:179–187.

Asbury AK. Uremic neuropathy. In: Dyck PJ, Thomas PK, Lambert EH, Bunge R, eds. Peripheral neuropathy. Vol 2, 2nd ed. Philadelphia: WB Saunders, 1984:1811–1825.

Asbury AK, Victor M, Adams RD. Uremic polyneuropathy. Arch Neurol 1963;8:413–428.

Babb AL, Popovich RP, Christopher TG, Scribner BH. The genesis of the square-meter–hour hypothesis. Trans Am Soc Artif Intern Organs 1971;17:81–91.

Bergstrom J, Furst P. Uraemic toxins. In: Drukker W, Parsons FM, Maher JF, eds. Replacement of renal function by dialysis. Amsterdam: Martinus Nijhoff, 1983:368–372.

Bittar EE. Maia muscle fibre as a model for the study of uraemic toxicity. Nature 1967;214:310.

Bolte HD, Riecker G, Rohl D. Measurements of membrane potential of individual muscle cells in normal men and patients with renal insufficiency. 2nd International Congress of Nephrology 1963;78:114.

Bolton CF. Electrophysiologic changes in uremic neuropathy after successful renal transplantation. Neurology 1976;26:152–161.

Bolton CF. Chronic dialysis for uremia. N Engl J Med 1980a;302:1980.

Bolton CF. Peripheral neuropathies associated with chronic renal failure. Can J Neurol Sci 1980b;7:89–96.

Bolton CF. Factors affecting the amplitude of human sensory compound action potentials. American Association of Electromyography and Electrodiagnosis. Minimonograph 17, October 1981.

Bolton CF, Baltzan MA, Baltzan RB. Uremic neuropathy during hemodialysis and following renal transplantation. Ann R Coll Physicians Surg Can 1970;3:37.

Bolton CF, Baltzan MA, Baltzan RB. Effects of renal transplantation on uremic neuropathy. A clinical and Electrophysiologic study. N Engl J Med 1971; 284:1170–1175.

Bolton CF, Carter K. Human sensory nerve compound action potential amplitude. Variation with sex and finger circumference. J Neurol Neurosurg Psychiatry 1980;43:925–928.

Bolton CF, Carter K, Koval JJ. Temperature effects on conduction studies of normal and abnormal nerve. Muscle Nerve 1982;5:S145–S147.

Bolton CF, Gilbert JJ, Hahn AF, Sibbald WJ. Polyneuropathy in critically ill patients. J Neurol Neurosurg Psychiatry 1984;47:1223–1231.

Bolton CF, Laverty DA, Brown JD, et al. Critically ill polyneuropathy: electrophysiological studies and differentiation from Guillain-Barré syndrome. J Neurol Neurosurg Psychiatry 1986;49:563–573.

Bolton CF, Lindsay RM, Linton AL. The course of uremic neuropathy during chronic hemodialysis. Can J Neurol Sci 1975;2:332–333.

Bolton CF, Lindsay RM, Linton AL. Uremic neuropathy in patients on different hemodialysis schedules. Neurology 1977;27:396.

Bolton CF, Sawa GM, Carter K. The effects of temperature on human compound action potentials. J Neurol Neurosurg Psychiatry 1981;44:407–413.

Boudet J, Man NK, Cueille G, et al. Relationship between plasma concentration of middle molecule weight fraction b, motor nerve conduction velocity, and plasma creatinine failure in rats. Artif Organs 1980;4(Suppl):115.

Bourgoignie J, Klahr S, Bricker NS. Inhibition of transepithelial sodium transport in the frog skin by a low molecular weight fraction of uremic serum. J Clin Invest 1971;50:303.

Braguer D, Chauvet-Monges AM, Sari JC, et al. Inhibition in vitro of the polymerization of tubulin by uremic middle molecules: corrective effect of isaxonine. Clin Nephrol 1983;20:149–154.

Brismar T, Tegner R. Experimental uremic neuropathy. Part 2. Sodium permeability decrease and inactivation in potential clamped nerve fibers. J Neurol Sci 1984;65:37–45.

Brown WF. The physiological and technical basis of electromyography. Boston: Butterworths, 1984:169–221.

Bundschu HD. Skelettmuskulatur bei terminaler Niereninsuffizienz. J Neurol Sci 1977;23:243.

Cadilhac J, Mion CH, Duday H, et al. Motor nerve conduction velocities as an index of the efficiency of maintenance dialysis in patients with end-stage renal failure. In: Canal N, Pozz G, eds. Peripheral neuropathies. New York: Elsevier/North-Holland, 1978:372–380.

Callaghan N. Restless leg syndrome in uremic neuropathy. Neurology 1966;16:359–361.

Castaigne P, Cathala H-P, Beaussart-Boulengé L, Petrover M. Effect of ischaemia on peripheral nerve function in patients with chronic renal failure undergoing dialysis treatment. J Neurol Neurosurg Psychiatry 1972;35:631–637.

Chaumont PJ, Lefévre J, Lérique JL. Explorations électrologiques au cours des insuffisances rénales graves. Rev Neurol 1963;108:199–201.

Chiu SY, Morse HE, Ritchie J. Anomalous temperature dependence of the sodium concentrate in rabbit nerve compared with frog nerve. Nature 1979; 279:327–328.

Chokroverty S. Proximal vs distal slowing in renal failure treated by longterm hemodialysis. Arch Neurol 1982;39:53–54.

Clements RS Jr, DeJesus PV Jr, Winegrad AI. Raised plasma-myoinositol levels in uraemia and experimental neuropathy. Lancet 1973;1:1137–1141.

Cole CH, Maletz R. Changes in erythrocyte membrane ouabain-sensitive adenosine triphosphatase after renal transplantation. Clin Sci Mol Med 1975;48:239–242.

Cole CH, Steinberg R, Guttmann R. Altered erythrocyte sodium following renal transplantation. Nephron 1978;28:248–257.

Cunningham JN, Carter NW, Rector FC Jr, Selding DW. Resting transmembrane potential difference of skeletal muscle in normal subjects and severely ill patients. J Clin Invest 1971;50:49–59.

Curtis JR, Eastwood JB, Smith EK. Maintenance hemodialysis. Q J Med 1969;38:49–89.

D'Amour ML, Dufresne LR, Morin C, Slaughter D. Sensory nerve conduction in chronic uremic patients during the first six months of hemodialysis. Can J Neurol Sci 1984;11:269–271.

DeJesus PV, Clements RS, Winegrad AI. Hypermyoinositolemic polyneuropathy in rats: a possible mechanism for uremic polyneuropathy. J Neurol Sci 1974;21:237–249.

Delbeke J, Kopec J, McComas AJ. Effects of age, temperature and disease on the refractoriness of human nerve and muscle. J Neurol Neurosurg Psychiatry 1978;41:65–71.

Del Campo M, Bolton CF, Lindsay RM. The value of electrophysiological studies in assessing peripheral nerve function during optimal hemodialysis. Muscle Nerve 1983:533–534.

Dinapoli RP, Johnson WJ, Lambert EH. Experience with a combined hemodialysis-renal transplantation program: neurologic aspects. Mayo Clin Proc 1966; 41:809–820.

Dinn JJ, Crane DL. Schwann cell dysfunction in uremia. Neurology 1970;20:649–658.

Dobblestein VH, Altmeyer B, Edel H, et al. Periphere Neuropathie bei chronischer Niereninsuffizienz, bei Dauerdialysebehandlung und nach Nierentransplantation. Med Klin 1968;63:616–622.

Dyck PJ, Johnson WJ, Lambert EH, et al. Detection and evaluation of uremic peripheral neuropathy in patients on hemodialysis. Kidney Int 1975a;7:S201–S205.

Dyck PJ, Johnson WJ, Lambert EH, O'Brien PC. Segmental demyelination secondary to axonal degeneration in uremic neuropathy. Mayo Clin Proc 1971;46:400–531.

Dyck PJ, Johnson WJ, Nelson RA, et al. Uremic neuropathy. III. Controlled study of restricted protein and fluid diet and infrequent hemodialysis versus conventional hemodialysis treatment. Mayo Clin Proc 1975b;50:641–649.

Dyck PJ, Karnes K, O'Brien PC, Zimmerman IR. Detection thresholds of cutaneous sensations in humans. In: Dyck PJ, Thomas PK, Lambert EH, Bunge R, eds. Peripheral neuropathy. Vol 1. Philadelphia: WB Saunders, 1984:chapter 49;1103–1138.

Eckbom KA. Restless leg syndrome. Neurology 1960;10:868.

Edmondson RPS, Hilton PJ, Jones NF, et al. Leucocyte sodium transport in uraemia. Clin Sci Mol Med 1975;49:213–216.

Egan JD, Wells IC. Transketolase inhibition and uremic peripheral sensory neuropathy. J Neurol Sci 1979; 41:379–395.

Eggers PW. Effect of transplantation on the medicare end-stage renal disease program. N Engl J Med 1988;318:223–229.

Evans RW, Manninen DL, Garrison LP, et al. The quality of life of patients with end-stage renal disease. N Engl J Med 1985;312:553–559.

Fleming LW, Lenman JAR, Stewart WK. Effect of magnesium on nerve conduction velocity during regular dialysis treatment. J Neurol Neurosurg Psychiatry 1972;35:342–345.

Funck-Brentano JL, Chaumont P, Vantelon J, Zingraff J. Polyneuritis during the course of chronic uremia. Follow-up after renal transplantation (10 personal observations). Nephron 1968;5:31–42.

Ganji SS, Mahajan S. Changes in sort-latency somatosensory evoked potentials during hemodialysis in chronic renal failure. Clin Electroencephalogr 1983;14:202–206.

Gilchrest BA, Rowe JW, Mihm MC Jr. Clinical and histological skin changes in chronic renal failure: evidence for a dialysis-resistant, transplant-responsive microangiopathy. Lancet 1980;2:1271–1975.

Gokal R. Continuous ambulatory peritoneal dialysis (CAPD)—ten years on. Q J Med [New Ser 63] 1987;242:465–472.

Goldstein DA, Chiu LA, Massry SG. Effect of parathyroid hormone and uremia on peripheral nerve calcium and motor nerve conduction velocity. J Clin Invest 1978;62:88–93.

Gonzales-Carillo M, Maloney A, Bewick M, et al.

Renal transplantation in diabetic nephropathy. Br Med J 1982;285:1713–1716.

Guihneuc R, Ginet J. The use of the H-reflex in patients with chronic renal failure. In: Desmedt JE, ed. New developments in electromyography and clinical neurophysiology. Vol 2. Basel: Karger, 1973:400–403.

Hansen S, Ballantyne JP. A quantitative electrophysiological study of uraemic neuropathy. Diabetic and renal neuropathies compared. J Neurol Neurosurg Psychiatry 1978;41:128–134.

Hegstrom RM, Murray JS, Pendras JP, et al. Two years' experience with periodic hemodialysis in the treatment of chronic uremia. Trans Am Soc Artif Intern Organs 1962;8:266–275.

Hollinrake K, Thomas PK, Wills MR, Baillod RA. Observations on plasma magnesium levels in patients with uremic neuropathy under treatment by periodic hemodialysis. Neurology 1970;20:939–941.

Ibrahim MM, Crossland J, Honigsberger L, et al. Effect of renal transplantation on uraemic neuropathy. Lancet 1974;2:739–742.

Jakobsen J. Peripheral nerves in early experimental diabetes. Expansion of the endoneural space as a cause of increased water content. Diabetologia 1978;14:113–119.

Jebsen RH, Tenckhoff H, Honet JC. Natural history of uremic polyneuropathy and effects of dialysis. N Engl J Med 1967;277:327–332.

Jennekens FGI, Dorhout Mees EJ, van der Most van Spijk D. Clinical aspects of uraemic polyneuropathy. Nephron 1971;8:414–426.

Jennekens FGI, Kemmelems-Schinkel AJ. Neurological aspects of dialysis patients. In: Drukker W, Parsons FM, Maher JF, eds. Replacement of renal function by dialysis, 2nd ed. Amsterdam: Martinus Nijhoff, 1983:732–741.

Kimura J. The F-wave. In: Kimura J, ed. Electrodiagnosis in diseases of nerve and muscle: principles and practice. Philadelphia: FA Davis, 1983a:353–377.

Kimura J. The H-reflex and other late responses. In: Kimura J, ed. Electrodiagnosis in diseases of nerve and muscle: principles and practice. Philadelphia: FA Davis, 1983b:379–398.

Kominami N, Tyler R, Hampers CL, Merrill JP. Variations in motor nerve conduction in normal and uremic patients. Arch Intern Med 1971;128:235–239.

Konishi T, Hiroshi N, Motomura S. Single fiber electromyography in chronic renal failure. Muscle Nerve 1982;5:458–461.

Konotey-Ahulu FID, Baillod R, Comty CM, et al. Effect of periodic dialysis on the peripheral neuropathy of end-stage renal failure. Br Med J 1965; 2:1212–1215.

Koppell JD, Dirige OV, Jacob M, et al. Transketolase activity in red blood cells in chronic uremia. Trans Am Soc Artif Intern Organs 1972;18:250–256.

Kumegawa M, Hiramatsu M, Yamada T, Yajima T. Effects of intermediate sized molecular components in uremic sera on nerve tissue in vitro. Brain Res 1980;198:234–238.

Kurtz SB, Wong VH, Anderson CF, et al. Continuous ambulatory peritoneal dialysis. Three years' experience at the Mayo Clinic, Mayo Clin Proc 1983; 58(10):633–639.

Lewis EG, Dustman RE, Beck EC. Visual and somatosensory evoked potential characteristics of patients undergoing hemodialysis and kidney transplantation. Electroencephalogr Clin Neurophysiol 1978;44:223–231.

Lindholm B, Tegner R, Tranaeus A, Bergstrom J. Progress of peripheral uremic neuropathy during continuous ambulatory peritoneal dialysis (CAPD). Trans Am Soc Artif Intern Organs 1982;28:263–268.

Lindsay RM, Bolton CF, Clark WF, Linton AL. The effect of alterations of uremic retention products upon platelet and peripheral nerve function. Clin Nephrol 1983;19:110–115.

Locke S, Merrill FP, Tyler HR. Neurologic complications of acute uremia. Arch Intern Med 1961; 108:519–530.

Lonergan ET, Semar M, Lange K. Transketolase activity in uremia. Arch Intern Med 1970;126:851–854.

Low PA, Tuck RR, Takeuchi M. Nerve Microenvironment in diabetic neuropathy. In: Dyck PJ, Thomas PK, Asbury AK, et al., eds. Diabetic neuropathy. Philadelphia: WB Saunders, 1987:266–278.

Lowitzsch K, Gohring U, Hecking E. Refractory period, sensory conduction and vibration before and after hemodialysis. Acta Neurol Scand 1979;60(Suppl 73).

Lowitzsch K, Gohring U, Hecking E, Kohler H. Refractory period, sensory conduction velocity and visual evoked potentials before and after hemodialysis. J Neurol Neurosurg Psychiatry 1981;44:121–128.

Lowrie EG, Laird NM, Parker TF, Sargent JA. Effect of the hemodialysis prescription on patient morbidity. Report from the National Cooperative Dialysis Study. N Engl J Med 1981;305:1176–1181.

Lowrie EG, Steinberg SM, Galen MA, et al. Factors in the dialysis regimen which contribute to alterations in the abnormalities of uremia. Kidney Int 1976;10:409–422.

Ludin H-P, Tackmann W. Examination techniques. In: Ludin H-P, Tackmann W, eds. Sensory neurography. Stuttgart: Thieme, 1981:26.

Lynch PG, Yuill GM, Nicholson JAH. Acute polyneuropathy complicating chronic renal failure. Nephron 1971;8:278–288.

Mallamaci F, Zoccali C, Ciccarelli M, Briggs JD. Autonomic function in uremic patients treated by hemodialysis on CAPD and in transplant patients. Clin Nephrol 1986;25:175–180.

Man NK, Cueille G, Zingraff J, et al. Investigations on clinico-chemical correlations in uraemic polyneuritis. Proc Eur Dial Transplant Assoc 1974;11:214.

Man NK, Cueille G, Zingraff, J, et al. Uremic neurotoxin in the middle molecular weight range. Artif Organs, 1980;4:116–120.

Man NK, Terlain B, Paris J, et al. An approach to "middle molecules" identification in artificial kidney dialysate, with reference to neuropathy prevention. Trans Am Soc Artif Intern Organs 1973;19:320–324.

Massry SG, Goldstein DA. The search for uremic toxin(s) "x" "x" = PTH. Clin Nephrol 1979;11:181–189.

Mathias CJ, Naik RB, Warren DJ, Frankel H. Autonomic neuropathy. Arch Intern Med 1983;143:1635.

Maynard FM, Stolov WC. Experimental error in determination of nerve conduction velocity. Arch Phys Med Rehabil 1972;53:362–372.

McGonigle RJS, Bewick M, Weston MJ, Parsons V. Progressive, predominantly motor, uraemic neuropathy. Acta Neurol Scand 1985;71:379–384.

Merrill JP, Hampers CL. Uremia. N Engl J Med 1970;282:953–961.

Nielsen VK. Sensory nerve conduction studies in uraemic patients. Proc Eur Dial Transplant Assoc 1967;4:279–284.

Nielsen VK. The peripheral nerve function in chronic renal failure. I. Clinical symptoms and signs. Acta Med Scand 1971a;190:105–111.

Nielsen VK. The peripheral nerve function in chronic renal failure. II. Intercorrelation of clinical symptoms and signs and clinical grading of neuropathy. Acta Med Scand 1971b;190:113–117.

Nielsen VK. The peripheral nerve function in chronic renal failure. IV. An analysis of the vibratory perception threshold. Acta Med Scand 1972;191:287–296.

Nielsen VK. The peripheral nerve function in chronic renal failure. V. Sensory and motor conduction velocity. Acta Med Scand 1973a;194:445–454.

Nielsen VK. The peripheral nerve function in chronic renal failure. VI. The relationship between sensory and motor nerve conduction and kidney function, azotemia, age, sex and clinical neuropathy. Acta Med Scand 1973b;194:455–462.

Nielsen VK. Sensory and motor nerve conduction in distal and proximal nerve segments in chronic renal failure. Electroencephalogr Clin Neurophysiol 1973c;34:809.

Nielsen VK. Sensory and motor nerve conduction in the median nerve in normal subjects. Acta Med Scand 1973d;194:435–443.

Nielsen VK. The peripheral nerve function in chronic renal failure. VII. Longitudinal course during terminal renal failure and regular hemodialysis. Acta Med Scand 1974a;195:155–162.

Nielsen VK. The peripheral nerve function in chronic renal failure. VIII. Recovery after renal transplantation. Clinical aspects. Acta Med Scand 1974b;195:163–170.

Nielsen VK. The peripheral nerve function in chronic renal failure. IX. Recovery after renal transplantation. Electrophysiological aspects (sensory and motor nerve conduction). Acta Med Scand 1974c;195:171–180.

Nielsen VK. The peripheral nerve function in chronic renal failure. X. Decremental nerve conduction in uremia? Acta Med Scand 1974d;196:83–86.

Nielsen VK. The peripheral nerve function in chronic renal failure: a survey. Acta Med Scand 1974e;(Suppl) 573:7–32.

Nielsen VK. The vibration stimulus effects of viscous-elastic resistance of skin on the amplitude of vibrations. Electroencephalogr Clin Neurophysiol 1975; 38:647–652.

Nielsen VK. Pathophysiological aspects of uraemic neuropathy. In: Canal N, Pozza G, eds. Peripheral neuropathies. New York: Elsevier/North-Holland 1978:197–210.

Nielsen VK, Winkel P. The peripheral nerve function in chronic renal failure. III. A multivariate statistical analysis of factors presumed to affect the development of clinical neuropathy. Acta Med Scand 1971; 190:119–125.

Obeso JA, Marti-Masso JF, Asin AL, et al. Conduction velocity through the somesthetic pathway in chronic renal failure. J Neurol Sci 1979;43:439–445.

Oh SJ, Clements R, Lee YW, Diethelm AG. Rapid improvement in nerve conduction velocity following renal transplantation. Ann Neurol 1978;4:369–373.

Panayiotopoulous CP, Laxos G. Tibial nerve H-reflex and F-wave studies in patients with uremic neuropathy. Muscle Nerve 1980;3:423–426.

Panayiotopoulous CP, Scarpalezos S. F-wave studies in the deep peroneal nerve. J Neurol Sci 1977;31:331–341.

Pendras JP, Erickson RV. Hemodialysis: a successful therapy. Ann Intern Med 1966;64:293–311.

Phadke AG, Mackinnon KJ, Dossetor JB. Male fertility in uremia: restoration by renal allografts. Can Med Assoc J 1970;102:607–608.

Pierratos A, Blair G, Khanna R, Quinton C, Oreopoulos, DG. Nerve electrophysiological parameters in patients undergoing continuous ambulatory peritoneal dialysis (CAPD) over two years. Ann CRMCC 1981;14:231.

Posen GA, Kaye M. Magnesium metabolism in patients on chronic hemodialysis. Proc Eur Dial Transplant Assoc 1967;4:224–228.

Preswick G, Jeremy D. Subclinical polyneuropathy in renal insufficiency. Lancet 1964;2:731–732.

Read DJ, Feest TG, Holman RH. Vibration sensory threshold: a guide to adequacy of dialysis? Proc Eur Dial Transplant Assoc 1982;19:253–257.

Reznek RH, Salway JG, Thomas PK. Plasma-myoinositol concentrations in uremic neuropathy. Lancet 1977;1:675–676.

Rossini PM, Treviso M, Di Stefano E, Di Paolo B. Nervous impulse propagation along peripheral and central fibres in patients with chronic renal failure. Electroencephalogr Clin Neurophysiol 1983;56:293–303.

Said G, Boudier L, Selva J, et al. Different patterns of uremic polyneuropathy: clinicopathologic study. Neurology 1983;33:567–574.

Savazzi GM, Buzio C, Migone L. Lights and shadows on the pathogenesis of uremic polyneuropathy. Clin Nephrol 1982;18:219–229.

Savazzi GM, Juvarra G, Marbini A, et al. Interrelazioni morfologiche e funzionali fra neuropatia e danno muscolare. Minerva Nefrol 1980;27:211.

Schaeffer K, Offermann G, Von Herrath D, et al. Failure to show a correlation between serum parathyroid hormone, nerve conduction velocity and serum lipids in hemodialysis patients. Clin Nephrol 1980;14:81–88.

Seneviratne KIV, Peiris OA. Peripheral nerve function in chronic liver disease. J Neurol Neurosurg Psychiatry 1970;33:609–614.

Serra C, D'Angelillo A, Facciolla Dietal. Somatosensory cerebral evoked potentials in uremic polyneuropathy. Acta Neurol (Napoli) 1979;34:1–14.

Solders G, Persson A, Gutierrez A. Autonomic dysfunction in non-diabetic terminal uraemia. Acta Neurol Scand 1985;71:321–327.

Solders G, Wilczek H, Gunnarsson R, et al. Effects of combined pancreatic and renal transplantation on diabetic neuropathy: a two year follow-up study. Lancet 1987;2:1232–1235.

Stewart WK, Fleming LW, Anderson DC, et al. Changes in plasma electrolytes and nerve conduction velocities during chronic haemodialysis without magnesium. Proc Eur Dial Transplant Assoc 1967;4:285–291.

Tackmann W, Ullerich D, Cremer W, Lehmann HJ. Nerve conduction studies during the relative refractory period in sural nerves of patients with uremia. Eur Neurol 1974;12:331–339.

Tegner R. The effect of skin temperature on vibratory sensitivity in polyneuropathy. J Neurol Neurosurg Psychiatry 1985;48:176–178.

Tegner R, Brismar T. Experimental uremic neuropathy. Part I. Decreased nerve conduction velocity in rats. J Neurol Sci 1984;65:29–36.

Tegner R, Lindholm B. Uremic polyneuropathy: different effects of hemodialysis and continuous ambulatory peritoneal dialysis. Acta Med Scand 1985a;218:409–416.

Terger R, Lindholm B. Vibratory perception threshold compared with nerve conduction velocity in the evaluation of uraemic neuropathy. Acta Neurol Scand 1985b;71:284–289.

Tenckhoff HA, Boen FST, Jebsen RH, Spiegler JH. Polyneuropathy in chronic renal insufficiency. JAMA 1965;192:1121–1124.

Tenckhoff HA, Curtis FF. Experience with maintenance peritoneal dialysis in the home. Trans Am Soc Artif Intern Organs 1970;16:90–95.

Thiele B, Stålberg E. Single fibre EMG findings in polyneuropathies of different aetiology. J Neurol Neurosurg Psychiatry 1975;38:881–887.

Thomas PK, Hollinrake K, Lascelles RG, et al. The polyneuropathy of chronic renal failure. Brain 1971;94:761–780.

Tyler HR. Neurologic disorders in renal failure. Am J Med 1968;44:734–748.

van der Most Van Spijk D, Hoogland RA, Dijkstra S. Conduction velocities and related degrees of renal insufficiency. In: Desmedt JE, ed. New developments in electromyography and clinical neurophysiology. Vol 2. Basel: Karger, 1973:381–389.

Van der Vliet JA, Navarro T, Kennedy WR, et al. Diabetic polyneuropathy and renal transplantation. Transplant proc 1986;19:3597–3599.

Vaziri D, Pratt H, Saiki JD, Starr A. Evaluation of somatosensory pathway by short latency evoked potentials in patients with end-stage renal disease maintained on hemodialysis. Int J Artif Organs 1981;4:17–21.

Versaki AA, Olsen KJ, McMain PB. Uremic polyneuropathy: motor nerve conduction velocities. Trans Am Soc Artif Intern Organs 1964;10:328–330.

Wehle G, Bevegard S, Castenfors J, et al. Carotid baroreflexes during hemodialysis. Clin Nephrol 1983;19:236–242.

Welt LG, Sachs JR, McManus TJ. An ion transport defect in erythrocytes from uremic subjects. Trans Assoc Am Physicians 1964;77:169–181.

Willett RW. Infectious neuronitis (Guillain-Barré syndrome) in association with chronic renal failure. NC Med J 1964;25:99–102.

Williams IR, Davison AM, Mawdsley C, Robson JS. Neuropathy in chronic renal failure. In: Desmedt JE, ed. New developments in electromyography and clinical neurophysiology. Vol 2. Basel: Karger, 1973:390–399.

Wright EA, McQuillen MP. Hypoexcitability of ulnar nerve in patients with normal conduction velocity. Neurology 1973;23:78–83.

Yatzidis H, Koutsicos D, Alaveras AG, et al. Biotin for neurologic disorders of uremia. N Engl J Med 1981;305:764.

B

Uremic Mononeuropathy

The dysfunction of peripheral nerve that occurs in a generalized fashion in chronic renal failure renders these nerves susceptible to local damage. The type of damage is compression, ischemia, or both. Such damage to the median nerve at the wrist, carpal tunnel syndrome, is now recognized as the commonest peripheral nerve disorder in chronic renal failure. However, compressive palsies also occur in the ulnar nerve at the elbow and in the common peroneal nerve at the fibular head. Severe ischemic neuropathies may develop as direct complications of arteriovenous fistulas or shunts. Finally, bleeding near peripheral nerves as a result of the bleeding diathesis in chronic renal failure may cause an acute, severe focal neuropathy.

Carpal Tunnel Syndrome

While the symptoms and signs of carpal tunnel syndrome in chronic renal failure are remarkably similar to those in otherwise healthy persons, the underlying etiology of the syndrome in renal failure has proven to be, until recently, remarkably complex.

The association was first described by Warren and Otieno in 1975. Subsequent studies revealed an incidence varying from five percent (Kenzora, 1978; Delmez et al., 1982; Bradish, 1985) to 12 percent (Spertini et al., 1984) to 31 percent (Halter et al., 1981).

The earliest symptoms are an intermittent numbness and tingling in various parts of the median distribution of the hand and an aching pain that may be experienced not only distally, but proximally as far as the neck. These symptoms are precipitated during the day by acts such as holding the steering wheel of a car, knitting, buttoning clothes, and so forth. They may be particularly bothersome at night. The distinctive feature in uremic patients, however, is that the symptoms often become most pronounced during the dialysis procedure itself. In more advanced cases, sensory loss and weakness within the median nerve distribution becomes unrelenting. Phalen's sign (having the patient continually flex the hand and wrist to precipitate symptoms) or Tinel's sign (gently percussing the median nerve at the wrist) may be positive, and in severe cases proximal thenar muscle wasting develops. In patients without renal failure, the syndrome is commonest on the side of the dominant hand, but in seven of 15 renal failure patients it occurred bilaterally (Halter et al., 1981).

As with nonuremic patients, electrophysiological studies aid greatly in clearly establishing the presence of carpal tunnel syndrome. The time for conduction through the area of the carpal tunnel is prolonged for both motor and sensory fibers (Halter et al., 1981).

It was originally suggested by Warren and Otieno in 1975 that carpal tunnel syndrome was due to the presence of a forearm arteriovenous fistula used for access during hemodialysis. They noted that venous pressure and hand volume were greater on the side of the fistula. However, it was recognized that nerve ischemia could also be a significant contributing factor. While forearm fistulas cause a local increase in forearm blood flow, xenon 133 blood flow studies (Lindstedt and Westling, 1975) showed that blood flow to the adductor pollicis muscle was greatly reduced, but such flow was increased when the fistula was occluded by direct compression or when the radial artery distal to the fistula was occluded. Engorgement of the carpal tunnel area, secondary to such shunts, could occur through dilatation of the veins and also through fluid extravasation as a result of the combination of high venous pressure and partial ischemia. Further evidence of such a mechanism was provided by Delmez et al. (1982), who noted that fistula flow rates were, as demonstrated angiographically, highest on the side with the carpal tunnel syndrome. Finally, it is known that with each dialysis procedure there is a fall in the partial pressure of the oxygen, as well as in blood pressure (Aurigemma et al., 1977), which would explain the transient development of symptoms during this procedure. Harding and Le Fanu (1977) noted in one of their patients that the symptoms improved when the radial artery was ligated distal to the fistula.

Uremic nerves respond differently than healthy nerves to ischemia. Castaigne et al. (1972) showed that the nerves of uremic patients rendered ischemic by tourniquet caused evoked sensory nerve action potentials to persist longer than in control subjects, an effect which could be reversed by macromolecular perfusion and enhanced by a single dialysis. This effect was likely related to plasma volume factors, suggesting an abnormality of cell membranes in uremia.

However, other studies have called into question the role of the forearm fistula in producing carpal tunnel syndrome. Delmez et al. (1982) noted no relationship between carpal tunnel syndrome, previous access surgery, or the type of vascular access. Halter et al. (1981)

made similar observations. Moreover, the patients of Halter et al. showed no evidence of edema or venous engorgement at surgery, simply thickening of the flexor retinaculum and flattening of the underlying median nerve as occurs in patients with carpal tunnel syndrome who are not uremic. Analysis of portions of the transverse carpal ligament taken at surgery revealed no evidence of amyloid deposits.

Decompressive surgery, with sectioning of the flexor retinaculum, has been found to be an effective method of treatment (Delmez et al., 1982; Halter et al., 1981; Harding and Le Fanu, 1977), but restoring peripheral nerve function by successful renal transplantation did not alone improve the symptoms of carpal tunnel syndrome (Delmez et al., 1982).

Until 1980, it was generally considered that carpal tunnel syndrome was due to a combination of factors: narrowing of the carpal tunnel due to age, susceptibility of uremic nerve to compression, ischemia in peripheral nerve induced by arteriovenous forearm fistulas, and engorgement of the carpal tunnel with resultant compression of the median nerve due to edema and venous congestion, again induced by the fistula. However, it was becoming obvious that the problem had not been solved, as exemplified by the following case report of a patient in our renal unit that we observed for several years.

A 58-year-old man gradually developed end-stage renal failure because of chronic glomerulonephritis. Regular hemodialysis was begun in 1972 via a Scribner shunt in the left forearm. In 1974, the shunt from the left arm was removed and dialysis was then achieved through a Brescia-Cimino fistula in the right forearm. At that time, he was placed on a home dialysis program in which he was dialyzed by a Gambro-Lundia machine with a Cuprophan membrane. Dialysis was performed three times weekly, six hours each time.

There was a mild subclinical polyneuropathy, demonstrated by nerve conduction studies. These studies were performed at yearly intervals. In 1979, he developed typical symptoms and electrophysiological signs of a right carpal tunnel syndrome, presumed to be a complication of the arteriovenous fistula. However, there was only transient clinical improvement, confirmed by repeat nerve conduction study two months later. On the chance that the use of the fistula during hemodialysis was, in some way, accounting for the problem, he was tried on CAPD for several months. This resulted in no improvement in carpal tunnel symptoms and in increasing generalized symptoms of uremic toxicity; he had to be placed again on chronic hemodialysis.

In 1981, carpal tunnel surgery was repeated on the right, and was done for the first time on the left. This failed to cause any improvement, and postoperative nerve conduction studies showed the presence of severe compressive palsies of both median nerves. However, there was also considerable slowing of conduction for both motor and sensory fibers in the forearm segments. Moreover, clinical and electrophysiological studies suggested that he had now developed a slightly worse, generalized uremic polyneuropathy.

The clinical picture at this point was striking. He complained of severe, aching pain involving the wrists and hands, on both dorsal and palmar aspects. These symptoms were more marked on the right, and the pain extended proximally to the shoulder and even into the base of the neck. There was an associated numbness and tingling diffusely throughout the right hand but particularly in the median nerve distribution. Of particular note was that the pains would come on within one hour of hemodialysis and would not disappear until the procedure was finished. The pains were also worsened by lying down and were partially relieved by sitting.

Examination revealed mild to moderate restriction of movements of the neck and all joints in both upper limbs. There were mild, fixed flexion contractures of the hand (Figure 5.11). There was severe proximal wasting of the right and left thenar eminences and wasting of the right interossei muscles. All of the pulses in the upper extremities were readily palpable, except for the left radial pulse, the artery having been ligated in 1974. A normally functioning arteriovenous fistula was present in the right forearm.

When he raised his arms above his head, within

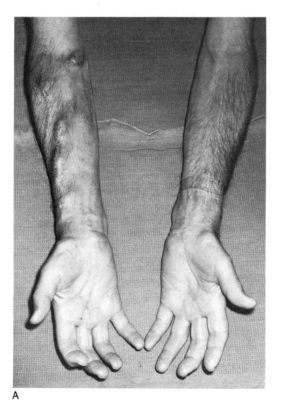
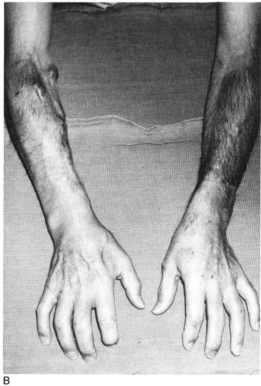

A   B

Figure 5.11. The upper limbs of a patient who had β_2 microglobulin amyloidosis. It caused bilateral carpal tunnel syndrome (note proximal thenar wasting) and a right ulnar neuropathy (note wasting of interosseus muscles). Tissue biopsied at the time of carpal tunnel surgery revealed infiltration of blood vessels by amyloid. The pain may have been due to an arthropathy (note thickening and flexion contraction of interphalangeal joints) and periodic nerve ischemia. Repeated surgery for carpal tunnel syndrome provided only transient relief. (The Brescia-Cimino forearm fistula caused the dilated veins of the right forearm.)

seconds, all of the painful symptoms in both upper limbs developed and seemed to intensify until he lowered his hands, when they promptly improved. With the arms elevated, the pulses did not disappear but some pallor of the hands developed.

These symptoms and findings suggested that there was a neuropathy involving the upper limbs, which likely had a prominent ischemic component, since symptoms were affected by hemodynamic variations caused by hemodialysis and by posturing of the body and upper limbs.

A biopsy was performed of the right superficial and deep peroneal nerves and adjacent muscle. These revealed no specific cause for a neuropathy. There was a moderate axonal degeneration of motor and sensory fibers, consistent with uremic polyneuropathy, and there was some associated chronic denervation of muscle.

A brief trial of oral steroids was unsuccessful. Ultimately, by 1984, life was so miserable he requested discontinuation of hemodialysis and died shortly thereafter. Autopsy was refused.

Initial conventional stains for amyloid were negative. However, the carpal tunnel and sural nerve were recently reexamined, and special stains for β_2 microglobulin were positive for the right carpal tunnel area (Figure 5.12); the results for the sural nerve were equivocal. Thus, he suffered from amyloidosis due to accumulation of β_2 microglobulin, causing intractable bilateral carpal tunnel syndrome and upper limb arthropathy. The ulnar neuropathy may also have been on this basis. Not commented upon in the literature, but present in this and two of our other patients, was upper limb pain that was worse during each hemodialysis procedure, most marked in the limb being dialyzed and worse according to body position. This suggests a periodic nerve is-chemia, the finding of amyloid infiltration of small blood vessels near the median nerve being consistent with this hypothesis. The amyloid infiltration of sural nerve may have produced the mild deterioration of clinical and electrophysiological signs in the lower limbs.

Role of Amyloid

A major breakthrough was made by Charra and colleagues in France (1984), who observed amyloid deposits in the carpal tunnel synovia and tendons in patients on long-term hemodialysis. Many also had shoulder pain and stiffness, and at autopsy, amyloid was found in the biceps tendon and shoulder joint synovia. They reviewed their experience with 52 patients who were operated on for carpal tunnel syndrome (Charra et al., 1984). The signs and symptoms were usually typical, and in only 14 cases were nerve conduction studies necessary to confirm the diagnosis. Median nerve compression was observed at surgery, and it was noted that symptoms and signs disappeared after the operation. The patients had been on chronic hemodialysis with the Kiil machine for a mean of 11 years. None had had renal transplantation or been on peritoneal dialysis for more than six months.

It is now recognized that this shoulder pain is much commoner in patients who have carpal tunnel syndrome due to amyloidosis than in

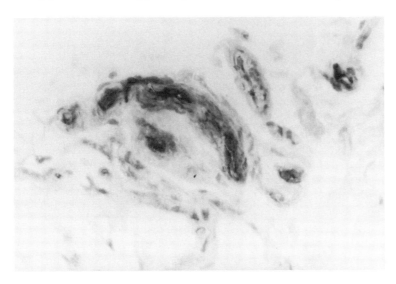

Figure 5.12. A section of the synovium from the right carpal tunnel in patient (Fig. 5.11) to show positive stain for β_2 microglobulin (appears black) within small blood vessels. (Original magnification ×400.)

those who are free of amyloid in the carpal tunnel region. Pain, stiffness, and swelling occur not only in the shoulder joints, but also in other joints of the upper and lower limbs. Bony radiolucencies may be seen on radiographs, particularly in the areas of the wrist and hip, and spontaneous fractures may occur (Bardin et al., 1986; Huaux et al., 1985). The spine may also be involved. Biopsy has frequently shown the presence of amyloid in such lesions. Whether these amyloid deposits are even more widespread is still speculative (Munoz-Gomez et al., 1985; Varga et al., 1986). Aspirates of abdominal fat and skin biopsy specimens have been negative, but deposits have been found in a few patients in the rectal mucosa (Shirahama et al., 1985; Morita et al., 1985).

Due largely to work in Japan (Shirahama et al., 1985; Gejyo et al., 1986), the amyloid material has been shown to be of low molecular weight and identical in amino acid composition to β_2 microglobulin. In direct immunofluorescence studies, anti–β_2 microglobulin reacted positively with the amyloid deposits. On electron microscopy, the amyloid deposits appear as tightly packed filaments that consist of two fine parallel fibrils, differing from the randomly oriented, rigid filaments generally observed in other types of amyloidosis (Morita et al., 1985).

β_2 microglobulin is normally present in small amounts in serum and other body fluids (Berggard and Bearn, 1968). In healthy persons, it is catabolized by the normally functioning kidneys, and consequently, it progressively rises in renal failure (Vincent et al., 1978), becoming abnormally elevated. Its concentration may be as much as 60 times the normal value. The levels are lower if some residual renal function has been preserved (Gejyo et al., 1986). The type of dialysis machine is also important. The levels are higher in patients who are being dialyzed with the standard Cuprophan membrane, in contrast to those who are dialyzed with an AN-69 polyacrylonitrile membrane (Zingraff et al., 1986; Blumberg and Burgi, 1987). Chandard et al. (1986) found that carpal tunnel syndrome was much commoner in patients being dialyzed with the Cuprophan membrane than in those using the AN-69

membrane. It has also been shown that the Cuprophan membrane induces transient leukopenia, complement activation, interleukin-1 production, generation of free radicals, and liberation of blood granulocyte proteases (Yamagami et al., 1986). This might initially damage tissue and predispose it to the deposition of amyloid.

It is of interest that the levels of β_2 microglobulin in patients on CAPD are just as high as those on intermittent hemodialysis (Blumberg and Burgi, 1987; Ballardie et al., 1986). However, to our knowledge, carpal tunnel syndrome has not yet been reported in patients receiving CAPD, perhaps because they have not been treated long enough for it to develop.

Therefore, the present evidence is that carpal tunnel syndrome in patients on long-term hemodialysis is, in most cases, due to amyloidosis resulting from the accumulation of β_2 microglobulin; this is a new and unique form of amyloidosis occurring only in such patients. The condition is most likely to occur in those being dialyzed with a Cuprophan membrane, and it may be that eliminating this form of dialysis and using methods that successfully clear the abnormal protein may ultimately result in reduced incidence of carpal tunnel syndrome. It may still be that the syndrome is due, in some patients, to factors discussed earlier, such as advanced age, edema, and ischemia induced by forearm arteriovenous fistulas. In practical terms, it is mandatory that at the time of carpal tunnel surgery, biopsies be taken and stained appropriately to determine the presence or absence of amyloid.

Table 5.4 shows the current classification of amyloidosis, with the newly discussed AB_2M type added. It is of interest that carpal tunnel syndrome occurs in 25 percent of patients who have type AL amyloidosis (Kelly, 1987) and also in patients who have AF prealbumin familial amyloid polyneuropathy (Thomas, 1987).

Mononeuropathy Associated with Arteriovenous Fistulas or Shunts

A percutaneous cannula introduced through either the femoral vein or the subclavian vein or an external arteriovenous shunt such as

Table 5.4. Classification of Amyloid

Biochemical Type	Clinical Form	Comment
AL	Primary amyloid Multiple myeloma associated amyloid	Homologous to N-terminal residue of variable region of κ or α light chain (or rarely whole chain). Varied molecular weight
AA	Secondary (reactive) amyloid Amyloid of familial Mediterranean fever	Serum protein SAA is putative precursor; Arg-Ser-Phe-Phe-Ser sequence to 76 amino acids
$AF_{prealbumin}$	Familial amyloid polyneuropathy (Japanese, Swedish, Portuguese)	Most with single amino acid substitution of methionine for valine at position 30; probably other variants exist
AE_{mct}	Amyloid-associated medullary carcinoma of thyroid	Probable calcitonin precursor; may be true of other endocrine-related forms of amyloid
AS_C	Senile cardiac	May be prealbumin
AP	P component	Distinct from amyloid fibril; found in all systemic forms. Serum SAP is the precursor
AB_2M	Carpal tunnel syndrome	Only in dialysis with a cuprophan membrane

Source: Reprinted with permission from Cohen AS. Amyloidosis. In: Braunwald et al., eds. *Harrison's Principles of Internal Medicine*, 11th ed., 1987:1404.

Quinton-Scribner shunt between the radial artery and cephalic vein are now used for access for hemodialysis only in acute renal failure. They are associated with a high incidence of infection or clotting when used over a more prolonged period of time, so they are not currently used for chronic hemodialysis. The preferred method for chronic hemodialysis is the arteriovenous fistula, the most common being a surgically created fistula between the radial artery and cephalic vein in the forearm (Brescia-Cimino). A fistula may also be created with an artificial conduit, such as a bovine graft between the cephalic vein and the brachial artery in the upper arm. However, these grafts are associated with a very high incidence of complications, particularly occult infection. The Brescia-Cimino fistula and the bovine shunt have both been associated with a significant incidence of mononeuropathy as a complication (Hackim and Lazarus, 1986).

The Brescia-Cimino arteriovenous fistula is usually created in the forearm some months before it is actually required for chronic hemodialysis. By that time, the veins become greatly distended, making the procedure of inserting the two needles for cannulation to and from the dialyzer as easy and as uncomplicated as possible. However, the procedure results in a relative arterial ischemia distal to the fistula and in venous engorgement. There

is also a tendency for extravasation of fluid extracellularly and the development of edema. The shunting of blood from the radial artery to the cephalic vein becomes even more pronounced during dialysis. Thus, there is a true tendency for ischemia to develop at either the median nerve or the median or ulnar nerves in the forearm.

Knezevic and Mastaglia (1984) studied 21 patients who had unilateral Brescia-Cimino arteriovenous fistulas and observed that seven patients had symptomatic median or ulnar neuropathy, all showing abnormalities of motor and sensory nerve conduction. Of the 14 asymptomatic patients, nine had electrophysiological evidence of median or ulnar neuropathy in the arm with the fistula. Evidence of subclinical median or ulnar neuropathy was found in the contralateral extremity in 11 of the 21 subjects. The symptoms consisted of pain, numbness, or paresthesias in the digits and palm within the median or ulnar nerve distributions. These symptoms often worsened during the hemodialysis procedure itself. In three patients, there were signs of median neuropathy, reduction in sensation in the hand, and a flattening of the thenar eminence and weakness of median-innervated hand muscles. Signs of ulnar neuropathy consisted of reduced sensation within the distribution of that nerve. Although the electrophysiological abnormalities reported were statistically significant in some instances, they did appear relatively mild in comparison to control values, even when comparing fistula and nonfistula arms.

It is likely, therefore, that clinical evidence of neuropathy in Brescia-Cimino fistulas is relatively uncommon. Neuropathy is not mentioned as a complication in the review by Hackim and Lazarus (1986). In the review of 83 patients by Ringden et al. (1976), looking particularly at vascular insufficiency, only one patient developed arterial insufficiency in the hand, which resulted in finger ulcerations, probably due to radial-steal syndrome. Four patients got very swollen hands because of venous thrombosis. These complications were reversed by closing the fistulas. Neuropathy was not described as a complication in these patients. Also, neuropathy was not mentioned as a complication in the 103 patients studied by Lindstedt (1972).

However, a very severe neuropathy may rarely result as a complication of shunts or fistulas created between the brachial artery and antecubital vein in the arm more proximally than the distal Brescia-Cimino fistula. Bolton et al. (1979) observed a very severe neuropathy of median, ulnar, and radial nerves developing distally to a bovine shunt. Electrophysiological studies revealed severe axonal degeneration of these nerves. After closure of the shunt in the first patient, recovery over a number of months was only partial and incomplete. A milder neuropathy of these nerves developed in a second patient, but with closure of the shunt there was considerable improvement. Wytrzes et al. (1987) observed three diabetic patients who developed pain, paresthesia, and weakness in the distribution of the median, ulnar, and radial nerves shortly after construction of a proximal brachial artery–antecubital vein fistula. As in Bolton's cases, these patients, in addition to experiencing severe weakness and loss of sensation, also had severe pain. Electrophysiological studies revealed marked axonal degeneration of motor and sensory fibers. However, with banding or ligation of the shunt, some improvement did occur over a number of months.

In practical terms, patients who develop symptoms and signs of neuropathy after the creation of these shunts should be evaluated immediately and if clinical examination shows clear-cut evidence of neuropathy, banding or ligation of this shunt should be performed in an attempt to prevent ischemic neuropathy. Electrophysiological studies are of little value in the acute stage, since it may take five to 10 days or more for nerve conduction and needle electromyography evidence of nerve damage to develop. Once such neuropathies develop, they are likely to be severe, and the recovery phase is prolonged and potentially incomplete.

Dysfunction of the Eighth Cranial Nerve

Cochlear and vestibular dysfunction may both occur in the course of chronic renal failure through several mechanisms. Certain genetic and congenital disorders, notably Alport's syndrome, may cause both nerve deafness and nephritis (Alport, 1927; Rosenberg et al., 1970; Bergstrom et al., 1979). Hearing loss and vestibular dysfunction may also occur as a result of erythromycin, aminoglycosides, and diuretics, all drugs that are commonly used in renal failure (Quick, 1976; Thompson et al., 1980; Matz and Naunton, 1968; Mathog and Klein, 1969; Fee, 1980; Oda et al., 1976; Gailiunas et al., 1978; Kusakari et al., 1978). However, it was realized that eighth nerve dysfunction could occur simply as a result of uremic toxicity itself. A major contributor to investigations in this area has been Bergstrom's group in Denver, Colorado (Bergstrom et al., 1973). They observed among 224 patients with chronic renal failure, many on hemodialysis or having had renal transplantation, that 91 (40 percent) had sensorineural hearing loss. In 11 percent, it was due to noise exposure; in seven percent it was of genetic etiology; in 20 percent it was due to multiple factors, including autotoxicity; in 41 percent it was due to autotoxic drug exposure; and in 11 percent it was of unknown etiology. They estimated that perhaps 20 percent had hearing loss purely on the basis of the renal failure itself. This group carried out histopathological studies of the temporal bone (Bergstrom et al., 1973; Bergstrom et al., 1980) and found diverse pathology, none of it necessarily related to renal failure per se.

In 1982, Hutchinson and Klodd reviewed the literature and performed a prospective study of their own. Of 74 patients, the majority were excluded because of drug or noise exposure and diabetes mellitus. Twenty-four were suitable for study, and all had audiometry, tests for acoustic reflex threshold and reflex decay, electronystagmography, and brainstem auditory-evoked response. The hearing loss tended to be of the high-tone variety. All tests argued against any retrocochlear lesion. The results of electronystagmography were essentially normal. So also were the results of brainstem auditory-evoked potentials. It was the final conclusion of Hutchinson and Klodd that there was no convincing evidence that renal failure per se caused eighth nerve dysfunction, when other causes had been excluded.

However, a recent case report and brief review of the literature by Lucien et al. (1987) suggest that renal failure may, in fact, be the cause of eighth nerve dysfunction. They report a case in which severe hearing loss occurred during acute uremia and then improved dramatically when the renal failure was successfully treated by intermittent hemodialysis for two weeks. They emphasized reports in the literature that improvement in hearing occurs after transplantation (Quick, 1976; Mitschke et al., 1975; Mitschke et al., 1977; Mcdonald et al., 1978) and after dialysis (Bergstrom et al., 1973; Johnson and Mathog, 1976; Rizvi and Holmes, 1980). The improvement in the eighth nerve dysfunction seemed to fit with observations after transplantation, in which polyneuropathy invariably improved (Bolton et al., 1971).

Dysfunction of the Facial Nerve

While patients in acute or chronic renal failure show no evidence of weakness of facial muscles on clinical examination, Taylor et al. (1970) have found slight, but statistically significant, prolongations in the latency of conduction of facial nerve fibers in such patients compared to a control group. This is likely a further reflection of the generalized toxicity of uremic toxins to peripheral nerve.

The blink reflex was studied comprehensively by Strenge (1980). This reflex provides information about the afferent fibers of the trigeminal nerve, synaptic connections within the brainstem, and the efferent fibers of the facial nerve. Abnormalities were found in 85 percent of the patients, consisting of delayed latencies, and there was a strong correlation in these abnormalities with reduced conduction velocity of the peroneal nerve. However, it could not be determined if the electrophysiological abnormalities were due primarily to a disorder of any one component of the blink reflex. These findings, like those in the eighth cranial nerve, suggest a diffuse disorder of neural conduction of the various components of the facial nerve.

Other Mononeuropathies

Patients in renal failure are particularly prone to focal compressive neuropathies. First of all, their nerves are particularly susceptible to damage by direct mechanical compression and ischemia, as already discussed. Thus, with the cachexia associated with chronic renal failure, the ulnar nerves at the elbow and the common peroneal nerve at the fibular head are more exposed and more likely to be traumatized. Moreover, at the time of transplant surgery, these nerves may be compressed inadvertently by operating room equipment, surgical personnel, etc. The brachial plexus and radial nerve are particularly susceptible to damage when the arm is kept in an abducted position. However, if the transplant is successful, nerve regeneration will likely occur, as it does in healthy persons who experience such perioperative complications. On the other hand, such compressive neuropathies may not recover as fully in patients who are on chronic hemodialysis.

In chronic renal failure, there is a bleeding diathesis due to uremic toxicity and this diathesis is worsened if anticoagulants or antiplatelet drugs are used in association with dialysis procedures, renal transplantation, and so forth. The peripheral nerves may be damaged by direct bleeding into the nerve, or perhaps more commonly by the "compartment syndrome" mechanism (Shields et al., 1986). In this syndrome, bleeding into the ileopsoas muscle, for example, may cause acute swelling in the fascial compartment enclosing the femoral nerve, causing an acute compressive neuropathy. In such a situation, electrophysiological studies will be of no value, since nerve conduction and needle electromyography abnormalities do not appear for several days. A computed tomographic scan will, however, confirm the presence and location of the hematoma (Emery and Ochoa, 1978). This is an emergency situation that may require surgical decompression.

Conclusion

Carpal tunnel syndrome is now the commonest disorder of peripheral nerves in chronic renal failure. Initially, it was thought to be an occasional complication of the forearm arteriovenous fistula used for access during chronic hemodialysis, but it is now recognized that the commonest cause may be accumulation of amyloid in the carpal tunnel. This is most likely to occur in patients who have been treated for many years with hemodialysis, particularly with the dialysis machine that uses a Cuprophan membrane. The abnormal protein has been identified as β_2 microglobulin, and it is unique to this disorder. Sectioning of the flexor retinaculum and biopsy of synovia and tendon to determine the presence of amyloid is the definitive procedure. However, carpal tunnel syndrome may later recur. Moreover, clinical and morphological study in our patients suggest generalized amyloid infiltration of blood vessels, particularly the vasa nervorum, which may produce more widespread neuropathic symptoms. Intensive investigation is now under way to develop dialysis machines that will

successfully clear this abnormal protein and may ultimately entirely prevent this distressing complication. Carpal tunnel syndrome may also occur in association with forearm arteriovenous fistulas.

More proximal upper limb shunts, notably bovine shunts between the cephalic vein and brachial artery, may rarely cause an acute, severe neuropathy of median, ulnar, and radial nerves. Banding or ligation of the shunt should be performed to prevent a severe, persisting neuropathy.

The eighth cranial nerve may be damaged, presumably by uremic toxins in both the cochlear and vestibular divisions. The process can be reversed by successful renal transplantation. While there are no signs or symptoms of facial nerve dysfunction, electrophysiological tests are mildly abnormal, presumably due to uremic toxicity.

Since nerves subject to uremic toxicity are susceptible to both compression and ischemia, patients may develop compressive palsies of the ulnar nerve at the elbow and the common peroneal nerve at the fibular head. The brachial plexus and radial nerves may also be damaged at the time of surgery for renal transplantation, as a result of compression by operating room equipment or prolonged abduction of the arm. Such palsies may not improve during chronic dialysis therapy, but may do so following successful renal transplantation.

References

Alport AD. Hereditary familial congenital hemorrhagic nephritis. Br Med J 1927;1:504–506.

Aurigemma NM, Feldman NT, Gottlieb M, et al. Arterial oxygenation during hemodialysis. N Engl J Med 1977;297:871–873.

Ballardie FW, Kerr DNS, Tennent G, Pepys MB. Haemodialysis versus CAPD. Equal predisposition to amyloidosis? Lancet 1986;1:795–796.

Bardin T, Zingraff J, Kuntz D, Drueke T. Dialysis-related amyloidosis. Nephrol Dial Transplant 1986;1:151–154.

Berggard I, Bearn AG. Isolation and properties of a low molecular weight β_2-microglobulin occurring in human biological fluids. J Biol Chem 1968;243:2095–4103.

Bergstrom L, Jenkins P, Sando I, English GM. Hearing loss in renal disease: clinical and pathological studies. Ann Otol Rhinol Laryngol 1973;82:555–576.

Bergstrom L, Thompson P, Wood RP II. New patterns in genetic and congenital otonephropathies. Laryngoscope 1979;89:177–184.

Bergstrom L, et al. Renal disease. Arch Otolaryngol 1980;106:567–572.

Blumberg A, Burgi W. Behavior of β_2-microglobulin in patients with chronic renal failure undergoing hemodialysis, hemodiafiltration and continuous ambulatory peritoneal dialysis (CAPD). Clin Nephrol 1987;27:245–249.

Bolton CF, Baltzan MA, Baltzan RB. Effects of renal transplantation on uremic neuropathy: a clinical and electrophysiologic study. N Engl J Med 1971;284: 1170–1175.

Bolton CF, Driedger AA, Lindsay RM. Ischemic neuropathy in uremic patients due to arteriovenous fistulas. J Neurol Neurosurg Psychiatry 1979;42:810–814.

Bradish CF. Carpal tunnel syndrome in patients on haemodialysis. J Bone Joint Surg [B] 1985;67:130–132.

Castaigne P, Cathala HP, Beaussart-Boulengé L, Petrover M. Effect of ischaemia on peripheral nerve function in patients with chronic renal failure undergoing dialysis treatment. J Neurol Neurosurg Psychiatry 1972;35:631–637.

Chanard J, Lavaud S, Toupance O, et al. Carpal tunnel syndrome and type of dialysis membrane used in patients undergoing long-term hemodialysis. Arthritis Rheum 1986;29:1170–1171.

Charra B, Calemard E, Uzan M, et al. Carpal tunnel syndrome, shoulder pain and amyloid deposits in long-term haemodialysis patients. Proc Eur Dial Transplant Assoc ERA 1984;21:291–295.

Delmez JA, Holtmann B, Sicard GA, et al. Peripheral nerve entrapment syndromes in chronic hemodialysis patients. Nephron 1982;30:118–123.

Emery S, Ochoa J. Lumbar plexus neuropathy resulting from retroperitoneal hemorrhage. Muscle Nerve 1978;1:330–334.

Fee WR Jr. Aminoglycoside ototoxicity in the human. Laryngoscope 1980;90:1–19.

Gailiunas P Jr, et al. Vestibular toxicity of gentamicin. Arch Intern Med 1978;138:1621–1624.

Gejyo F, Homma N, Suzuki Y, Arakawa M. Serum levels of beta-2 microglobulin as a new form of amyloid protein in patients undergoing longterm hemodialysis. N Engl J Med 1986;314:585–586.

Hackim MR, Lazarus MJ. Medical aspects of hemodialysis. In: Brenner BM, Rector FC, eds. The kidney. Philadelphia: WB Saunders, 1986:1799–1802.

Halter SK, DeLisa JA, Stolov W. Carpal tunnel syndrome in chronic renal dialysis patients. Arch Phys Med Rehabil 1981;62:197–201.

Harding AE, Le Fanu J. Carpal tunnel syndrome related to antebrachial Cimino-Brescia fistula. J. Neurol Neurosurg Psychiatry 1977;40:511–513.

Huaux JP, Noel H, Bastien P, et al. Amylose articulaire, fracture du col fémoral, et hémodialyse périodique chronique. Rev Rhum Mal Osteoartic 1985;52:179–182.

Hutchinson JC, Klodd DA. Electrophysiologic analysis of auditory, vestibular and brain stem function in chronic renal failure. Laryngoscope 1982;92:833–843.

Johnson DW, Mathog RH. Hearing function and chronic renal failure. Ann Otol Rhinol Laryngol 1976;85:43–49.

Kelly JJ. Polyneuropathies associated with malignancies and plasma cell dyscrasias. In: Brown WF, Bolton CF, eds. Clinical electromyography. Boston: Butterworths, 1987:305–325.

Kenzora JE. Dialysis carpal tunnel syndrome. Orthopedics 1978;1:195–203.

Knezevic W, Mastaglia FL. Neuropathy associated with Brescia-Cimino arteriovenous fistulas. Arch Neurol 1984;41:1184–1186.

Kusakari J, Ise I, Comegys TH, et al. Effect of ethacrynic acid, furosemide and ouabain upon the endolymphatic potential and upon high energy phosphates of the stria vascularis. Laryngoscope 1978; 88:12–37.

Lindstedt E. Studies in therapeutic arteriovenous fistulae. Scand J Urol Nephrol 1972;Suppl 14.

Lindstedt E, Westling H. Effects of an antebrachial Cimino-Brescia arteriovenous fistula on the local circulation in the hand. Scand J Urol Nephrol 1975;9: 119–124.

Lucien JC, Anteunis MA, Jacob MVM. Hearing loss in a uraemic patient: indications of involvement of the VIIIth nerve. J Laryngol Otol 1987;10:492–496.

Mathog RH, Klein WJ Jr. Ototoxicity of ethacrynic acid and aminoglycoside antibiotics in uremia. N Engl J Med 1969;280:1223–1224.

Matz GJ, Naunton RF. Ototoxic drugs and poor renal function. JAMA 1968;206:2119.

Mcdonald TJ, Zincke H, Anderson CF, Ott NT. Reversal of deafness after renal transplantation in Alport's syndrome. Laryngoscope 1978;88:38–42.

Mitschke H, Schmidt P, Kopsa H, Zazgornik J. Reversible uremic deafness after renal transplantation. N Engl J Med 1975;292:1062–1063.

Mitschke H, Schmidt P, Zazgornik J, et al. Effect of renal transplantation on uremic deafness. A long-term study. Audiology 1977;16:530–534.

Morita T, Suzuki M, Kammimura A, Hirasawa Y. Amyloidosis of a new type in patients receiving long-term hemodialysis. Arch Pathol Lab Med 1985;109:1029–1032.

Munoz-Gomez J, Bergada-Barado E, Gomez-Perez R,

et al. Amyloid arthropathy in patients undergoing periodical hemodialysis for chronic renal failure: a new complication. Ann Rheum Dis 1985;44:729–733.

Oda M, Preciado MC, Quick CA, Paparella MM. Labyrinthine pathology of chronic renal failure patients treated with hemodialysis and kidney transplantation. Laryngoscope 1976;84:1489–1506.

Quick CA. Hearing loss in patients with dialysis and renal transplants. Ann Otol Rhinol Laryngol 1976;85:776–790.

Ringden O, Fagrell B, Friman L, Lundgren G. Subcutaneous arteriovenous fistulas for dialysis with special emphasis on vascular insufficiency. Scand J Urol Nephrol 1976;10:73–79.

Rizvi SS, Holmes RA. Hearing loss from hemodialysis. Arch Otolaryngol 1980;106:751–756.

Rosenberg AL, Bergstrom L, Troost BT, et al. Hyperuremia and neurologic deficits. N Engl J Med 1970;282:992–997.

Shields RW, Root KE, Wilbourn AJ. Compartment syndromes and compression neuropathies in coma. Neurology 1986;36:1370–1374.

Shirahama T, Skinner M, Cohen AS, et al. Histochemical and immunohistochemical characterization of amyloid associated with chronic hemodialysis as β_2 microglobulin. Lab Invest 1985;53:705–709.

Spertini F, Wauters JP, Poulenas I. Carpal tunnel syndrome: a frequent, invalidating, long-term complication of chronic hemodialysis. Clin Nephrol 1984;21:98–101.

Strenge H. The blink reflex in chronic renal failure. J Neurol 1980;222:205–214.

Taylor N, Jebsen RH, Tenckhoff HA. Facial nerve conduction latency in chronic renal insufficiency. Arch Phys Med Rehabil 1970;259–263.

Thomas PK. Classification and electrodiagnosis of hereditary neuropathies. In: Brown WF, Bolton CF, eds. Clinical electromyography. Boston: Butterworths, 1987:177–207.

Thompson P, Wood RP II, Bergstrom L. Erythromycin ototoxicity. J Otolaryngol 1980;9:60–62.

Varga J, Felson D, Skinner M, Cohen AS. Absence of amyloid in fat aspirates of long-term dialysis patients (abstract). Arthritis Rheum 1986;29:514.

Vincent C, Revillard JP, Galland M, Traeger J. Serum beta-2 microglobulin in hemodialyzed patients. Nephron 1978;21:260–268.

Warren DJ, Otieno LS. Carpal tunnel syndrome in patients on intermittent hemodialysis. Postgrad Med 1975;51:450–452.

Wyrtzes L, Markley HG, Fisher M, Alfred HJ. Brachial neuropathy after brachial artery–antecubital vein shunts for chronic hemodialysis. Neurology 1987;37:1398–1400.

Yamagami S, Yoshihara H, Kishimoto T, et al. Cuprophan membrane induces interleukin-1 activity. Trans Am Soc Artif Intern Organs 1986;32:98–101.

Zingraff J, Beyne P, Bardin T, et al. Dialysis amyloidosis and plasma β_2-microglobulin. In: Abstracts of the 33rd Congress of the European Dialysis and Transplant Association, Budapest, Hungary, June 29–July 3, 1986.

Chapter 6

Associated Disorders of the Nervous System

Contents

Acronyms

CNS   central nervous system
CSF   cerebrospinal fluid
CT   computed tomography

DIC   disseminated intravascular coagulation
EEG   electroencephalogram
MRI   magnetic resonance imaging
NMDA   *N*-methyl-D-aspartate
PAN   periarteritis nodosa
SLE   systemic lupus erythematosus
TTP   thrombotic thrombocytopenic purpura

This chapter is devoted to those diseases in which the nervous system is affected by mechanisms other than the accumulation of neurotoxins or the complications of the treatment of renal disease. These disorders can be grouped into two broad categories: vascular disease of the nervous system secondary to renal hypertension, and diseases that commonly affect the kidney and nervous system independently of each other.

Both the central and peripheral nervous systems may be affected by the second category mentioned above at any time during the various stages of renal failure. However, these conditions are considered before advanced renal failure and its treatment complicate the picture. At this stage, the nervous system dysfunction is less likely to directly relate to the renal disease.

This chapter presents these conditions mainly according to the primary disease. The selection has been somewhat eclectic, reflecting the perspectives and experience of the authors. We have not discussed a number of pediatric diseases, including those associated with hereditary deafness and renal disease, hereditary metabolic disorders such as the oculocerebrorenal syndrome of Lowe, hereditary connective tissue disorders, the association of berry aneurysms with polycystic kidney disease, or pregnancy-induced hypertension and eclampsia. Also, conditions that uncommonly affect the nervous system and kidney independently have been omitted. Finally, we have described these conditions only as they relate to kidney disease. The reader who wishes a more encyclopedic knowledge should consult other sources.

A

Vascular Disorders

Stroke

Strokes are arterial events that cause enduring damage to the brain or retina. They can be divided into ischemic and hemorrhage subgroups. Ischemic strokes comprise those in which the arterial or arteriolar occlusion occurs *in situ* and those in which occlusion is a result of thrombotic or atheromatous material arising from another site being carried by the blood to occlude the vessel, an embolic event. Small, deep, ischemic brain infarcts called "lacunes" are closely linked to hypertensive small arteriolar disease (Mohr, 1983).

Large-Vessel Ischemic Stroke

Large-vessel ischemic stroke is usually due to atherosclerotic disease of an artery to the brain, in which thrombosis occurs or hemorrhage into the wall develops, or from which an embolus may arise. The other major source of emboli to the brain is the heart. Although a number of cardiac conditions may be responsible, in our population atherosclerotic and hypertensive heart disease prevail: poor ventricular contractility, mural thrombus after myocardial infarction, and atrial fibrillation are usually responsible. Lesions of the mitral or aortic valves or annuli may also be worthy of consideration in some individuals (Barnett et al., 1986).

Atherosclerosis can affect the brain vasculature either directly or indirectly through effects on the heart, aorta, or great vessels. Major risk factors for atherosclerosis include hypertension, lipid abnormalities, and hyperglycemia. β Thromboglobulin (see Hemodialysis and Stroke, below) may play an important role, but this needs to be further defined.

Atheromas occur in three degrees of severity (Moore, 1983). The mildest lesion is the fatty streak, which consists of raised lesions in the inner walls of arteries, with the long axis parallel to the direction of blood flow (Haust, 1971). These show lipid droplets in smooth muscle cells and a variable number of foam cells and lipid in interstitial tissue. The intermediate lesion is the fibrous plaque, again with axis parallel to the blood flow. Such plaques show increased interstitial tissue containing collagen, elastica, and proteoglycans, with a variable amount of intra- and extracellular lipid. Complicated lesions are similar to fibrous plaques but show ulceration of the intimal lining of the arterial lumen overlying the lesion, in association with thrombus formation. Such lesions are thought to arise because of injury to the endothelial lining, with formation of a neointima that fosters the deposition of lipid. Platelet-derived growth factor, from the platelet reaction following the initial endothelial loss, and the binding of lipids to the increased glycosaminoglycans in the interstitium play a role. A reduced ratio of high-density to low-

or very low-density lipoprotein contributes to the endothelial injury (Nordoy, 1980).

Hypertension probably damages the endothelial lining through mechanical stress. In addition, serum lipid values tend to be higher in hypertensives than in nonhypertensives, and experimentally induced hypertension aggravates diet-induced atherosclerosis (Bronte-Stewart and Heptinstall, 1954; Robertson and Strong, 1968). Mitchell and Schwartz (1965) found that diastolic blood pressure during life correlated with the surface area of the great vessels occupied by yellow streaks and fibrous plaques. Robertson and Strong (1968) found that hypertension accelerated the natural progression of atherosclerosis.

About 20 percent of ischemic strokes arise as cardiogenic emboli (Castaigne et al., 1970; Lhermitte et al., 1968). In older individuals, this is often due to mural thrombi resulting from myocardial infarction. The proportion of cardiogenic strokes is higher for younger individuals, but in only a minority of these is premature atherosclerosis the cause (Hachinski and Norris, 1985).

Lacunes

Lacunes are small infarcts deep in the cerebral hemispheres of the brainstem that result from the occlusion of penetrating end arteries with lumina varying from 100 to 400 μm. Such infarcts range in size from 2 to 15 mm in diameter. The pathogenesis of lacunar infarcts is closely linked to hypertension and also to atherosclerosis of large arteries. Lesions in the arteries are most commonly microatherosclerosis, with lipohyalinosis a close second (Mohr, 1983). Both of these are strongly associated with hypertension. Microembolism has been suggested as the cause in some cases in which the vessels in the region of the infarction appeared undiseased (Fisher, 1979). Lacunar infarctions are often multiple, but have the same relative frequency of site of distribution as spontaneous hypertensive hemorrhage mentioned in the previous section. The computed tomographic (CT) scanner is limited in detecting lacunes; the ones commonly missed are those under 2 mm and those in the brainstem. Nuclear magnetic resonance imaging (MRI) has higher resolution and less associated artifact, making it the test of choice.

The particular manifestations of lacunes depend on the site of infarction. Some, e.g., in basal ganglia, may be silent. Lacunar strokes may have a slower mode of onset than other ischemic strokes. Up to 30 percent develop over 36 hours (Mohr, 1983). One of the most common lacunar syndromes is pure motor hemiplegia, related to occlusion of a lenticulostriate branch of the middle cerebral artery supplying the posterior limb of the internal capsule. Individuals with this syndrome have paresis of the contralateral face, arm, and leg but no neuropsychological disturbance such as aphasia, no visual field defect, and no sensory disturbance. Occasionally, pure motor hemiplegia can result from an infarct in the basis pontis or medulla, due to occlusion of a paramedian branch of the basilar artery. Rarely, the infarct may be in the corona radiata or in the cerebral peduncle (Mohr, 1983).

If the perforating branch of the posterior cerebral artery going to the posterior thalamus is occluded, this can result in "pure sensory" stroke. Like pure motor hemiplegia, the patient has an isolated loss or reduction of sensation from the opposite face, arm, and leg, unassociated with any visual field defect or abnormal mental status. Further, motor strength is preserved, but, because of loss of sensory feedback, motor function can be compromised.

Brainstem lacunar infarcts have a variable picture, depending on the site of involvement. One of the most common is ataxic hemiparesis, originally described in association with a lesion in the basis pontis (Fisher and Cole, 1965). The paretic limbs show a degree of incoordination beyond that produced by the motor weakness. The dysarthria–clumsy hand syndrome (Fisher, 1967) includes dysphagia, facial weakness, and modest unilateral upper-limb weakness, with an ipsilateral extensor plantar response. It is likely a variant of the ataxic hemiparesis syndrome.

Patients with severe or accelerated hypertension may have multiple lacunar infarctions, with resultant pseudobulbar palsy, gait apraxia, multifocal upper motor deficits, and dementia (Hughes et al., 1954).

Parenchymal Brain Hemorrhage

In the general population, brain hemorrhage, including subarachnoid hemorrhage, accounts for 19 percent of strokes (Kinkel and Jacobs, 1976). Coagulation disorders play a role, but the major underlying cause is damage to the arterial wall from hypertension (Stehbens, 1972). Since patients with renal failure are commonly hypertensive, they are clearly at increased risk of such hemorrhages. The arterial lesion responsible was linked by 19th-century physicians Charcot and Bouchard to small arteries in the brain that showed aneurysmlike dilatations (Pickering, 1968). The media of such arterioles show necrosis, hyaline change, lipohyalinosis, or replacement of the media and elastic tissue with collagenous connective tissue (Fisher, 1959; Russell, 1963). Russell (1963) showed that the Charcot-Bouchard aneurysms coincided with common sites of intracerebral hemorrhage and that their presence correlated with hypertension during life. Such sites of involvement include, in order of prevalence: putamen and adjacent internal capsule (which accounts for about half the cases); a variety of regions in the deep, central white matter; thalamus, cerebellar hemispheres; and the pons. The aneurysms were 200 to 900 μm in diameter and arose mainly at branching points of the penetrating arteries (Russell, 1963). These areas are affected in hypertensive renal failure patients with or without dialysis treatment.

There have been no prospective studies of vascular events that occur in uremic patients, but several retrospective studies indicate that hemodialyzed patients have increased risk of intracranial hemorrhage, while posttransplant patients suffer a significant increase in ischemic strokes.

Hemodialysis and Stroke

Rotter and Roettger (1973) reviewed the autopsy reports on 326 patients with chronic renal failure who had been hemodialyzed. Comparisons were made with three autopsy control groups: victims of accidents, deaths from other diseases, and patients who suffered from essential hypertension without renal insufficiency. The authors found that 7.5 percent of dialyzed patients had intracerebral hemorrhages of variable size; 5.8 percent (19 cases) showed abundant, fatal parenchymal hemorrhage. Ischemic stroke was found in about five percent of uremic patients; this was considerably lower than the 20 percent figure previously found by the same authors on autopsies of patients with essential hypertension without renal failure.

A retrospective clinical study of maintenance hemodialysis patients was conducted by Onoyama et al. (1986) involving 10,364 patient-years. The findings were similar to those of Rotter and Roettger (1973): cerebral hemorrhage developed in 66 patients, ischemic infarction in 16 patients, subarachnoid hemorrhage in 3 patients, and unclassified stroke in 5 patients. The incidence of cerebral hemorrhage was five times, and that of ischemic stroke only one-third, that in the general population in Japan.

It is clear that the hemodialyzed uremic population is at increased risk of developing intracranial hemorrhage. Intracranial, particularly brain parenchymal hemorrhages, may occur for a number of reasons in uremia. Since they were much more likely in patients on hemodialysis than in other uremic patients, this procedure must contain some risk factors. The most obvious is the anticoagulation with heparin used to prevent thrombosis in the apparatus. The coagulopathy of uremia could be additive.

As far as ischemic stroke is concerned, the reported incidence, as noted above, is lower than expected, despite an increased incidence of risk factors. There are a number of possible explanations for this paradox. It is possible that the coagulation defects of uremia and the heparin used in dialysis have a protective role for ischemic stroke. It is also possible that the low incidence of ischemic stroke is an artifact of the study. In the Japanese study, the patient data was derived from observation during 13 years, yet the normative data for the general population was likely derived from a much longer duration. Patients with preexisting stroke would have been excluded from Onoyama's study (1986), producing some selection bias. Moreover, other diseases may have prevented the development of stroke. Uremic patients are at considerably higher risk for dying of causes other than ischemic stroke than is the general population. For example, of 113 deaths in patients with chronic renal failure who were followed for 13 years, six died of stroke (Higgins et al., 1977). Cardiac problems and infections were the major killers. Also, the study group was not age-matched with the general population with which it was compared. Finally, the controls were derived from earlier studies (Robins and Baum, 1981; Ueda et al., 1981; Tanaka et al., 1982), and ischemic stroke has shown a declining incidence with time (Garraway et al., 1979). However, one retrospective study does suggest an increased incidence of ischemic stroke (Thomas and Lee, 1976). In the following discussion it will be emphasized that dialyzed patients have a large number of risk factors for ischemic stroke. If these are controlled, there is probably no increase in ischemic cerebrovascular disease in uremic patients, dialyzed or not (Lundin and Friedman, 1978; Bernardi et al., 1986).

Ross et al. (1977) consider uremia to be a cause of endothelial damage. Atherosclerosis is accelerated in patients with renal failure (Lindner et al., 1974), probably because of an increased prevalence of hypertension, hyperlipidemia, and to a lesser extent, hyperglycemia.

Hypertension was documented during life in 59 percent of patients dying while under treatment for chronic renal failure (Clyne et al., 1986).

Bagdade et al. (1968) found elevated plasma triglyceride levels in dialyzed and nondialyzed, nonnephrotic patients with uremia, a type IV hyperlipidemia. Plasma immunoreactive insu-

lin levels were elevated, despite absence of obesity. In the hemodialyzed patients, the plasma triglycerides correlated with increased levels of immunoreactive insulin. Hypotryptophanemia, a possible cause of hypertriglyceridemia in nephrotic syndrome, was present in 58 percent of the chronic renal failure population of Kaladelfos and Edwards (1976). Both this group of uremic patients and that of Bagdade et al. (1968) showed decreased heparininduced lipoprotein lipase activity. These factors clearly contribute to stroke or heart disease (Meyer et al., 1987).

Hyperglycemia is also more common in patients with renal failure: insulin resistance occurs in uremia (see Diabetes Mellitus, below); also, because diabetes mellitus is a common cause of renal failure, the two conditions often coexist. There is good clinical and experimental evidence that diabetes mellitus is associated with increased atherosclerosis in the form of fatty streaks, fibrous plaques, and complicated atherosclerotic lesions (Robertson and Strong, 1968). These factors clearly contribute to stroke or heart disease (Meyer et al., 1987).

β Thromboglobulin is a constituent of platelet alpha granules. It causes increased reactivity of platelets and may be associated with increased atherosclerosis. Kubisz et al. (1985) found increased levels of β thromboglobulin in patients with renal failure. However, only 12 percent of these showed increased platelet aggregability with an in vitro test, and this did not correlate with β thromboglobulin levels. It is possible that increased β thromboglobulin levels play a minor role in promoting atherosclerosis in patients with renal failure who are treated conservatively or with maintenance hemodialysis.

Heart disease is prevalent in uremia. While ischemic heart disease was no more common in uremics than in the general population in the autopsy series of Clyne et al. (1986), hypertensive heart disease was common, and congestive heart failure was the leading cause of death. Such cardiac failure tended to occur terminally. Other studies show increased coronary artery disease in uremics (Brunner et al., 1979; Kaladelfos and Edwards, 1976). Rabbits with experimental chronic uremia have moderate coronary and mild carotid athero-sclerosis, compared to controls (Tvedegaard et al., 1985). Another factor of interest is the development of premature aortic and mitral annular calcification in uremia (Maher et al., 1987). Either can serve as a source of emboli to the brain.

Posttransplant Strokes

The principal causes of morbidity and mortality following renal transplantation are continuation of the primary disease, immune reactions, and immunosuppression (Lindstrom, 1977). With better immunological management, vascular complications affecting the heart and brain are becoming more important. Thromboembolic disease, primarily affecting the heart or the brain, is a common cause of death in post–renal transplant patients, coming second only to sepsis in several retrospective series (Ibels et al., 1974; Blohme and Ahlmen, 1977; Rao et al., 1976; Mahony et al., 1982). In the series of Mahony et al. (1982), 119 renal transplant patients were considered. Fifty-two (44 percent) survived for 10 years. Of the 67 who died, 16 (24 percent) of the deaths were from vascular complications; cerebral infarcts led the group with eight, followed by five myocardial infarcts and three pulmonary emboli. Of the survivors, 14 patients (30 percent) had vascular complications: seven had myocardial infarctions, three had angina, three had strokes, one had transient ischemic attacks, and five had intermittent claudication. The major risk factor was hypertension following transplantation, which was usually nephrogenic. In the series of Rao et al. (1976), 25 of 100 consecutive renal transplant patients developed thromboembolic complications, nine of whom died. Occlusive cerebrovascular disease developed in four patients aged 28 to 48 years. Three cases were due to atherosclerosis, while one was related to disseminated intravascular coagulation. Adams et al. (1986) conducted a retrospective study of 467 patients for a follow-up period of a mean of 4.6 years after renal transplantation. Cerebrovascular events occurred in 44 patients

(9.4 percent). These were more common in older individuals and those with diabetes mellitus, polycystic kidney disease, and systemic lupus erythematosus. Eleven patients had transient ischemic events, transient neurological events of vascular etiology lasting less than 24 hours (Hachinski and Norris, 1985). Twenty-nine patients had cerebral infarctions (6.2 percent), but in eight these were related to causes other than atherosclerosis: systemic lupus, subacute bacterial endocarditis, coagulation disorders, or fat embolism. Deaths from stroke occurred in six patients (25 percent of deaths): three from intracerebral hemorrhage, two from ischemic infarction, and one from spontaneous subdural hemorrhage. Dintenfass and Ibels (1975) studied 29 patients, aged 24 to 55 years, who had received renal transplants four to 48 months previously. Nineteen (66 percent) had arterial disease on examination; 10 (34 percent) were symptomatic. Six patients had myocardial infarction, and four had ischemic stroke. The period of greatest risk of posttransplant stroke is uncertain: two studies (Rao et al., 1976; Ibels et al., 1975) suggest that the first three months are the most dangerous, but Adams et al. (1986) found that most cerebrovascular events occurred more than six months posttransplant.

Successful renal transplantation should, one would think, slow the atherosclerotic process by reducing blood pressure and normalizing serum lipids (Higgins et al., 1977). This is not usually the case, however. Hypertension, lipid abnormalities, steroid diabetes, and increased blood viscosity are all incriminated.

Hypertension in the posttransplant period can have many causes. It occurs as a manifestation of renal allograft rejection, but it can occur independently of the latter. Ingelfinger et al. (1981) found that 80 percent of renal transplant children and adolescents had elevated blood pressure in the absence of rejection or intercurrent disease. Hypertension was more common if there had been previous nephritis, even if the native kidneys were removed prior to transplantation. The etiology in these patients was not clear. In other series, recurrent nephritis, volume overload, and high-dose corticosteroids are important. More recently, cyclosporine has been associated with posttransplant hypertension. This may relate to increased sympathetic activity related to the drug, which increases activity of the renin-angiotensin-aldosterone system, and to inhibition of renal postaglandin synthesis (Siegl et al., 1983). In older patients or individuals with accelerated atherosclerosis, stenosis of the artery to the transplanted kidney may cause severe hypertension associated with hypertensive encephalopathy or a decline in renal function (Lacombe, 1975; McGonigle et al., 1984).

Lipid abnormalities are present after transplantation but show some differences from those found in dialysis patients. Cassaretto et al. (1973) found significantly elevated serum triglyceride and cholesterol levels in their patients. This was associated with significantly increased levels of immunoreactive insulin which, in turn, may have been due to exogenous corticosteroids. These authors found normal levels of lipoprotein lipase, suggesting the increased lipid levels were due to increased hepatic production and release into the plasma, secondary to the augmented activity of insulin on the liver. Others have implicated insulin resistance (Bagdade et al., 1968) or elevated growth hormone levels producing increased release of fatty acids from adipose tissue (Ibels et al., 1975) as causes of hyperlipidemia. More detailed analysis of the lipid abnormalities in post–renal transplant patients was performed by Ibels et al. (1975), who found consistent positive correlations of hypercholesterolemia with age and of hypertriglyceridemia with prednisone dosage and serum creatine. These authors did not find immunoreactive insulin levels to be elevated. Although dialysis patients tended to have type IV hyperlipidemia, the lipid profile of the allograft recipients was more variable. The most prevalent types were IIa and IIb. Cholesterol elevation was more common, and hypertriglyceridemia less so, in transplanted than in dialyzed uremic patients. Elevated serum glucose may result from corticosteroid usage (Ibels et al., 1975; Cassaretto et al., 1973). It appears that atherosclerosis is above normal in incidence and progression in renal failure patients (Lindstrom, 1977).

Secondary polycythemia may follow renal transplantation (Makovi et al., 1980). Dintenfass and Ibels (1975) found that posttransplant patients with arterial disease had significant elevations in plasma viscosity, aggregation of red blood cells measured at 37° and 20°C, and fibrinogen and erythrocyte sedimentation rates, when compared to transplant patients who did not have vascular disease. There were also more frequent elevations of serum lipids in the arterial disease group; hypertension was not assessed. It is thus difficult to know how much weight to attach to these observations. However, it is likely that viscosity factors are additive to hypertension and lipid disturbances in producing premature vascular disease in these patients.

A recent case of cerebral angiitis apparently restricted to the brain was reported in a 53-year-old patient following renal transplantation for polycystic kidney disease (Rothenberg, 1985). The patient suffered a multi-infarct dementia while on immunosuppressive therapy with prednisone and azathioprine. The transplanted kidney was unaffected. The patient had concomitant infection with cytomegalovirus, herpes simplex virus type 2, and Epstein-Barr virus. It was speculated that she may have developed immune complexes related to these infections and that this caused the cerebral vasculitis.

Prognosis and Management of Stroke

The prognosis for hemodialyzed patients who develop intraparenchymal brain hemorrhage is poor. Onoyama et al. (1986) found that 49 of 59 (83 percent) of such individuals died; their mean duration of survival was 72 days, with a range of two to 720 days.

Management of lacunar strokes is supportive; when they are single, patients often make excellent recoveries. Hypertension should be controlled. Unfortunately, in the living patient there is no reliable test to determine the type of vascular lesion responsible for the lacune. Anticoagulation, in most cases, would be hazardous. In selected cases, e.g., those in which

there were preceding transient ischemic attacks and angiography reveals considerable
atherosclerosis of a parent vessel, aspirin therapy or anticoagulation may be reasonable
(Mohr, 1983).

Hypertensive Encephalopathy

Hypertensive encephalopathy is a neurological
syndrome that occurs in association with malignant or accelerated hypertension (Oppenheimer and Fishberg, 1928). (Diffentiation
from acute uremic encephalopathy is discussed
in Chapter 4.) Accelerated hypertension is a
significant increase in blood pressure, usually
above 200/140 mm Hg, with evidence of vascular damage on funduscopic examination.
These changes include segmental arteriolar
narrowing, microhemorrhages, and infarctions. If frank papilledema is present, the condition is referred to as malignant hypertension
(Williams and Braunwald, 1987). Accelerated
hypertension affects between one and two percent of patients with preexisting severe essential hypertension. Hypertensive encephalopathy
is considered rare by most authors, but precise
epidemiological data are lacking.

Patients with renal disease, especially those
with renovascular hypertension and glomerular disease, are at risk for hypertensive encephalopathy because of the higher prevalence
of hypertension. Furthermore, advanced hypertension and its treatment can cause worsening of renal status. The hypertensive
population in general has a potential to develop accelerated or malignant hypertension
and, thus, hypertensive encephalopathy. Most
patients with hypertensive encephalopathy
originally had essential hypertension. Blacks
with essential hypertension are probably at
greater risk for developing hypertensive encephalopathy than whites. Pheochromocytoma
should always be looked for in any case of
severe, rapidly worsening or rapidly developing hypertension. In pregnancy, toxemia is
often responsible.

Since dialysis itself tends to control hypertension and water overload, hypertension is a
rare occurrence during dialysis. However, the
occurrence is greater after renal transplantation, particularly if renal artery stenosis is present or if the patient, especially a child, is
receiving cyclosporine (see Chapter 9).

Clinical Features

Hypertensive encephalopathy occurs in the
context of a sustained rise in blood pressure.
Frank neurological deficits or positive phenomena such as seizures are heralded by headache in almost all cases, which correlates
strongly with diastolic blood pressure over 140
mm Hg (Badran et al., 1970). The neurological
symptoms and signs relate to focal or multifocal brain dysfunction, but a metabolic encephalopathy due to acute worsening of renal
function may complicate the picture (see
Chapter 4A).

Cerebral seizures are prominent in most
descriptions, ranging in incidence from nine to
41 percent (Oppenheimer and Fishberg, 1928;
Jefferson, 1955; Clarke and Murphy, 1956;
Kinkaid-Smith et al., 1958). They may be a
more prominent complication of hypertensive
encephalopathy in children, in which they were
the presenting feature of 12 to 55 cases in the
series of Still and Cottom (1967). By definition, they are universally present in eclampsia.
Simple or complex partial seizures or generalized convulsions may occur. Seizures with
olfactory auras and absence seizures do not
occur (Jefferson, 1955).

Visual disturbance is also extremely common. In Jefferson's series (1955), 25 percent
of patients complained of deterioration in vision. This can vary from blurred vision to transient loss of vision. It probably relates to the
grade III or IV retinopathy found funduscop-
ically in most patients, but in some patients
the blindness may be cortical or central. Jellinek et al. (1964) described several cases of
cortical blindness in association with severe
hypertension without striking retinal abnormalities and with preserved pupillary reflexes.
Two of the three patients had other clinical
evidence of cerebral dysfunction. The visual
disturbance is usually reversible, as are the

funduscopic abnormalities, unless infarction occurs. The funduscopic findings and visual disturbances relate to the vascular disease at a small arteriolar and capillary level, and are not due to raised intracranial pressure (Taylor et al., 1954).

Stupor or coma in the absence of acute uremia, electrolyte disturbance, a postictal state, or a stroke is said to be extremely rare in hypertensive encephalopathy (Ziegler et al., 1965). These conditions, in various combinations, are commonly present, however.

Focal mental status disturbances, such as aphasia or hemiparesis, and multifocal deficits with dementia are associated with multiple, small vascular lesions, infarcts, or small hemorrhages in the brain at postmortem. Binswanger's disease, a rare subcortical demyelinative clinicopathological syndrome, is discussed separately. Some patients may show pathological emotionality in association with pseudobulbar palsy (Hughes et al., 1954) as a complication of multiple cerebral infarctions, often lacunar. Organic psychoses, including paranoid behavior, depression, and carelessness, may uncommonly occur (Clarke and Murphy, 1956; Hughes et al., 1954) and may relate to multiple vascular lesions or associated metabolic disturbance.

Cranial nerve dysfunction, especially facial palsy, is not uncommon. In most cases, it likely relates to vascular lesions of the brainstem (Chester et al., 1978). In some cases the facial palsy may be peripheral: hemorrhage within the Fallopian canal, through which the facial nerve runs in the skull, has been described (Monier-Vinard and Puech, 1930). Interestingly, facial palsies may recur with other bouts of severe hypertension (Griffith, 1933).

Pathology

The only comprehensive pathological study of hypertensive encephalopathy is that of Chester et al. (1978). On gross examination the brain weights were normal, and increased atherosclerosis affected the arteries of the circle of Willis. Multiple petechial hemorrhages, usually microscopic, were found in eight of their 20 cases. Multiple microscopic ischemic lesions were found with highest density in the basis pontis, followed by the basal ganglia, cerebral white matter, and spinal cord. The arterioles and small arteries showed focal and segmental irregularities in all 20 cases, fibrinoid necrosis in 13 (65 percent), and fibrin thrombi in 12 (60 percent). The magnitude and severity of the damage was closely related to the neurological deficit and degree of hypertension.

There has been an uncommon occurrence of cerebral, especially white matter, edema in some series. Of the 100 cases of hypertensive cerebrovascular disease in the autopsy series of Hudson and Hyland (1958), there was edema in only one. Furthermore, in cases of eclampsia, gross cerebral edema is not a feature (Levitt and Altchek, 1965). Adachi et al. (1966) found that the water content of the brains of 12 hypertensive patients was significantly higher than those of controls. Some authors have found histological changes in the cerebral white matter that may have been due to previous vasogenic cerebral edema (Feigin and Popoff, 1963). These white-matter changes are discussed separately under Binswanger's encephalopathy, but there may be a spectrum of white-matter change in hypertensive individuals.

Pathogenesis

An elegant set of experiments was performed by Byrom in 1954. He excised the right kidney and clamped the left renal artery of rats and recorded behavior, intracranial pressure, capillary permeability of the brain, and the appearance of pial arteries as seen through cranial windows. When blood pressures rose to very high levels nine days to nine months after surgery, rats developed seizures, myoclonus, weakness, apathy, and ultimately coma. The smaller pial arteries showed narrowing, while in larger arteries the narrowing, which he called spasm, alternated with dilated areas. The encephalopathic brains showed staining with trypan blue that had been injected into the systemic circulation, indicating vasogenic cerebral edema.

Other authors have performed similar studies on animals made hypertensive experimentally. One of the most definitive was that of

Mackenzie et al. (1976). These authors showed that the caliber of the pial arteries narrowed in a linear fashion with increasing blood pressure in order to maintain constant cerebral blood flow (autoregulation). At very high blood pressures, alternating constriction and dilatation of the arteries, like sausages in a string, occurred and cerebral autoregulation was impaired; cerebral blood flow increased with further increases in blood pressure. However, the caliber of the apparently constricted areas was in keeping with the degree of hypertension. It was the dilated segments that were behaving abnormally. With the marked hypertension and loss of autoregulation, the capillary beds of the brain were subjected to the higher pressures, and cerebral edema occurred. The principal mechanism for increased capillary permeability, which leads to cerebral edema in these animals, was shown by Nag et al. (1977) to be increased pinocytosis by cerebral capillary endothelial cells.

The histological findings of fibrinoid necrosis, thrombi in small vessels, and hemorrhages of various sizes are likely due to mechanical damage to cells in the vessel wall produced by the extreme hypertension.

Management

Malignant hypertension is a medical emergency. The main aim should be to reduce the diastolic blood pressure to lower values, but not below 90 mm Hg. (The latter is primarily to avoid the development of "watershed infarcts" in the brain. These are ischemic lesions at the boundary zones of the anterior, middle, and posterior cerebral arteries.) Diazoxide is the easiest antihypertensive agent to administer. A bolus dose of 300 mg can be given intravenously, but as the blood pressure drop in some patients is excessive, some physicians use 150 mg rapidly intravenously. This can be followed by a second dose of 150 mg in five minutes if the first dose produced only minimal effect. Intravenous nitroprusside can be more carefully titrated to the blood pressure response. Patients started on these short-acting drugs will require maintenance drugs to prevent rebound severe hypertension. Such drugs

include methyldopa or hydralazine, which can be given intravenously and later switched to oral preparations. The diuretics furosemide and ethacrynic acid are helpful in maintaining the sodium diuresis and in relieving the workload on the heart.

In some patients, especially those with renal failure, a period of peritoneal or hemodialysis is helpful and often necessary to remove fluid. Blood pressure control may be facilitated, and further deterioration in renal status may be avoided.

The neurological complications such as cerebral seizures should be treated symptomatically. A suitable regime is to stop the seizures with a short-acting benzodiazepine such as diazepam or lorazepam given intravenously. Five to 10 mg of diazepam given no faster than 2 mg/min or 4 mg of lorazepam given over 5 minutes is usually effective. Patients are then given phenytoin intravenously as a loading dose of 15 to 20 mg/kg. This should not be given faster than 50 mg/min. Phenytoin should not be used in patients with heart failure or cardiac conduction defects because of the risk of hypotension or precipitation of heart block or cardiac arrest. An alternative technique that is as effective as the benzodiazepine-phenytoin regimen is that of phenobarbital alone. The drug is given intravenously in a dose of 15 to 20 mg/kg at a rate of 100 mg/min (Delgado-Escueta et al., 1983).

Once stabilized, patients should be investigated to determine the cause of the hypertensive crisis. Renal status should be carefully evaluated, especially for primary renal disease or renal artery stenosis. Pheochromocytoma, Cushing's disease, and hyperaldosteronism should be excluded. Drug history should be taken, especially for withdrawal from antihypertensives such as clonidine or abuse of drugs such as amphetamines, phenylpropanolamine, or cocaine.

Binswanger's Disease

Binswanger's disease (Binswanger, 1894), also known as subcortical arteriosclerotic encephalopathy, is a rare disorder that is closely associated with hypertension. The predominant involvement is the deep cerebral white matter. There are a number of good reviews of the pathology, along with hypotheses for the pathogenesis of this condition (Feigin and Popoff, 1962; 1963; de Reuck et al., 1980; Hachinski et al., 1974; Loizou et al., 1982; Earnest et al., 1974).

Patients develop a *gradual* accumulation of deficits with superimposed stepwise progression due to multiple strokes (Caplan and Schoene, 1978). A slowly developing dementia occurs along with multifocal neurological symptoms and signs (Caplan and Schoene, 1978; White, 1979). Partial or secondary generalized convulsive seizures occur in a minority of patients (Caplan and Schoene, 1978; Loizou et al., 1982).

The CT and MRI scans show extensive symmetrical disease and cerebral white-matter hypodensity with enlarged ventricles. Microinfarcts are frequently seen (Zeumer et al., 1980). Electroencephalograms (EEGs) are usually abnormal (Caplan and Schoene, 1978) and may show prominent delta (slow-wave) activity, as described in white-matter diseases (Gloor et al., 1968). Periodic activity was found in one

case (White, 1979). This could cause confusion with Creutzfeldt-Jakob disease, in which periodic sharp-wave complexes are characteristic (Chiappa and Young, 1978).

Given the strong clinical association of hypertension and vascular disease found pathologically in Binswanger's disease, the obvious treatment is to achieve optimal control of hypertension and other risk factors for vascular disease.

Vasculitis

There are many types of inflammatory disease of blood vessels. These have been traditionally classified according to the size and type of involved blood vessels, the histological features, and the sites of predilection in the body. The principal types and their features are given in Table 6.1.

There are many perplexing aspects to the vasculitides and connective tissue syndromes. The blood vessel disease is clearly not the whole story, as will be seen. Furthermore, the role of immune complexes and antibodies against various tissues, proteins, etc. with re-

Table 6.1. Classification of Vasculitides

Clinical Type	Size and Type of Involved Blood Vessels	Histology and Stage of Lesions	Anatomic Predilections
Periarteritis nodosa	Medium and small arteries and veins	Necrotizing inflammation, coexistence of acute and healing lesions, no giant cells	Widespread, common to branching points of arteries, lungs rarely involved
Allergic granulomatosis	Medium and small arteries, adjacent veins, arterioles, capillaries	Necrotizing inflammation with extravascular granulomas, coexistence of acute and healing lesions, giant cells in granulomas, abundant eosinophils	Widespread, lungs frequently involved
Wegener's granulomatosis	Small arteries, arterioles, venules, some capillaries	Necrotizing inflammation with granulomas, coexistence of acute and healing lesions, giant cells in granulomas	Upper and lower respiratory tract involved, necrotizing glomerulitis
Hypersensitivity vasculitis (e.g., SLE)	Arterioles, venules, capillaries	Necrotizing inflammation, all lesions at same stage, no giant cells	Widespread, common to skin, serosal surfaces, and glomeruli
Giant-cell arteritis	Large and medium arteries	Inflammation without necrosis, giant cells present, no neutrophils	All large arteries including aorta, vertebral, and carotid

Source: Modified from Mannik and Gilliland, 1983.

spect to their pathogenesis is incompletely defined. For the vasculitis itself, the initiating damage may be to the endothelium (Bacon, 1985). Free radicals released from leukocytes, release of lymphokines from lymphocytes, and antigen-antibody complexes can all damage vascular endothelium.

Because of important strides in treatment, especially the use of aggressive immunosuppressive therapy early in the course of these diseases, it is vital to make an accurate diagnosis. Renal angiography and biopsy can greatly facilitate this (Bacon, 1985). Biopsy of involved organs can also be useful.

We shall review diseases that may affect the nervous system and the kidney together. Renal disease may then affect the nervous system, either through the effects of renal failure or through the development or aggravation of hypertension.

Periarteritis Nodosa

In periarteritis nodosa (polyarteritis nodosa), medium and small arteries, adjacent arterioles and venules, but not capillaries, are involved. There is a predilection for the bifurcation of vessels. Segments of vessels are involved with inflammatory infiltrate that consists mainly of lymphocytes, eosinophils, plasma cells, and some polymorphonuclear leukocytes in the early stages. More important than inflammation is fibrinoid necrosis in the tunica media, which extends to involve the intima and adventitia; this may precede the inflammatory infiltrate (Kernohan and Woltman, 1938). Later, granulation and chronic scar formation occur. Fibroblasts proliferate around the vessel, the internal elastic lamina is separated, and the lumen is narrowed. This narrowing to the point of occlusion or the development of thrombosis may result in infarction of tissue. Granulation and scarring may lead to aneurysm formation; such aneurysms may rupture. Vascular lesions are widespread throughout the body, including the kidney and nervous system.

The kidney is the organ most commonly affected in periarteritis; at least 80 percent of patients have significant involvement (Hollenberg, 1983). Arteriolar narrowing, with resultant ischemic lesions, or glomerulonephritis are found. Hypertension, often accelerated, occurs in about 50 percent of those with renal involvement.

Periarteritis is chiefly a disease of adult males. Systemic symptoms of early involvement include fever, weakness, anorexia, myalgias, arthralgias, and weight loss. Gastrointestinal complaints, related to celiac and mesenteric arterial involvement as revealed on angiography, are frequent. Cutaneous disease may be manifested by subcutaneous aneurysms and infarctions with ulcerations or gangrene of digits. Renal disease occurs in half the patients. Hepatic dysfunction may occur, and massive hepatic infarction has been reported.

The peripheral nervous system is more commonly involved than the central nervous system (CNS). In the discussion, however, we shall adhere to the format of first discussing the CNS complications.

Central Nervous System Involvement

Clinically, the CNS is involved in at least eight percent of patients (Arkin, 1930), but careful clinical, neuropsychological, EEG, cerebrospinal fluid (CSF) examinations reveal CNS disease in about 80 percent (Lewis et al., 1954). Pathological studies have shown an intermediate value from 30 to 69 percent. Almost any parts of the CNS may be involved in various combinations, with different degrees of reversibility, so the possibilities are endless. However, some syndromes are more common than others.

Foster and Malamud (1941) found meningeal signs in 22 percent of their patients with polyarteritis. Patients had headache, photophobia, neck stiffness, and positive Kernig's and Brudzinski's signs. The CSF may show xanthochromia due to subarachnoid hemorrhage or increased protein. Alternatively, there may be a pleocytosis with neutrophils (occasionally over 1,500/mm^3) or with a small number of lymphocytes. CSF pressure and/or protein may be elevated.

A toxic delirium with hallucinations, mania, and paranoia has been described in 23 percent of the series of Ford and Siekert (1965). Depression or mild agitation are less common (Goetz, 1980). The second major global syndrome is dementia. Unlike most other dementing illness, there may be periods of remission (Goetz, 1980). The last general presentation is one of impaired level of consciousness. This may be due to multifocal dysfunction from the polyarteritis, or it may relate to acute uremic or hypertensive encephalopathy as a result of renal involvement.

The arteries involved in periarteritis are the smaller cortical and penetrating vessels, rather than the larger ones of the circle of Willis. Bleeding is commonly into the brain, as well as into surrounding CSF. Thus, there are usually signs of focal brain dysfunction as well as of subarachnoid hemorrhage. Small petechial hemorrhages or areas of infarction may occur in the cerebral hemispheres or brainstem; hemiplegia, various aphasias, visual field defects, and sensory disturbances and brainstem syndromes with cranial nerve signs may occur.

Seizures, partial or focal, with or without secondary generalization as a grand mal convulsion, occur in about 15 percent of cases (Ford and Siekert, 1965). Status epilepticus, which may be fatal, may also develop. It should be remembered that seizures can arise as a result of uremia in periarteritis.

Optic nerve lesions and extraocular muscle palsies from cranial nerve involvement presumably relate to small vessel involvement. Other ocular complications include hypertensive retinopathy, scleritis, conjunctivitis, iritis, uveitis, and the syndrome of orbital pseudotumor (Sheehan et al., 1958).

The fifth, seventh, and eighth cranial nerves are the most frequently involved (Goetz, 1980). Cogan's syndrome (interstitial nonsyphilitic keratitis, bilateral deafness, and vestibular dysfunction) occurs as a complication of periarteritis (Cheson et al., 1976). Ford and Siekert (1965) felt that the cranial nerve palsies often were peripheral, i.e., outside the brainstem, as they often occurred in an isolated manner. This hypothesis has not been pursued with pathological studies.

Cord involvement does occur but is uncommon. Spinal arterial involvement may result in cord infarction as a hemicord syndrome or, occasionally, as an acute transverse myelopathy (Goetz, 1980). A cauda equina syndrome and a syndrome that mimicked motor neuron disease as an initial presentation of periarteritis nodosa have been reported (Goetz, 1980).

Neuromuscular Complications

Polyarteritis nodosa and other connective tissue diseases, such as Churg-Strauss vasculitis, Wegener's granulomatosis, and cranial arteritis may affect both peripheral nerves and the kidney at the same time. However, the clinical features of the peripheral nerve involvement and the fact that end-stage renal disease is unlikely to have been reached allow these conditions to be differentiated from uremic polyneuropathy.

The peripheral nervous system is more commonly involved than the CNS. This often occurs at or near the start of the illness. Between 19 and 50 percent of cases show clinical involvement, while pathologically studied cases show a 76 percent incidence (Goetz, 1980). This usually takes the form of either mononeuritis multiplex or symmetrical polyneuropathy. Other, less common, presentations are discussed separately.

Mononeuritis multiplex is the most common type of peripheral nerve involvement; it is the initial clinical feature of 50 percent of the cases in which it appears (Conn and Dyck, 1984; Lovshin and Kernohan, 1948). Pain, usually an abrupt, shooting type, is prominent but not universal with neuropathy. Paralysis of individual nerves may be very abrupt in onset, but rapid remission is also characteristic. A waxing and waning course is usual. Lower limbs are more commonly affected than upper limbs, and distal nerves are more likely to be involved than proximal ones (Goetz, 1980). The common peroneal nerve is the one most often affected.

Symmetrical polyneuropathy is usually heralded by sensory symptoms; legs are more involved than arms, with associated pain and tenderness. Paresis with atrophy of muscles may be striking. Some cases begin as mono-neuritis multiplex and evolve into a more symmetrical polyneuropathy (Goetz, 1980). Although the symmetrical polyneuropathy can occur with "pure" periarteritis, care should be taken that it is not due to a complication, e.g., renal failure or diabetes mellitus, the latter from pancreatic involvement or steroid therapy.

Other neuropathic patterns may be seen. A Guillain-Barré syndrome of subacute, sym-metrical, ascending, motor-sensory polyneu-ropathy has been described (Goetz, 1980). Glaser (1963) pointed out that in this situation the CSF protein is only occasionally elevated, in contrast to typical Guillain-Barré syndrome, in which it is characteristically raised in the absence of pleocytosis.

Radiculopathies or plexopathies may also occur, and are probably variants of mononeu-ritis multiplex.

Muscle Involvement

Muscle involvement in periarteritis is com-mon; frank myopathy is considerably less than histological disease. Myopathy has to be dif-ferentiated from neuropathy and from arthri-tis. A polymyositis-like syndrome may occur, with predominant proximal muscle disease. Muscle enzymes such as creatine kinase are elevated, and myoglobinuria may develop in the acute syndrome (Adams, 1975).

Confirmatory Tests

Hepatitis B surface antigen is present in about 40 percent of polyarteritis patients. The diag-nosis is largely based on the clinical picture along with laboratory evidence of involvement of various systems. Histopathological evidence from a biopsy of muscle or another involved organ, e.g., the kidney, is the most definitive. Angiography may help in showing aneurysm formation in various viscera in the early phases of the disease.

Pathology and Pathogenesis

While vascular involvement, perhaps related to antigen-antibody complex deposition, is the obvious explanation for many of the neurolog-ical syndromes in periarteritis, some cases of CNS involvement have failed to show lesions at autopsy (Goetz, 1980). It is possible that the CNS may be affected by antineuronal an-tibodies, as has been postulated for a similar syndrome in systemic lupus erythematosus (see Systemic Lupus Erythematosus, below). This may apply to some of the symmetrical periph-eral nervous manifestations as well, but this has not been resolved.

Treatment

The waxing and waning course requires careful judgment regarding timing of immunosuppres-sive therapy, which is the definitive treatment. Corticosteroids are still the main therapy. Other immunosuppressive agents and techniques may prove useful.

Complications such as hypertension, cere-bral seizures, diabetes, heart failure, etc. each require specific supportive therapy.

Systemic Lupus Erythematosus

Systemic lupus erythematosus (SLE) has been defined as "an inflammatory, remitting and exacerbating, often lifelong disease affecting mostly young women, sharply delineated against other polyarthritic diseases by the fol-lowing triad: (1) multisystem involvement of kidneys, brain, skin, hair, lungs, plurae, pericardium, arterioles, etc.; (2) nonerosive, usually nondeforming, polyarthritis or polyar-thralgias; (3) prominent autoimmunity of a wide spectrum usually with demonstrable an-tinuclear serology" (Bitter, 1974). The 1982 criteria set by the American Rheumatism As-sociation for the diagnosis of SLE are shown in Table 6.2. Of the eleven criteria, the patient must fulfill at least four for the diagnosis of SLE. The relative sensitivities and specificities of the criteria are given in Table 6.3.

SLE has been traditionally placed in the category of hypersensitivity or small vessel vas-culitis (see Table 6.1). When vessels are in-

Table 6.2. 1982 American Rheumatism Association Criteria for Systemic Lupus Erythematosus

Criterion	Definition
Malar rash	Fixed erythema, flat or raised, over malar eminences
Discoid rash	Erythematous, raised patches with adherent keratotic scaling and follicular plugging; atrophic scarring may occur in older lesions
Photosensitivity	Skin rash as result of reaction to sunlight
Oral ulcers	Oral or nasopharyngeal ulceration, usually painless
Arthritis	Nonerosive arthritis involving two or more peripheral joints
Serositis	(a) Pleuritis, or
	(b) Pericarditis
Renal disorder	(a) Persistent proteinuria greater than 0.5 g/day or greater than 3+, or
	(b) Cellular casts—may be red cell, tubular, or mixed
Neurological disorder	(a) Seizures—in the absence of offending drugs or known metabolic derangements, e.g., uremia or electrolyte imbalance, or
	(b) Psychosis—in the absence of offending drugs or known metabolic disturbance
Hematological disorder	(a) Hemolytic anemia—with reticulocytosis, or
	(b) Leukopenia—less than 4,000/mm^3 total on two or more occasions, or
	(c) Lymphopenia—less than 1,500/mm^3 on two or more occasions, or
	(d) Thrombocytopenia—less than 100,000/mm^3 in the absence of offending drugs
Immunological disorder	(a) Positive lupus erythematosus cell preparation, or
	(b) Anti-DNA—antibody to native DNA in abnormal titer, or
	(c) Anti-Sm—presence of antibody to Sm nuclear antigen, or
	(d) False positive serologic test for syphilis known to be positive for at least 6 months and confirmed by *Treponema pallidum* immobilization or fluorescent treponema antibody absorption test
Antinuclear antibody	An abnormal titer for antinuclear antibody by immunofluorescence or an equivalent assay at any point in time and in the absence of drugs known to be associated with "drug-induced lupus" syndrome

Source: From Tan et al., 1982.

volved, small arteries (less than 100 μm in diameter) show fibrinoid necrosis or proliferative thickening. Inflammatory cell infiltration may occur but is uncommon (Richardson, 1980). However, venous and arterial events are usually due to mechanisms other than vasculitis per se (see Pathology and Pathogenesis).

Although the emphasis will be placed on neurological manifestations, it should be clear that SLE is a systemic disease with a propensity to involve many organ systems. Renal, especially glomerular, involvement occurs in about one-half of the patients with SLE; this can vary from laboratory detection of proteinuria and red blood cell casts to massive hematuria or proteinuria or frank nephrotic syndrome. In some, this may progress to total renal failure (Mannik and Gilliland, 1983). There is often a dissociation of nervous and renal involvement, but they may coexist. Ure-

mia may cloud the issue by contributing to global CNS dysfunction, cerebral seizures, peripheral neuropathy, or altered drug handling. Accelerated hypertension from renal disease may also affect the CNS. Other mechanisms in which the CNS is indirectly affected in SLE include increased coagulability (e.g., lupus anticoagulant) and complications of immunosuppressive therapy.

Central Nervous System Involvement

CNS involvement is common in SLE. It may occur in the context of active systemic disease, but often there is a striking dissociation. Systemic disease may be unaccompanied by CNS dysfunction, and focal, multifocal, or diffuse brain dysfunction may appear and progress when other organ systems are stable or when

Table 6.3. Sensitivity and Specificity of 1982 SLE Criteria

Criterion	Sensitivity (percent)	Specificity* (percent)
Malar rash	57	96
Discoid rash	18	99
Photosensitivity	43	96
Oral ulcers	27	96
Arthritis	86	37
Serositis	56	86
Renal disorder	51	94
Neurological disorder	20	98
Hematological disorder	59	89
Immunological disorder	85	93
Antinuclear antibody	99	49

*Controls for specificity aspect were patients with other connective tissue disorders (weighted for rheumatoid arthritis).

Source: From Tan et al., 1982.

various immunological tests on the blood have reverted to a normal or near-normal status. The commonest neurological problems are personality change, seizures, and headaches.

The picture of aseptic meningitis can occasionally be a presenting or early feature of SLE (Richardson, 1980). This is usually brief and may respond to steroid treatment. The meningitic picture may herald the later development of parenchymal, especially brainstem, disease. The CSF shows normal pressure, lymphocytic pleocytosis of less than 200 cells/mm³, elevated protein concentration, and normal glucose level. Such CSF abnormalities may also be seen in SLE without a frank meningitic picture.

"Organic psychosis" or abnormal behavior and thought to the point of disintegration and loss of contact with reality occurs in from 12 percent (Dubois and Tuffanelli, 1964) to over 50 percent (O'Connor, 1959) of patients with SLE. Depression is the most common type, but mania and schizophrenia-like states may occur with hallucinations, paranoia, or even catatonic features (Richardson, 1980). Typically, florid psychiatric syndromes last less than six weeks. Richardson (1980) maintains that it

is rare for permanent mental disability or dementia to arise from such psychotic episodes, but persistent cognitive impairment may occur (Bresnihan, 1982).

Seizures occur at some time in the course of SLE in about 14 percent of cases (Johnson and Richardson, 1968; Grigor et al., 1978). In children, they are reported to occur in over 50 percent of cases (Johnson and Richardson, 1968). They tend to occur early in the course, even as the initial presentation. Simple or partial complex with or without secondary generalization may occur. Absencelike seizures have been reported, but are rare (Richardson, 1980).

Seizures from cerebral lupus should be differentiated from metabolic or toxic seizures related to renal involvement. Difficulty arises when phenytoin is used in treatment, as this drug can induce a lupuslike state. Theoretically, SLE may be aggravated by phenytoin; seizures could worsen as a result.

Focal signs and symptoms have been reported to occur in six (Grigor et al., 1978) to 20 percent of cases of SLE (Richardson, 1980). These are usually abrupt and stroke-like in onset and frequently resolve quickly and completely (Richardson, 1980). Occasionally they resemble typical transient ischemic attacks (Haas, 1982). They may improve and plateau, with a limited but permanent deficit. We have observed patients with multifocal disease, with different degrees of reversibility. There is increasing evidence that persistent CNS lesions, including cerebral infarction, retinopathy, retrobulbar neuritis, and myelopathy, relate to elevated anticardiolipin antibodies and lupus anticoagulant (Harris and Hughes, 1984; Oppenheimer and Hoffbrand, 1986). Presumably, vascular occlusions are responsible.

Retinal lesions are of interest in that they are common and clinically visible, unlike the rest of the CNS. Cytoid bodies are round, white exudates in the nerve fiber layer. They sometimes coalesce to form large, fluffy areas. Circumpapillary edema, superficial retinal hemorrhages, and choroidal degeneration are also described.

Virtually any type of focal dysfunction may occur. Sometimes these behave like large cortical, subcortical white-matter, or even deep gray-matter (especially thalamic), lesions (Richardson, 1980). Among the more frequently reported are hemiparesis or monoparesis, postchiasmal visual field defect—either homonymous hemianopsia or quadrantanopsia, and aphasia.

The most characteristic movement disorder to develop in SLE is chorea. This occurs in about two to four percent of cases (Grigor et al., 1978). This may be unilateral (hemichorea) or bilateral. The face, arm, and leg may be involved, with involuntary, irregular movements. A few patients have hemiballismus, a more proximal, unilateral movement disorder, or features of both hemiballismus and hemichorea. Mean duration is about eight weeks (Richardson, 1980). Immunosuppressive therapy may help the problem resolve more quickly (Richardson, 1980).

Tremors may occur in a few patients. This can be a postural action tremor or a rest tremor, as seen in Parkinson's disease (Richardson, 1980).

The brainstem and cerebellum are commonly involved, producing a variety of combinations of lower or supranuclear cranial nerve palsies, long tract signs, and ataxia. Cogan et al. (1950) reported a case of unilateral internuclear ophthalmoplegia due to infarction of one medial longitudinal fasciculus. In fact, this may be a helpful differentiating feature from multiple sclerosis, in which the internuclear ophthalmoplegia is almost always bilateral. Of interest, we have observed some patients in whom multiple sclerosis and SLE were shown at autopsy to have coexisted. In contrast to periarteritis, cranial nerve palsies are usually due to intrinsic brainstem disease rather than to involvement of the peripheral part of the nerve (Johnson and Richardson, 1968).

Headache is common in the course of SLE and may accompany parenchymal involvement. The headache is usually of a vascular type, sometimes even classical migraine (Richardson, 1980).

Benign intracranial hypertension (pseudotumor cerebri), consisting of raised intracranial pressure without signs of parenchymal brain dysfunction, has been reported rarely with SLE. The condition requires treatment to prevent secondary optic atrophy from the associated papilledema. It responds promptly to corticosteroid therapy in SLE (Richardson, 1980).

Clinically significant spinal cord involvement is infrequent in SLE (Richardson, 1980). The most common presentation is one of acute transverse myelopathy (Andrianakos et al., 1975). Myelopathy in SLE is usually not as transient and reversible as in other CNS syndromes; permanent paraplegia may occur.

Occasionally, the syndrome of inappropriate antidiuretic hormone release may occur in SLE (Bresnihan, 1982). This may be due to hypothalamic involvement. Hyponatremia relates to decreased free water clearance and may result in impaired consciousness and seizures as the usual clinical manifestations. Intracranial pressure may be increased.

Neuromuscular Complications

SLE, a relatively rare illness, is an even rarer cause of end-stage renal disease—less than two percent of the time (Evans et al., 1985). Among all patients who have SLE, whether they have kidney disease or not, the peripheral nervous system is affected in only 11 percent (Hansen and Ballantyne, 1978). Thus, it would be a rare cause of peripheral neuropathy among patients with renal disease.

The pathology consists of multifocal ischemia of peripheral nerves secondary to small vessel vasculitis. The nerves may be affected at various sites. As expected, the onset of symptoms and signs is acute; these later potentially resolve. The long-term effect may be a more generalized polyneuropathy. Compressive neuropathies of the ulnar nerve at the elbow and of the median nerve at the carpal tunnel, acute monophasic polyneuropathy typical of Guillain-Barré syndrome (Albers, 1987), and chronic inflammatory polyneuropathy (Albers, 1987) also occasionally occur. Polymyositis is exceptionally rare. In fact, a myopathy in SLE is more likely to be secondary to steroids. Peripheral neuropathy normally suggests a poor prognosis, since it is indicative of a widespread vasculitis (Goetz, 1980), but steroids may effect a substantial improvement in the neuropathy.

Confirmatory Tests

A large variety of hematological and immunological abnormalities may be found in SLE (see Tables 6.2 and 6.3). The most helpful diagnostically are autoantibodies. Antinuclear antibodies are the most helpful. Antibodies to native (double-stranded) DNA are the most specific and are associated with active systemic disease. Anti-Sm (an acidic nuclear protein) antibodies are specific for SLE but are present in a minority of cases. Depressed serum complement levels correspond to active systemic disease. The finding of other antibodies—e.g., a positive Coombs's test or rheumatoid factor—are of some support in the diagnosis.

Neuroradiological tests, especially CT and MRI tests of the brain, are often abnormal in SLE but are nonspecific. The most common abnormality is cortical atrophy, with widened cortical sulci. Much less commonly, areas of infarction or hemorrhage are found. Electroencephalograms are often abnormal in SLE, but the findings are very nonspecific; the test is rarely helpful.

Pathology and Pathogenesis

The largest neuropathological series are those of Devinsky et al. (1988) (50 cases) and Johnson and Richardson (1968) (24 cases). Three-quarters of each series had psychiatric and/or neurological disease during life. Vasculitis involving the brain was found only in the form of two possible old, healed lesions in two of the patients of Devinsky et al. (1988) and in active form in three patients in the series of Johnson and Richardson (1968).

Johnson and Richardson (1968) found four cases of intraparenchymal hemorrhage and four with multiple small infarcts. In some, they probably related to hypertension, and in others, to necrosis in the walls of small vessels. Twenty of their 24 cases had multiple microscopic infarcts. The small size implied disease of small arterioles and capillaries. In some cases, it was uncertain whether the small lesions would have produced symptoms during life. Fibrin thrombi were found in small vessels of those who died with active CNS lupus. Five of the 24 cases showed necrosis of the walls

of small arterioles. The vascular lesions and their etiologies were studied in more detail by Devinsky et al. (1988). Among their 50 cases, embolic brain infarction was found in 10 (related to Libman-Sacks endocarditis in five, chronic vasculitis in two, and mural thrombus in two cases), and lacunar infarction was found in one. Platelet-fibrin thrombi were found in six cases. Seven of the patients with embolic infarcts also had evidence of thrombotic thrombocytopenic purpura as a terminal illness. Venous infarction was found infrequently in the brain or retina of lupus patients (Johnson and Richardson, 1968).

Thus, although SLE has traditionally been considered a vasculitis or collagen vascular disease, vasculitis is rarely found in the brain, even with well-documented focal, multifocal, or diffuse symptoms and signs. The pathogenesis of microinfarcts and other vascular and perivascular alterations is uncertain, but there is a strong association of cerebral infarction, venous thrombosis, and pulmonary emboli with elevated immunoglobulin G or M anticardiolipin levels (Harris et al., 1983). Cardiolipin is a complex phospholipid antigen that shares antigenic properties with phospholipids in platelets and with prothrombin activator complex. Anticardiolipin antibodies may promote coagulation by activating the coagulation cascade, promoting platelet release, and acting upon the endothelium to reduce prostacyclin release (Harris et al., 1983). These antibodies share many features with lupus anticoagulant and, at high titers, are responsible for a false-positive Venereal Disease Research Laboratory test (Harris et al., 1983). Since there is some correlation with clinical CNS disease, these changes must play a role in CNS dysfunction.

It is of interest that immune complex deposits similar to those found in renal glomeruli have been described in the choroid plexus of the brain in SLE (Lampert and Oldstone, 1973). Siebold et al. (1982) have also detected such complexes in the CSF of patients with CNS lupus. The role of these complexes has yet to be defined. They may play a role in altered blood-brain barrier function.

Another finding of uncertain significance is that of autoantibodies in the serum of SLE patients that cross-react with neurons (Bluestein and Zvaifler, 1976). If there is damage to the blood-brain barrier, such antibodies could gain access to the CNS and contribute to the neurological dysfunction, even if infarction of tissue does not occur. The role of autoantibodies in SLE is unproven, but this is a promising area for further research.

Cerebral hemorrhages probably relate to necrosis in the walls of small blood vessels. Severe hypertension secondary to renal disease or therapy, or autoimmune thrombocytopenia may be responsible in a few patients.

Small vessel disease is usually the cause of lupus myelopathy, but one case described by Richardson (1980) and two cases in the series of Devinsky et al. (1988) showed a peculiar vacuolating myelopathy of the white matter similar to that found in subacute combined degeneration.

Treatment

Management of neurological involvement in SLE is very difficult, and requires continuous or frequent reassessment. Accurate diagnosis that the neurological features are related to SLE, and not to a complication of the treatment or to an indirect effect of the disease or some other condition, is the first mandatory step. The mainstay of treatment is immunosuppression. Corticosteroids have been used with incomplete but definite effectiveness for decades. For active disease, treatment should be prompt and vigorous—intravenous methylprednisolone, one gram intravenously daily for five days is combined with cyclophosphamide. Dosages of prednisone range from 20 to 60 mg/day or more. Alternate day therapy may be suitable as the disease becomes more quiescent. Other cytotoxic drugs such as azathioprine are worthy of consideration in aggressive cases of SLE.

Plasmapheresis, in which three or four liters of plasma are exchanged weekly, can be helpful in systemic as well as active neurological disease but has not achieved widespread use.

Wegener's Granulomatosis

Wegener's granulomatosis is a vasculitis affecting small arteries, arterioles, venules, and some capillaries. The vessels show necrotizing inflammation with granulomata and giant cells. To make the diagnosis, both granulomas and necrotizing vasculitis must be found.

Wegener's granulomatosis usually affects males between 40 and 50 years of age. It is a very aggressive disease, which is fatal unless vigorously treated. Symptoms begin in the upper respiratory tract with blood-stained, offensive nasal discharge, but accompanied by severe systemic malaise. Following this, there may be erosion of bones of the nose, paranasal sinuses, and orbits. Saddle-nose deformity may occur. Otitis media is common, as is superinfection of the upper or lower airway. Involvement of the oral cavity, larynx, and lungs is common. Rounded, necrotizing lesions are found on chest radiographs. Renal involvement occurs in more than 90 percent of cases and is universal in the generalized form of the disease. This may take the form of an acute glomerulonephritis or nephrotic syndrome. Renal involvement is associated with a high mortality. The eyes are involved in 50 percent of cases, usually as an iritis, scleritis, or conjunctivitis. Cardiac involvement may occur with coronary arteritis or pericarditis. Skin lesions are found in 50 percent of cases: petechiae, vesicles, and necrotic ulcerations.

Nervous System Involvement

The nervous system is involved in more than half the cases (Drachman, 1963). The peripheral nervous system is more commonly involved than the CNS (Walton, 1958; Drachman, 1963). The former tends to be involved earlier in the course of the illness, while CNS complications, which are in themselves often fatal, occur later or terminally. There is often a tendency for hypertensive encephalopathy to occur; typical arteriolar changes may be found in the brain (Drachman, 1963). Death from renal failure, myocardial infarction, or the neurological complications may occur in one to three months from onset, but more commonly ensues after one to two years.

The meninges and cranial nerves are involved in 26 percent of cases (Drachman, 1963). This occurs from direct invasion of the inflammatory process. Orbital involvement with exophthalmos, which may or may not be accompanied by meningeal disease, occurs in about 12 percent of the total group (Drachman, 1963). This results in ophthalmoplegia from oculomotor nerve or extraocular muscle involvement and blindness because of granulomatous or vascular injury to the optic nerve or retina (Haynes et al., 1977).

The intracranial portion of the optic nerves, the chiasm, or the tracts are involved in about seven percent of cases, from direct upward extension of the erosive disease intracranially (Drachman, 1963). The cavernous sinus region may be involved, with resultant palsy of the third, fourth, sixth, and the first division of the fifth cranial nerves in any combination. Proptosis, chemosis, and venous obstruction may simulate cavernous sinus thrombosis.

Basal meningitis may cause palsy of virtually any cranial nerve, as well as a meningitic syndrome. (Less commonly, cranial nerve involvement may arise due to "remote" or noncontiguous inflammatory or vascular lesions.) With bony erosion, the natural barriers against infection are destroyed and patients not uncommonly have bacterial superinfections, especially meningitis, from nasal microorganisms. Another complication of bony involvement is invasion of the inner ear, with vertigo and end-organ deafness (Drachman, 1963).

The base of the brain, especially the hypothalamus, may be directly invaded from meningeal disease. Diabetes insipidus has been reported in several cases (Drachman, 1963). The brainstem may also suffer infiltration from meningeal disease.

Other brain lesions may be due to remote granulomatous lesions or to vasculitis. Cerebral granulomata may be multiple (Drachman, 1963). Vasculitic involvement may produce ischemic damage, the territory and volume of infarction dependent on the vessel, or hemorrhage in the brain or subarachnoid space.

The development of bacterial brain abscess or subdural or epidural empyema is an ever-present danger because of the frequently associated paranasal sinusitis, the breakdown of skull barriers, and possibly the opportunity for venous infection.

Diagnosis

The clinical, radiological, and histopathological findings on biopsy should present no difficulty with diagnosis. The condition needs to be differentiated from malignancy involving the nose, especially malignant lymphomas, and from Stewart's granuloma (see following section). This is usually possible histologically, if not clinically. Other immunological conditions, such as Goodpasture's syndrome and polyarteritis nodosa, may occasionally cause diagnostic confusion in the early stages.

Stewart's Granuloma

When pathological changes are limited to the nose and paranasal space, the condition is referred to as Stewart's granuloma (or midline granuloma, lethal midline granuloma, or granuloma gangrenescens). This appears to be a limited form of Wegener's granulomatosis; in the latter, granulomatous disease is found in other structures as well (Anderson et al., 1975). This view is controversial, however. Some authorities feel that the two entities are pathologically and pathogenetically distinct (Wolff, 1983). The "splitters" argue that Stewart's granuloma is rarely, if ever, associated with a true vasculitis. Recommended treatments of Wegener's and Stewart's syndromes differ as well; this last point, in particular, justifies the separation from Wegener's granulomatosis. Stewart's granuloma is treated with local radiotherapy; corticosteroids are ineffective and cytotoxic drugs are of unproven value.

Treatment

Recently, there has been a dramatic change in the outlook for patients with Wegener's granulomatosis. The disease was previously uniformly fatal, but with the advent of modern chemotherapy, the course has been altered and remissions have been produced. The drug of choice is cyclophosphamide. This drug is given orally, beginning at 2 mg/kg/day. The white blood count is followed to determine subsequent dosages. Treatment continues until the patient has been in remission for one year (Wolff, 1983). Azathioprine could also be used. Prednisone is an adjunctive drug. Complications such as superinfections have to be treated separately.

Other Vasculitides

Other vasculitides less commonly produce simultaneous, significant involvement of the kidney and the nervous system. Furthermore, it should be recognized that many times vasculitic syndromes cannot be adequately fitted into traditional classifications. These have been called "polyangiitis overlap syndromes" (Leavitt and Fauci, 1986). They will not be discussed here.

Scleroderma

Scleroderma (progressive or diffuse systemic sclerosis), listed with the vasculitides as the primary lesion, is thought to be endothelial cell injury in vessels ranging from small arteries to capillaries (Gilliland, 1987). The cause of the initial injury is unknown. Platelet aggregation then leads to myointimal cell proliferation and fibrosis, causing narrowing of vessel lumina. Increased vascular permeability leads to interstitial edema, fibroblast stimulation, and tissue fibrosis.

Scleroderma is a multisystem disorder involving the skin and a variety of other organs, especially the gastrointestinal tract, kidney, lungs, and heart. Although the kidneys are involved in nearly half the cases, this occurs later in the course of the illness; renal failure contributes to or causes 40 to 50 percent of the deaths. Accelerated hypertension may be the first sign of renal disease; this may lead to hypertensive encephalopathy. Alternatively,

proteinuria and a more gradual onset of uremia is found. Hypertension almost always accompanied renal involvement in scleroderma.

Both the central and peripheral nervous systems may be affected in scleroderma, either as part of the disease or as a complication of the uremia. In some cases, CNS disease related to renal hypertension may apply.

Central Nervous System Involvement

Psychotic illness appears as a late neurological complication in 10 percent of patients with scleroderma (Piper and Helwig, 1955). These may take the form of paranoid delusions with or without obvious dementia. Hallucinations are rare. Mental changes related to frontal lobe dysfunction may be especially prominent (Binder and Gerstenbrand, 1980). Occasionally, complications due to malnutrition related to gastrointestinal disease, may cause neurological problems: Wernicke's encephalopathy, pellagra, or vitamin B_2 neuropathy.

Often the brain is involved in a multifocal fashion, with added deficits over time (Binder and Gerstenbrand, 1980). Initially, there may be a hemiparesis, hemianopsia, hemisensory defect, or aphasia. A parkinsonian syndrome with akinesia and rigidity may occur (Binder and Gerstenbrand, 1980). Various vascular brainstem syndromes have been described (Gordon and Silverstein, 1970). Herniation of the brain may occur from edema or bleeding (Gordon and Silverstein, 1970).

Epileptic seizures of a generalized nature are usually related to uremic encephalopathy. There is a syndrome of focal Jacksonian seizures, circumscribed scleroderma (morphea), and facial hemiatrophy (Gordon and Silverstein, 1970).

Myelopathy

Subacute combined degeneration from deficiency of vitamin B_{12} may develop (Binder and Gerstenbrand, 1980). Vascular lesions of the spinal cord could produce acute hemicord syndromes or acute transverse myelopathy (Binder and Gerstenbrand, 1980). Pseudotabetic features have been described (Lee and Haynes,

1967). Spinal fluid examination is always normal (Binder and Gerstenbrand, 1980).

Diagnosis

The diagnosis is usually dependent on characteristic skin changes. Firm, taut, and bound-down skin proximal to the metacarpophalangeal joints is the major criterion. (Similar changes *distal* to these joints, termed sclerodactyly, are not diagnostic.) Less than five percent of cases have visceral but no skin involvement with the histological features described under Pathology and Pathogenesis. Nailfold capillaroscopy is helpful in early cases. Further support is given by positive autoimmune serology and increased plasma beta-thromboglobulin levels.

The differential diagnosis includes mixed connective tissue disease (polyangiitis overlap syndrome), in which characteristic features of more than one vasculitic illness are present. Eosinophilic fasciitis is an inflammation of the skin and deeper tissues of the trunk and proximal limbs of younger individuals. There is a variable progression to visceral involvement; the condition then shows a close resemblance and, probably, relationship to scleroderma.

Pathology and Pathogenesis

Vascular disease is responsible for focal lesions of the brain and spinal cord, including the parkinsonian syndrome. Fibrinoid degeneration of the collagen, with proliferation of endothelial cells may directly occlude the vessel or there may be superimposed thrombosis (Binder and Gerstenbrand, 1980). The penetrating arteries or the major arteries, including the anterior, middle, and posterior cerebral arteries, the internal carotid artery, and the basilar artery may become occluded, with resultant brain infarction (Lee and Haynes, 1967).

Demyelination of the posterior and lateral columns are found in subacute combined degeneration. Vascular lesions, or sometimes no abnormality, can be found in some cases with apparent spinal involvement (Binder and Gerstenbrand, 1980). It is unclear why some cases fail to show appropriate lesions, but it has been speculated that this may be due to spinal ischemia short of frank infarction (Binder and Gerstenbrand, 1980). Pseudotabes, as in diabetes, may be due to peripheral neuropathy.

Treatment

Treatment has been hard to evaluate because of the highly variable course of the disease. Corticosteroids have mainly been used in acutely progressive scleroderma or when myositis is present. A number of treatments have been used for the skin disease itself, which will not be discussed here.

It is important to treat complications of scleroderma. Vitamin supplements, given parenterally, may be necessary. Treatment of the renal disease and hypertension may help avoid some CNS complications.

Thrombotic Thrombocytopenic Purpura

Thrombotic thrombocytopenic purpura (TTP, thrombotic microangiopathy, Moschcowitz's disease, or thrombotic angiothrombosis) is an acute illness characterized by intravascular hemolysis, producing a microangiopathic anemia, thrombocytopenia, and organ dysfunction from disturbance of microcirculation. The brain and kidney are characteristically involved.

Clinical Features

The first case was described by Moschcowitz (1925) in a 16-year-old girl who developed a subacute febrile illness with initial complaints of limb weakness and arthralgias in association with marked pallor and constipation. Thirteen days later, while still febrile and pale, she developed a left hemiparesis followed by pulmonary edema. Although the latter improved, she lapsed into coma and died the next day.

The above description typifies TTP. The victim is usually an adolescent or young adult female. The patient acutely develops a fever, anemia, and symptoms of renal, cerebral, and sometimes hepatic disease. Petechiae in the skin and conjunctivae are common. Symptoms and signs may fluctuate, but develop in a step-wise fashion. The condition has a high associated mortality. If patients do survive, there is a significant risk of recurrence.

Central nervous system dysfunction may occur in a multifocal or diffuse fashion. Headache is common. Most patients develop an incomplete motor paresis. Aphasia, blurred vision, various agnosias, and virtually any focal sign or symptom could develop. Focal or generalized convulsive seizures are common. Any of these features could resolve to various degrees. Mild to severe obtundation is described: patients often become restless and confused; coma is commonly terminal.

In the series of Adams et al. (1948), areflexia in a limb or both lower limbs was found in three of the four cases. This could reflect either spinal cord or peripheral nerve involvement. In almost all cases, the brain involvement dominates the clinical picture.

Investigations

The combination of anemia with fragmented red blood cells on the peripheral blood smear, thrombocytopenia, renal failure, and clinical neurological deficits is pathognomonic of TTP. The anemia is severe, often yielding positive results on Coombs's test and associated with an increased reticulocyte count and nucleated red blood cells in the peripheral blood, but the fragmented helmet cells are the main feature of the microangiopathic hemolytic anemia; thus, the smear is vital. Platelet counts are reduced to 5,000 to 100,000/mm³, due to increased consumption. Tests of coagulation are normal and the screening tests for disseminated intravascular coagulation are negative. Bilirubin may be elevated from hemolysis or hepatic failure. Serum urea and creatinine are elevated.

Biopsy is not required, but typical vascular changes (see next section) in the skin or gingivae are supportive. Similar vascular changes may be seen, however, in disseminated intravascular coagulation and in the hemolytic-uremic syndrome.

Pathology and Pathogenesis

The terminal arterioles, capillaries, and even venules of virtually all organs show occlusion with hyaline material, presumably platelets and fibrin. Endothelial cells may be swollen or increased in number. The thrombosed vessels, depending on age, show various degrees of organization. The parenchymal pathology in the brain and other organs is secondary to these microvascular changes. In the brain, this includes areas of microinfarcton, edema, and small or confluent hemorrhages. No area is consistently involved or spared. The spinal cord may be similarly involved (Adams et al., 1948).

The etiology and pathogenesis are incompletely understood. Immunofluorescent studies show complement and immunoglobulin in arterioles. These features, and the association in some patients with underlying SLE, scleroderma, or Sjögren's syndrome suggest an immunologic cause (Cooper and Bunn, 1983). There is evidence that TTP may be due to a deficiency in von Willebrand's monomers. Support for this is the correction of TTP by administration of plasma.

Treatment

TTP should be regarded as a medical emergency. Diagnosis is usually not difficult but should be prompt. Differential diagnosis includes idiopathic thrombocytopenic purpura, which is not a microangiopathic condition.

Previously, the disease was almost universally fatal. It still has a high mortality. Variable successes have been reported with a variety of therapies, including corticosteroids, antiplatelet drugs, heparin, splenectomy, and plasmapheresis. Administration of plasma, which restores the deficient von Willebrand monomers, has been successful and should be tried first. Exchange transfusion with fresh frozen plasma may be even better. None has yet been found to be uniformly successful, but these modalities separately or in various combinations are worth trying in such a desperate condition.

Symptomatic therapy is necessary for epileptic seizures, impaired level of consciousness, and renal failure.

When the condition has been controlled, maintenance therapy with antiplatelet agents, such as aspirin and dipyridamole, should probably be continued for several months.

Hemolytic-Uremic Syndrome

Hemolytic-uremic syndrome is similar to TTP, and criteria separating the two conditions are not absolute. The following characteristics of hemolytic-uremic syndrome are usually used to separate them: it is more common in children than in adults; there is often a preceding viral illness; there may be a familial tendency; the nervous system is less commonly involved; and the mortality is lower, except in adults.

Clinical Features

Hemolytic-uremic syndrome is said to be the most common cause of acute renal failure in young children (Behrman and Vaughan, 1987). Most cases occur in children under 4 years of age.

Central nervous system involvement has been reported in 30 to 50 percent of cases (Rooney et al., 1971; Gianantonio et al., 1973; Bale et al., 1980). Children may show a stroke-like onset of focal neurological deficits such as hemiparesis, generalized or multifocal CNS dysfunction with coma and decerebrate posturing, or focal or generalized convulsive seizures. If the child survives, there may be complete or partial recovery (Steinberg et al., 1986) or severe disability with the need for chronic institutionalization (Mendelsohn et al., 1984). The syndrome rarely recurs (Behrman and Vaughan, 1987).

Investigations

The hematological and biochemical abnormalities are identical to those described for TTP. The CT scan in those with neurological involvement may show areas of infarction or extensive cerebral edema (Steinberg et al., 1986; Mendelsohn et al., 1984). Mendelsohn et al. (1984) described one case with a peculiar pattern of enhancement at the gray–white matter interface. The patient later developed cerebral atrophy in association with severe mental and motor handicap, as well as seizures.

Pathology and Pathogenesis

There is no essential difference in the microvascular pathology between this condition and TTP. Children may develop cerebral edema more readily (Mendelsohn et al., 1984), as with other brain insults. Areas of cerebral infarction may be larger than with TTP. The underlying etiology and pathogenesis are poorly understood, as with TTP. There is presumably endothelial injury as the initiating event.

Treatment

With aggressive therapy, 90 percent of children survive the acute illness (Behrman and Vaughan, 1987). Various modalities of treatment have been employed, as with TTP. It is difficult to weigh these individually.

B

Independent Kidney and Nervous System Disorders

Hematological Disorders

Multiple Myeloma

Multiple myeloma is a widespread malignancy of plasma cells usually associated with the production of monoclonal protein in one of the immunoglobulin classes or monoclonal light chains (Bence Jones protein) in the urine.

Myeloma usually causes renal damage by affecting the renal tubules. This is thought to occur because of precipitation of protein, especially Bence Jones protein, in the distal nephron or through a toxic effect of the Bence Jones protein on the tubular cells. The kidney may be indirectly affected by hypercalcemia or hyperuricemia, which commonly accompany myeloma.

The neurological complications of multiple myeloma can be divided into three main groups (Table 6.4): those from direct nervous tissue compression, those from infiltration by myeloma, and associated or indirect complications. Those from compression are the most common. Clarke (1956) found that 20 percent of patients with multiple myeloma had problems with spinal compression at some time.

Because of the manner of neurological involvement, the various syndromes will be reviewed sequentially, using Table 6.4 as a guide.

Compressive Lesions

Spinal compression occurs most commonly in the thoracic region, followed by the lumbar and then the cervical area (Spaar, 1980). Compression may be due to protruding vertebral tumors, bony collapse, primary epidural tumor, expanding hematoma, or a large amyloid deposit. There is usually local pain, followed by nerve root pain or dysfunction and then signs and symptoms of cord or cauda compression, depending on the site.

Compression of cranial nerves or the brain is rare in comparison with spinal compression. Myeloma masses may compress cranial nerves near their exit foramina. Any of the cranial nerves may be involved (Spaar, 1980), but those most frequently affected are II, III, V, VI, and VII. Those bordering on the sella or near the sphenoid bones are more likely to be affected by basal myeloma. Some authors (Dolin and Dewar, 1956; Someren et al., 1971) propose that these plasmacytomas arise from the nasopharynx or paranasal sinuses.

Involvement of the brain by external compression is very rare, despite the frequency of skull involvement. This may reflect the tendency of extraencephalic myeloma to grow in sheets or to infiltrate, rather than to form a rounded mass.

Table 6.4. Neurological Complications of Myelomatosis

Compression of nervous tissue by tumor or displaced bone
  Spinal: cord, roots, cauda equina
  Skull: cranial nerves, brain (base)
  Intracranial: brain, meninges (dura, venous sinuses), cranial nerves
Infiltration by or metastases from myeloma
  Dura and leptomeninges
  Central nervous system
  Peripheral nerves
Associated
  Remote effects: polyneuropathy, toxic myelopathy (?)
  Metabolic: hypercalcemia, uremia
  Hematological: anemia—anoxia if severe, bleeding, hyperviscosity
  Opportunistic infections of the CNS: herpes zoster, progressive multifocal leukoencephalopathy, toxoplasmosis, cryptococcus
  Amyloidosis: polyneuropathy, carpal tunnel syndrome, "tumorous amyloid," e.g., epidural
  Complications of therapy: corticosteroids, chemotherapy, radiation

Source: Adapted from Silverstein and Doniger (1963) and Spaar (1980).

Infiltration by Myeloma

There are three categories of infiltrative CNS myeloma (Spaar, 1980): direct invasion through dura mater and leptomeninges from adjacent bony involvement, metastatic disease as a general intracranial invasion with infiltration of the brain and subarachnoid space, and discrete nodular metastasis. Patients often show signs of raised intracranial pressure, as well as signs relevant to the brain region involved. Adams (1973) described a case with infiltration of the leptomeninges and expanding tumor nodules compressing the brain. Occasionally, such infiltration will cause palsies of multiple cranial nerve and spinal roots, hydrocephalus, and malignant cells and low glucose concentration in the CSF, similar to meningeal carcinomatosis (Spaar, 1980). There may be infiltration of the brain or optic nerves from the subarachnoid space. A most unusual case was described by Weiner et al. (1966) in which a temporal lobe plasmacytoma was associated with myeloma protein in the CSF.

Associated Complications of Myeloma

Polyneuropathy and amyloid involvement of the peripheral nervous system or carpal tunnel as remote effects of myeloma are not uncommon. These entities are discussed in Chapter 5.

Hypercalcemia may reach levels above 11.5 mg/dL (2.8 mmol/L), due to increased bone resorption. Levels occasionally are high enough to cause encephalopathy if disease is very extensive. Uremia may cause an acute encephalopathy. Occasionally, patients may present with acute uremic encephalopathy if they develop acute renal failure during dehydration in unsuspected multiple myeloma (e.g., patient fasting before an intravenous pyelogram). A hyperviscosity syndrome is not common with myeloma, but is more often a feature of macroglobulinemia associated with Waldenström's disease. Bleeding problems have been reported in association with acquired van Willebrand's disease with myeloma (Mohri et al., 1987).

Other indirect effects of multiple myeloma are listed in Table 6.4. They will not be further discussed in this section.

Treatment

The treatment of multiple myeloma has not changed significantly in years. It is aimed at treatment of complications and making an effort to reduce the number of neoplastic plasma cells. Adequate hydration is important to prevent or limit renal involvement.

Local spinal cord compression by myeloma may be treated by radiotherapy. If the compression is from bony collapse, surgical laminectomy or extensive reconstructive surgery is indicated. Radiotherapy of cranial or other spinal lesions may be beneficial. The intracranial lesions probably require biopsy beforehand to make a histological diagnosis and to exclude other etiology such as an opportunistic infection.

Plasma cell reduction is achieved by chemotherapy with vincristine, cyclophosphamide, and doxorubicin, along with prednisone. Persistent elevations of paraproteins after this should be treated with intermittent melphalan and prednisone, which are maintained until relapse occurs. Then doxorubicin is reinstituted.

Plasma Cell Dyscrasia

Peripheral neuropathy may occur in association with monoclonal gammopathy of undetermined significance; amyloidosis, light-chain type; multiple myeloma; osteosclerotic myeloma; Waldenström's macroglobulinemia; and gamma heavy-chain disease. All of these conditions may cause varying amounts of myeloma protein in the serum or urine. Bone marrow aspiration often reveals a plasma cell dyscrasia. Bone marrow biopsy may afford a tissue diagnosis of amyloidosis in light-chain disease, multiple myeloma, or osteosclerotic myeloma. The polyneuropathy is usually of a motor and sensory, distal, symmetrical variety that leads a chronic course, shows variable increase in CSF protein, and usually is associated with fairly marked slowing of conduction velocity. Thus, the underlying pathology is most often a segmental demyelination. Polyneuropathy and other manifestations are not usually associated with serious or end-stage renal disease (Kelly, 1987).

Hereditary Amyloidosis

Peripheral neuropathy and renal failure commonly coexist in certain types of hereditary amyloidosis. These types are dominantly inherited, and signs and symptoms usually begin in middle life. In the type I variety, there is a motor and sensory polyneuropathy in which pain and temperature sensation are particularly affected. Autonomic signs are also prominent. There is associated renal, cardiac, and ocular (vitreous opacities) involvement. In the type II variety, carpal tunnel syndrome is a prominent early feature, but a more diffuse polyneuropathy later develops, again with autonomic involvement, as well as heart disease and vitreous opacities. The type III variant has prominent renal involvement and peptic ulceration, and there is an associated motor and sensory polyneuropathy, particularly affecting pain and temperature. In the type IV variety, a cranial neuropathy presents initially, often accompanied by an ocular corneal lattice dystrophy. Other body systems are only mildly affected (Thomas, 1987).

Waldenström's Macroglobulinemia

This condition is briefly mentioned, because there is sometimes confusion with myeloma (Takahashi et al., 1986). Waldenström's macroglobulinemia is a rare lymphoproliferative disorder associated with a monoclonal immunoglobulin M peak on immunoelectrophoresis. Most patients have an underlying lymphoma, chronic lymphocytic leukemia, or a combination of these conditions. Middle-aged and elderly persons are affected, with males slightly outnumbering females. Renal failure is rare in Waldenström's macroglobulinemia, probably because Bence Jones proteinuria is not present. In contrast to multiple myeloma, most patients with Waldenström's macroglobulinemia show lymphadenopathy and enlargement of the liver and/or spleen. Hyperviscosity syndrome is much more strongly associated with Waldenström's macroglobulinemia, while lytic bone lesions and renal impairment are more common in myeloma. Patient survival tends to be longer with Waldenström's macroglobulinemia. Some similarities between Waldenström's macroglobulinemia and multiple myeloma include anemia and constitutional symptoms.

Neurological complications, which occur in 25 percent of patients (Solomon, 1965), are mainly due to the production of large quantities of macroglobulin, which may polymerize. Hyperviscosity from the hyperproteinemia probably accounts for many of the manifestations, but a hemorrhagic diathesis may also cause problems (Silberstein et al., 1987).

The principal CNS manifestations, in approximate order of descending frequency, are retinopathy, often with papilledema; generalized encephalopathy; focal or multifocal strokes; meningitis; and cerebellar ataxia.

Fabry's Disease

This disorder may be manifest as both peripheral neuropathy and renal failure. It is due to a deficiency of the enzyme α-galactosidase and is inherited through an X-linked, recessive pattern. The enzyme deficiency causes faulty breakdown of glycolipids, resulting in their deposition in tissues throughout the body. The skin becomes scaly and telangiectatic—so-called angiokeratoma corporis diffusum, chiefly present over the lower trunk and buttocks. While the patient rarely has visual symptoms, careful ophthalmological examination may reveal a corneal dystrophy and dilated conjunctival blood vessels. Ultimately, usually in later adult life, renal failure dominates the clinical picture and chronic dialysis or renal transplantation may ultimately be necessary. The peripheral nerve involvement is quite distinctive, consisting of persistent aching in the limbs and exacerbations of burning pain, sometimes induced by emotional disturbances. There may be lack of sweating and resulting episodes of hyperthermia. Nerve biopsy shows a deposition of glycolipid in the perineurial and capillary endothelial cells and the dorsal root ganglion cells. Small myelinated and unmyelinated fibers are selectively lost. Thus, standard nerve conduction studies may reveal only mild abnormalities. The pain may respond to phenytoin.

Sepsis

Sepsis can be defined as a systemic reaction to the presence of microorganisms or their toxins in the blood or tissues (Sanford, 1985). The brain, peripheral nerves, and kidneys are often involved, either together or separately, as part of the systemic reaction of multiple organ failure.

The general clinical features of sepsis are well known. There is commonly a febrile response. Cardiovascular changes include increased cardiac output and decreased peripheral resistance. The respiratory rate is increased. Other manifestations relate to the site of the septic focus and to those organs that are involved in the syndrome of multiorgan failure (Borzotta and Polk, 1983).

Septic Encephalopathy

In our recent prospective study (Young et al., in press), we found that two-thirds of patients with sepsis, defined as positive results on blood culture or well-defined bacterial infection in the body, had evidence of encephalopathy. Of these, two-thirds had severe disturbance in brain function. The clinical picture was that of a metabolic encephalopathy. The level of consciousness varied from a confusional state to coma. Delirium infrequently occurred. There was often considerable fluctuation in those patients with mild to moderate degrees of encephalopathy, with confusion occurring mainly at night. There was impairment of attention, concentration, memory, and writing in the encephalopathic patients who were testable. Paratonic rigidity, or gegenhalten, was universal in the encephalopathic patients. Tremor, asterixis, and multifocal myoclonus occurred in 10 to 25 percent of noncomatose, encephalopathic patients. Pupils were always spared.

Focal signs and seizures occasionally are found in sepsis. In our previous retrospective series of patients who died of sepsis, hemiparesis or gaze palsy was found in six, and focal or generalized convulsive seizures occurred in five, of the 12 patients (Jackson et al., 1985). In contrast, our prospective study contained only two patients with transient focal signs and one patient, who had severe renal failure, with generalized convulsions. The difference may relate to the more severe, protracted septic illness of the patients in the retrospective study.

Investigations

The EEG is sensitive to septic encephalopathy, reflecting the severity with accuracy

(Young et al., 1986). It often reveals features compatible with a metabolic encephalopathy, such as triphasic waves or intermittent, rhythmic delta waves superimposed on a slow background. We found (Young et al., in press) that the clinical severity of the encephalopathy and the degree of EEG abnormality significantly correlated in a linear fashion with serum urea, creatinine, and bilirubin levels. Thus, the brain appears to fail in parallel with the other organs. There was also a strong association of severe septic encephalopathy with adult respiratory distress syndrome.

The CSF examinations in both our retrospective and prospective studies were unremarkable, except for a modest elevation of protein in less than half of the patients. CT scans of the brain were unremarkable.

Other laboratory features include respiratory alkalosis in early sepsis, combined with or followed by lactic acidosis. The white blood count is elevated in proportion to the severity of the sepsis (Young et al., in press).

Pathology and Pathogenesis

In our autopsy series (Jackson et al., 1985), eight of the 12 cases had disseminated microabscesses in the CNS, chiefly in the cerebral cortex and subcortical white matter. The microabscesses did not appear to be merely agonal phenomena, as there was some reaction in the brain tissue surrounding them.

Four of the above 12 patients in the retrospective (autopsy) series also had an increase in protoplasmic astrocytes, as described in metabolic encephalopathies (Cavanagh, 1974). Three patients had central pontine myelinolysis, a complication of overcorrection of hyponatremia (see Chapter 8). Vascular lesions were found in six patients: five had multiple small cerebral infarcts (one terminal), and one had thrombocytopenia with brain purpura. In our prospective study of 68 patients (Young et al., in press), postmortem examinations were done on only four of the 19 patients who died; none of these showed any acute pathology related to the septic illness.

The significance of the microabscesses is unclear. It is likely that they occur mainly in protracted, severe sepsis. It seems unlikely that they play a role in the shorter duration, reversible encephalopathy, in which our data supports a metabolic pathogenesis.

Experimental data indicate that endotoxin is unlikely to directly act on the brain, at least in adults (Mela, 1981).

Significant hypotension occurred in only four of our 48 encephalopathic patients (Young et al., in press). Disturbed microcirculation could occur in sepsis, with disseminated intravascular coagulation. This may have been responsible in two of our patients. Bihari et al. (1987) showed that prostacyclin infusion increased oxygen uptake by tissues in patients with very severe sepsis. The mechanism is uncertain. This could be due to deaggregation of platelets, inhibition of attachment of leukocytes to damaged endothelium, vasodilation, or a combination of these mechanisms.

Although we found that the severity of the encephalopathy was correlated with serum bilirubin, urea, and creatinine levels, we could not necessarily attribute the brain dysfunction to hepatic or renal failure. It has been shown experimentally, however, that within five hours of the onset of sepsis, the liver shows impaired ability to clear indocyanine green from the blood (Chaudry et al., 1982). Serum urea may rise in part because of the hypercatabolism of amino acids in sepsis. Frank renal impairment in sepsis could be due to disseminated intravascular coagulation or to hypotension, in a few patients. The main mechanism is probably a reduced distribution of blood to the juxtaglomerular apparatus (Lucas, 1976). We found renal impairment to be severe enough to require dialysis in only one of our 68 patients; in most cases, the renal impairment, based on serum creatinine levels and creatinine clearances in a few patients, was not of sufficient severity to *cause* the encephalopathy.

Another mechanism for the encephalopathy could be related to altered metabolism of amino acids producing a reduction in the ratio of branched-chain to unbranched and aromatic amino acids. Freund et al. (1979) correlated the severity of septic encephalopathy in humans with the quantitative alteration of the above ratio. These authors suggest that the amino acid imbalance in the blood is reflected in the brain. As has been proposed in hepatic failure, in which a similar amino acid disturbance occurs, this could lead to altered neurotransmitter function, including increased serotonin levels or the production of false neurotransmitters such as octopamine (Fisher, 1974). Neuroendocrine alterations represent an unexplored area for septic encephalopathy.

In some patients, iatrogenic factors play a role in causing impaired consciousness: sedative drugs, including opiates, are commonly used in intensive care units to aid in managing patients on respirators. Total parenteral nutrition can be associated with hyperosmolality and hypophosphatemia. High doses of penicillin can cause seizures, especially if there is renal impairment. As we have seen, overcorrection of electrolyte disturbances can cause central pontine myelinolysis.

Management

The treatment of sepsis and its attendant complications is beyond the scope of this book. A few points should be made, however. Eradication of the responsible infection is foremost. In some cases, this requires surgery. In the syndrome of "occult sepsis," multiorgan (including the brain) failure occurs and persists or worsens until the intra-abdominal infection is properly treated (Polk and Shields, 1977). Also, we have found that the severity of the nervous system dysfunction, as assessed clinically or with EEG, electromyography, or nerve conduction tests, cannot be used as an indication that the condition is hopeless. We have had patients recover to useful lives who have been in deep coma with burst-suppression EEG patterns or very severe axonal neuropathy. From the nervous system point of view the main management is supportive and preventive; it is imperative that other causes of coma with sepsis, such as bacterial meningitis and bacterial endocarditis, are excluded.

Critical Illness Polyneuropathy

Critical illness polyneuropathy (Bolton et al., 1984; Zochodne et al., 1987) develops in at least 50 percent of patients in critical care units who suffer from sepsis and multiple organ failure. However, the degree of renal failure is usually mild, hemodialysis not often being required. (When it is, the prognosis is often poor [Cameron, 1986].)

Because of the severe systemic disease and other factors, the polyneuropathy may be overlooked and can only be reliably demonstrated by electromyography and nerve conduction studies. Occasionally, however, the neuropathy is so severe that there is a generalized, flaccid quadriplegia with sparing of cranial musculature that is obvious on clinical examination alone. The first clue to the diagnosis is failure of weaning from the ventilator as the sepsis and multiple organ failure seem to be coming under control.

Since the underlying pathology is a primary axonal degeneration of motor and sensory fibers, conduction velocity is little affected and the chief manifestations are reductions in the amplitudes of muscle and sensory compound action potentials and signs of denervation on needle electromyography—positive sharp waves and fibrillation potentials. Should the patient survive this severe systemic illness, as happens in 40 percent of the cases, the polyneuropathy will gradually resolve, in mild cases over a matter of weeks and in severe cases over a matter of months (Bolton et al., 1984; Zochodne et al., 1987).

Disseminated Intravascular Coagulation

Disseminated intravascular coagulation (DIC) is a condition that arises in a number of syndromes (Nossel, 1983). The pathogenesis is complex, but the key factor is the generation of thrombin in the circulating blood.

The sequence of events in DIC is shown in Figure 6.1. Following some kind of insult, or commonly sepsis, the coagulation system is activated, and thrombin is released. Thrombin acts as an enzyme on fibrinogen to form polymers (reaction 2). The fibrin polymer absorbs and activates plasminogen to form plasmin. Plasmin then cleaves the polymer to form fragment X and Bβ 1-42. Thrombin acts on the

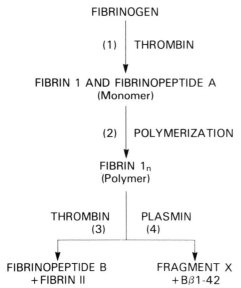

FIBRINOGEN

(1) | THROMBIN

FIBRIN 1 AND FIBRINOPEPTIDE A
(Monomer)

(2) | POLYMERIZATION

FIBRIN 1_n
(Polymer)

THROMBIN   PLASMIN
(3)   (4)

FIBRINOPEPTIDE B   FRAGMENT X
+ FIBRIN II   + Bβ1-42

Figure 6.1. The sequence of changes that result from fibrinogen proteolysis. (From Nossell, 1983.)

fibrin polymer as well to form fibrin II and fibrinopeptide B. In addition, thrombin activates and then inactivates factors V and VIII; which of these two actions predominates depends on the concentration of the factors and kinetics of the reactions. Thrombin also activates platelets to aggregate and degranulate. Thus, in DIC, one often finds reduced levels of fibrinogen, fibrin split products, and thrombocytopenia.

Thromboses in veins and arteries may develop in DIC. This could lead to ischemic damage in various organ systems, including the CNS and kidney. Furthermore, there is a tendency for hemorrhage which could particularly affect the brain.

DIC occurs in some patients with severe sepsis. It may complicate shock of any cause. It may follow trauma, burns, surgery, near drowning, an incompatible blood transfusion, or anaphylaxis. Certain obstetrical conditions, such as retained dead fetus, placental separation, or amniotic fluid embolism, may be followed by intravascular coagulation. Malignant neoplasia, especially carcinoma of the prostate, may be complicated by DIC.

The treatment is primarily the correction of the underlying condition. Hematological therapy includes replacement of blood compo-

nents. Giving more fibrinogen, however, may aggravate the DIC. Heparin deactivates thrombin, but there is a risk of hemorrhage. Deficient blood factors and elements, especially platelets, might be replaced after the coagulation has ceased.

Diabetes Mellitus

Diabetes mellitus is the most common serious metabolic disease in humans, affecting about one percent of the population (Foster, 1983). There are some six million cases in the United States. The disease consists of hyperglycemia along with various hormonal abnormalities. Complications include blood vessel involvement, ranging from thickening of the basement membranes of small vessels to accelerated atherosclerosis, and end-organ involvement, especially the eyes, kidneys, and nerves. Diabetes can be divided into a primary form and a secondary type due to pancreatic disease, hormonal abnormalities, deficient insulin receptors, and some genetic and less common syndromes. The primary variety can be further divided into insulin-dependent (type 1) and the non–insulin-dependent (type 2) categories.

Peripheral insulin antagonism occurs in at least a subpopulation of uremic patients. Also, in some uremic patients, insulin secretions may be reduced. Together, these may cause significant carbohydrate intolerance or frank diabetes in some uremic patients. The mechanisms are uncertain, but the problem may improve with reduced dietary protein, improved dialysis, or renal transplantation (De Fronzo et al., 1973).

In the classic study by Fagerberg (1959) of 356 Swedish patients with diabetes mellitus, 70 percent suffered from neuropathy, of whom 89 percent also had a retinopathy, 93 percent a nephropathy, and 66 percent peripheral vascular disease. It is now apparent that his original supposition that vascular abnormalities might be the underlying cause in all three areas of the body is turning out to be true. In all diabetics, whether they have neuropathy or not, renal disease is a complication in 50 percent, and diabetes is the second leading cause of end-stage renal disease in the United States (Evans et al., 1985). In patients with end-stage renal disease, there is an increase in the number who are now considered for dialysis or renal transplantation, due to improved methods of management, even though uremia accelerates atherosclerosis in diabetes mellitus, particularly after these procedures.

We shall first review the nephrological complications of diabetes and then the central nervous complications, using the model of an approach to coma in the diabetic. Finally, we shall consider the special case of diabetic retinopathy.

Complications of Diabetes

Diabetic Nephropathy

The nodular intraglomerular lesion of the kidney described by Kimmelstein and Wilson (1936) is the most specific renal lesion associated with diabetes. Diffuse thickening of the glomerular basement membrane is also part of diabetic nephropathy (Thomsen, 1965). Arteriosclerosis of the renal artery and its branches, larger vessel complications of diabetes, may be responsible for renal failure in some patients. Peritubular deposits of glycogen, fat, and mucopolysaccharides may cause nephropathy in other diabetics. In addition, chronic pyelonephritis, arterial and arteriolosclerosis and renal pupillary necrosis occur as complications of diabetes. It has been argued that the progression to renal failure in type I diabetes is related to the age of onset of the diabetes: the interval to progression is shorter for those with onset of diabetes after puberty (Krolewski et al., 1985; Wetzels et al., 1986).

Acute renal failure in diabetics can occur in the following situations or conditions (Garber et al., 1974): severe hyperglycemia in association with hyperglycemic, hyperosmolar coma or with diabetic ketoacidosis; exposure to radiocontrast media; renal papillary necrosis; glomerulonephritis; and septicemia.

The management of the diabetic uremic patient is not essentially different from the management of the two conditions independently.

It is sometimes difficult to adequately control serum glucose. Although uremia is associated with carbohydrate intolerance, there is often an increased tendency for hypoglycemia and thus a decrease in the safety factor with insulin administration (Garber et al., 1974). Insulin requirements in a diabetic who develops renal failure are often considerably reduced (Garber et al., 1974).

Special problems may occur with hemodialysis of diabetic uremics. Vascular access is a problem. Ischemic pain and gangrene of a limb are not uncommon. It is thus important to choose more proximal vessels. Hypotension may develop because of fluid shifts or a diabetic autonomic neuropathy. Serum glucose may be difficult to control; it is often necessary to use a continuous infusion of insulin intravenously, at least in the situation of acute uremia (Garber et al., 1974). Hemodialysis is preferable to peritoneal dialysis if the patient is hypercatabolic (Garber et al., 1974).

Peritoneal dialysis has some advantages over hemodialysis in diabetics. Access is not a problem, and rapid fluid shifts are not as likely.

Renal transplantation is a realistic option in diabetic renal failure (Kjellstrand et al., 1974; Khauli et al., 1986). However, this may apply only to those patients who do not have significant preexisting atherosclerotic vascular disease (Rimmer et al., 1986). In some centers, pancreatic and renal transplants are being performed together.

Diabetic Coma

It is instructive to review an approach to coma in the diabetic, as it gives a comprehensive overview of CNS complications, with or without the addition of renal impairment. Table 6.5 is a practical classification of coma in diabetes mellitus (Green, 1976). These various categories will be reviewed in turn.

Hypoglycemia must be considered first in the treated diabetic patient. Uremic diabetics may be more subject than others to insulin- or drug-induced hypoglycemia (see Hypoglycemia in Renal Failure, below). Also, severe hypoglycemia is more damaging to the CNS in the acute situation. Hypoglycemia is dealt

Table 6.5. Coma in Diabetes Mellitus

Coma related to diabetes and its treatment
  Hypoglycemia (treatment induced)
  Ketoacidosis
  Nonketotic hyperosmolar coma
  Lactic acidosis
Indirect causes from complications of diabetes
  Uremia
  Stroke
  Infection—sepsis
Unrelated

with in more detail later in this chapter (see Hypoglycemia in Renal Failure).

Ketoacidosis occurs in the context of insulin deficiency; hyperglycemia is an essential component, but the production of ketoacids is dependent on high levels of glucagon, which promotes oxidation in the liver of the mobilized fatty acids from the fat stores of the body.

Ketoacidosis has not decreased in frequency over the years. It is the leading cause of death in young diabetics and results in 4,000 deaths annually in the United States (Holman et al., 1983). Electrolyte abnormalities, shock, superinfection, and myocardial infarction can be produced by diabetic ketoacidosis; in addition, death may result from cerebral edema. Krane et al. (1985) found subclinical brain swelling on CT scans of all six of the children they studied immediately following treatment for diabetic ketoacidosis. This was originally thought to occur because of an osmotic shift of water from the vascular to the brain compartment during treatment. Originally, it was thought that idiogenetic osmoles in the brain were responsible. Arieff and Kleeman (1974), however, found that idiogenetic osmoles were not present in the brain during treatment of diabetic ketoacidosis. These authors suggested that cerebral edema likely arises because of a shift of potassium and water intracellularly during treatment. This finds some support in Tornheim's (1981) experiment in which he could not produce cerebral edema in the diabetic rat by hydration alone. The addition of insulin, however, was associated with cerebral edema. The practical message is that it is probably best to lower the serum glucose gradually.

Hyperglycemic, hyperosmolar, nonketotic coma accounts for between 10 and 33 percent of episodes of diabetic coma (Keller et al., 1975; Podolsky, 1978). It most commonly occurs after 75 years of age in individuals without a history of diabetes or in non–insulin-dependent diabetics (Grenfell, 1986). A variant occurred in the early days of hemodialysis and peritoneal dialysis (Potter, 1966). The use of phenytoin, which reduces the level of circulating insulin, or of corticosteroids, immunosuppressive drugs, or diuretics, which antagonize insulin's actions, may also be responsible in some patients. The serum glucose is usually greater than 50 mmol/L and the patients are seriously dehydrated; 30 percent are hypotensive (Grenfell, 1986).

In the treatment of this condition, it is important to replace fluid volume and to restore urine flow. This is best done with normal saline (Grenfell, 1986). The serum osmolality should not be lowered abruptly, as this will cause a shift of fluid from the vascular into the tissue compartment and a further drop in circulating blood volume (McCurdy, 1970). Once the volume has been replaced, the serum osmolality can be gradually returned to normal over 24 to 48 hours (Grenfell, 1986). Small doses of insulin should be used.

Lactic acidosis used to occur as a complication of phenformin, an oral hypoglycemic agent. This condition most commonly, but not exclusively, occurred in older individuals and carried a high mortality. Now lactic acidosis is most likely to occur as a complication of sepsis or circulatory failure.

The occurrence of uremia in diabetes is discussed under Diabetic Nephropathy, above. It is important to not be too parsimonious in the approach to the diabetic patient, in view of this association.

Diabetes mellitus is a widely accepted risk factor for ischemic stroke (Kannel, 1976; Schoenberg et al., 1980). For stroke to produce coma, the lesions should be in the vertebrobasilar territory, affecting the ascending reticular activating system from the midpontine tegmentum rostrally. Alternatively, there would have to be large, independent, bicerebral strokes. More commonly, hemispheric strokes are single and not coma producing in themselves unless complicated by brain swelling and herniation. According to Pulsinelli et al. (1982), the severity of the infarct is increased in the presence of hyperglycemia. It is probable that diabetes can act synergistically with the hypertension and lipid disturbances of renal disease (not necessarily renal failure) to aggravate atherosclerosis.

Diabetic Retinopathy

From a clinical (ophthalmological) viewpoint, diabetic retinopathy can be classified into simple and malignant categories. In simple diabetic retinopathy, there are microaneurysms, hemorrhages, waxy and cotton wool exudates, and venous abnormalities. Malignant retinopathy is largely dependent on neovascular formation. This can lead to proliferation of preretinal hemorrhage, fibrous tissue proliferation, retinal detachment, and secondary glaucoma (Beisswenger, 1976).

Hypoglycemia in Renal Failure

In addition to treatment-induced hypoglycemia mentioned under Diabetic Coma above, there are a number of reports of spontaneous hypoglycemia in patients with renal failure. In their series of 137 cases of hypoglycemia in 94 hospitalized adults, Fischer et al. (1986) found that renal insufficiency *unassociated* with diabetes was the second most frequent diagnosis to be associated with hypoglycemia. This may be severe enough to produce coma and convulsions and to cause permanent cerebral damage or death (Avram et al., 1984). Levels as low as 0.05 mmol/L (1 mg/dL) have been recorded (Fischer et al., 1986).

Clinical Features

The hypoglycemia is usually of the fasting (especially early morning) type, rather than reactive (Garber et al., 1974). Patients may be found in unexplained coma or may have altered mental status or drowsiness. As with other metabolic encephalopathies, the pupils and extraocular movements are spared, even if the patient shows decerebrate posturing (Plum and Posner, 1980). Recurrent attacks are common (Avram et al., 1984; Garber et al., 1974).

Clinical features or conditions associated with the development of hypoglycemia in uremic patients include septicemia (Miller et al., 1980; Walsh, 1984), cachexia and malnutrition (Block and Rubenstein, 1970; White and Kurtzman, 1971; Peitaman and Agarwal, 1977), and the concomitant use of a drug such as propranolol or metoprolol that can impair hepatic gluconeogenesis (Avram et al., 1984). Alcohol, aspirin, disopyramide and, of course, oral hypoglycemic agents used in the treatment of diabetes may also predispose to hypoglycemia (Editorial, 1986). It may occur immediately following hemodialysis when high glucose levels are used in the dialysate (Rigg and Bergu, 1967). Hypoglycemia may occur in uremic patients in the absence of these predisposing conditions, however. Improved control of the uremic condition by improved hemodialysis or renal transplantation may prevent further hypoglycemic episodes (White and Kurtzman, 1971).

The diagnosis depends on awareness of the entity. The differential diagnosis includes all the conditions that may cause impairment of consciousness or seizures in the uremic patient: uremic encephalopathy itself, fluid and electrolyte disturbances including dialysis dysequilibrium and hyponatremia, sepsis, hyperglycemia, altered drug handling, dialytic encephalopathy, subdural hematoma, stroke, and unrelated conditions.

Pathogenesis

There is considerable evidence that hepatic gluconeogenesis is impaired in uremia. Ritsky et al. (1978) reported four patients with chronic renal failure who developed hypoglycemia in association with a metabolic acidosis due to lactate, rather than the uremia. This was responsive to the administration of glucose, rather than to what should be glucose precursors for the liver, namely alanine, glycerol, and galactose. This is consistent with a hepatic defect in gluconeogenesis (Editorial, 1986).

An alternative or additional proposal is that there is a failure of substrate generation in uremia. Garber et al. (1974) describe a patient with diabetes mellitus and renal failure who developed profound hypoalaninemia followed by hypoglycemia. This patient was shown to have abnormally low rates for generation of alanine, which serves as a major substrate for glucose production (Felig et al., 1969).

Impaired glycogenolysis may play an added role in causing hypoglycemia in some patients with uremia (White and Kurtzman, 1971).

Although there is still some controversy about the relative importance of impaired hepatic gluconeogenesis, glycogenolysis, and substrate generation for hypoglycemia in uremia, it is possible each could play a role with variable emphasis in different patients. However, given an underlying predisposition for hypoglycemia, it is not difficult to see how sepsis, malnutrition, liver disease, and certain drugs may make hypoglycemia likely to occur.

Propranolol appears to cause a blockade in hepatic gluconeogenesis, which occurs despite normal receptor and normal cyclic adenosine monophosphate generation. Pun et al. (1984) found that serum glucose responses to glucagon were low in uremic patients treated with propranol. With metoprolol, this inhibition is relieved by dialysis, and the authors (Pun et al., 1985) suggest that an active metabolite of metoprolol was responsible, since metoprolol itself is not dialysable.

The hypoglycemia that occurs following hemodialysis with high glucose levels in the dialysate appears to be a different matter. It is likely a reactive type of hypoglycemia (Rigg and Bergu, 1967).

The mechanism for hypoglycemic brain dysfunction has been better clarified in recent years. It does not depend on reduced levels of high-energy phosphate compounds in the brain (Ferrendelli, 1974). The pattern of hypoglycemic brain damage with localization to the cerebral cortex and gray matter near CSF spaces has suggested the possibility of a neurotoxin. It has recently been shown that hypoglycemic brain damage in the rat striatum

can be prevented by blocking a particular type of glutamate receptor, the NMDA receptor (named after the ligand N-methyl-D-aspartate) (Wieloch, 1985). This gives support to the theory that excitotoxic transmitters are produced in hypoglycemia. There may be implications for limitation of brain damage using blockers of NMDA receptors that cross the blood-brain barrier.

Management

It is vital to consider hypoglycemia in uremic patients with CNS dysfunction. Because of the risk of recurrence of hypoglycemia and its significant morbidity and mortality, it is very important to look for predisposing factors such as drugs, malnutrition, and sepsis.

Diabetic Polyneuropathy

There is mounting evidence that the mechanism of diabetic neuropathy is multifocal ischemia to peripheral nerves. Dyck et al. (1985) have shown that the number of endothelial nuclei and the percentage of endoneurial capillaries that were closed were higher in nerves in diabetic patients with neuropathy than in those in diabetics without neuropathy. Moreover, these changes were clearly related to the severity of the neuropathy. In addition, a series of experiments on the microenvironment of the peripheral nerve by Low et al. (1987) has indicated that hyperglycemia generates increased endoneurial vascular resistance and reduced nerve blood flow. Whether this induces the pathological changes in capillaries is speculative. Nonetheless, endoneurial hypoxia, that is, lack of oxygen within the immediate environment of nerve fibers, is secondary to this decreased blood flow and increased endoneurial vascular resistance. This may impair axonal transport and sodium-potassium adenosine triphosphatase activity. Conduction velocity in peripheral nerves would thereby be reduced through either of these two mechanisms. It is felt that these pathological changes account for the generalized symmetrical motor and sensory polyneuropathy that is perhaps the commonest type of neuropathy in these patients.

However, many will also experience focal or multifocal neuropathies (Asbury, 1987). These may affect the cranial nerves, particularly the third cranial nerve. In the limb, the various components of the lumbosacral plexus, particularly the femoral nerve, may be involved. However, focal neuropathy may also occur in the distribution of the various nerve roots involving the trunk. The peripheral nerves are also unusually susceptible to compression. This is most likely to occur for the median nerve at the carpal tunnel, but also can occur for the ulnar nerve at the elbow and the common peroneal nerve at the fibular head.

Several quite distinct syndromes may occur. Diabetic amyotrophy (Asbury, 1987) presents with fairly rapidly progressive pain and weakness involving the thigh muscles. There is a syndrome of small fiber neuropathy (Asbury, 1987), in which very severe pain is accompanied by loss of pain and temperature sensation, with relative preservation of the other modalities but particular involvement of the autonomic nervous system. The latter may be manifest as a widespread disorder involving the heart and the various viscera, including the bladder and bowel. In the limbs, there may be patchy decreases or increases in sweating, and vascular autonomic changes.

We now know that all of these manifestations are potentially reversible to varying degrees. Diabetic amyotrophy is particularly likely to show substantial improvement. Moreover, the compressive neuropathies may be relieved by specific treatment, such as sectioning of the flexor retinaculum of the wrist for carpal tunnel syndrome. However, to what extent the achievement of relatively normal blood glucose levels truly affects the course of the neuropathy is not yet known.

Diabetic Polyneuropathy Versus Uremic Polyneuropathy

There are a number of differences between diabetic polyneuropathy and uremic polyneuropathy. The former is particularly likely to be manifest by focal neuropathy, compressive

palsies, and autonomic neuropathy. In contrast, uremic polyneuropathy is a relatively symmetrical disorder of motor and sensory fibers involving only the limbs and, except for a mild tendency to compressive neuropathies, usually without focal manifestations. However, standard motor and sensory nerve conduction studies may show similar abnormalities in the two neuropathies, since both show a combination of axonal degeneration and segmental demyelination in peripheral nerves. Thus, in both there will be mild to moderate reductions in conduction velocities and moderate reduction in the amplitudes of muscle and sensory compound action potentials. In diabetic neuropathy, however, there will more likely be evidence of focal or multifocal denervation of muscle in the limb and trunk muscles, but in uremic polyneuropathy any denervation will be present or most marked in the distal muscle groups. Electrophysiological signs of compression of the median nerve at the wrist, the ulnar nerve at the elbow, and the peroneal nerve at the fibular head are more likely in diabetic polyneuropathy. Formal tests of autonomic function have not shown the widespread and severe abnormalities in uremic patients that are found in diabetic patients.

A much more complex problem has been the effect on peripheral nerve of both diabetes mellitus and end-stage renal disease occurring in the same patient. Until recently, it was rare for this situation to arise, since the results of treating diabetic patients with chronic hemodialysis or intermittent peritoneal dialysis were quite poor. The results of transplantation were good if the kidney was from identical related donors, but in cadaveric transplantation the results have not been as good in diabetics as in nondiabetics (Najarian et al., 1979). However, recently it has been shown that diabetic patients do quite well on continuous ambulatory peritoneal dialysis (Amair et al., 1982). Good control of uremia and hypertension are obtained, and moreover, insulin can be administered reliably by the intraperitoneal route. Among 20 diabetics, Amair et al. (1982) found that, while this was a good form of treatment, in general the retinopathy, neuropathy, and osteodystrophy remained unchanged. Clinical observation and nerve conduction studies showed evidence of neuropathy in 15 of 20 patients, one of whom had severe polyneuropathy.

While both diabetic and uremic polyneuropathy have in common a combination of axonal degeneration and segmental demyelination in peripheral nerve, detailed electrophysiological studies have shown differences between the two neuropathies. Vibratory perception threshold increases with warming of the extremity in diabetic patients, but decreases in uremic patients (Tegnér, 1985). Also, collateral reinnervation of peripheral nerve is likely to occur as a reparative process in diabetic neuropathy but fails to occur in uremic neuropathy (Hansen and Ballantyne, 1978; Thiele and Stålberg, 1975; Konishi et al., 1982). On the other hand, both types of neuropathies show prolonged refractory periods and a "resistance" to nerve ischemia (Lowitzsch et al., 1979; Tackmann et al., 1974; 1975; Castaigne et al., 1972). Both vibratory perception and sensory compound action potentials tend to persist longer with nerve ischemia in both types of neuropathies. Mitz et al. (1984) found conduction velocities to be lower in chronic renal failure patients who had diabetes mellitus in comparison to such patients who did not.

The differences between these two neuropathies become especially clear when the effects of transplantation are considered. As discussed in Chapter 5, Solders et al. (1987), in a well-controlled study, showed that the polyneuropathy in diabetic patients with end-stage renal disease failed to improve not only in patients who had had renal transplantation, but in those who had combined renal and pancreatic transplantation. Thus, the polyneuropathy in such patients is presumably due almost entirely to the diabetes mellitus, and would seem to be remarkably resistant to treatment, even to restoration of normal blood glucose levels.

Defects of Neuromuscular Transmission

Defective neuromuscular transmission does not occur as a direct manifestation of uremic toxicity. However, it is an uncommon form of toxicity of aminoglycoside antibiotic drugs, which are frequently given for renal and other infections. The signs are those of generalized limb weakness, with reduced deep tendon reflexes. Repetitive stimulation studies of peripheral nerves will show an incrementing response, typical of a presynaptic defect in neuromuscular transmission (Swift, 1981). The condition will quickly resolve when the drug is discontinued.

An even rarer circumstance is the development of myasthenia after administration of high dosages of carnitine to lower elevated triglyceride levels (Bazzato et al., 1979). Elevated levels of magnesium may cause stupor, cardiac arrhythmias, and generalized muscle weakness, due to a presynaptic defect in neuromuscular transmission (Swift, 1979). The condition can be quickly resolved by stopping the drug. Intravenous calcium or 3,4-aminopyridine may be helpful, but dosages should be carefully regulated because of the renal failure.

Myopathy in Uremia

During renal failure in which there is a significant water-electrolyte disturbance, muscle weakness may develop, particularly in association with either hypo- or hyperkalemia. In those situations, muscle weakness occasionally occurs in acute attacks reminiscent of periodic paralysis, but in the former the serum potassium is abnormal between attacks, in contrast to the familial varieties of periodic paralysis (Jablecki, 1987).

Tetany is the result of lowered serum levels of calcium or magnesium, or of respiratory alkalosis. Hypocalcemia may occur in chronic renal failure from elevated levels of serum phosphate, which, in turn, induce calcium entry into bone and elevate parathyroid hormone levels. Hypocalcemia also occurs as a result of the kidney's inability to synthesize 1,25-dihydroxyvitamin D_3, leading to impaired reabsorption of calcium from the gut. In chronic renal failure, there is also poor mobilization of calcium salts from bone. However, tetany is rarely manifest in renal failure, possibly due to the associated acidosis; the condition is only likely to become manifest if patients are treated with large amounts of alkali. Serum levels of magnesium tend to be elevated in chronic renal failure, eliminating hypomagnesemia as a potential cause of tetany in these patients.

Tetany is clinically manifest as paresthesia, numbness and tingling, and light-headedness. The distal muscles go into sustained flexor, carpal, or pedal spasm. Laryngospasm may also occur and, in the most severe form, tetany is manifest as opisthotonic posturing of the body. Direct percussion of a peripheral nerve will induce contracture of the muscle it supplies (Chvostek's sign). Needle electromyography of muscle reveals spontaneous repetitive discharges appearing as double or triple discharges or multiple discharges whose components are typical of motor unit potentials. The reduction in extracellular calcium concentration induces excitability of the axonal membrane and decreased accommodation. Correction of hypocalcemia and the attendant alkalosis is the method of treatment.

Steroids may be used to treat various forms of primary renal disease, and in such a situation, myopathy may occur as a complication of treatment. Steroid myopathy is most likely to occur with the use of high dosages of steroids, particularly when halogenated synthetic steroids are used. Muscle weakness may be only mild, and the creatinine phosphokinase serum levels are not elevated. Needle electromyography reveals normal findings, except for some increase in the incidence of low-amplitude, polyphasic motor unit potentials. Muscle biopsy will reveal atrophy of type II fibers and accumulation of lipid droplets in type I fibers (Jablecki, 1987). There are a number of other medications (Lane and Mastaglia, 1978) and toxic substances that may induce myopathy, but these are unlikely to be encountered in renal failure.

Patients in end-stage renal disease may develop severe, generalized muscle wasting. This may be on the basis of cachexia (Jennekins, 1982). However, if sepsis has occurred, it may be on the basis of critical illness polyneur-opathy (Zochodne et al., 1987). Thus, electrophysiological studies and muscle biopsy may be required for diagnosis. If the myopathy is on the basis of cachexia, atrophy of type II fibers would be found. Critical illness polyneuropathy causes scattered or grouped small atrophic fibers to appear, typical of denervation of muscle.

The bone disease of end-stage renal disease, either due to secondary hyperparathyroidism or aluminum accumulation, may produce a distinctive myopathy. This is characterized by a painful wasting of muscles, usually in the proximal lower limbs, but occasionally in the proximal upper limbs (Figure 6.2). Needle electromyography reveals no clear-cut abnormalities. Creatine phosphokinase levels may be slightly increased, possibly due to cardiac disease (Medeiros et al., 1987). The muscle biopsy reveals atrophy of type II muscle fibers (Figure 6.3), as revealed in an excellent study and review of the literature by Bautista et al. (1983). This change is commonly seen in disuse atrophy of muscle (Banker and Engel, 1986). A similar myopathy is produced in patients with primary hyperparathyroidism (Patten et al., 1974). The myopathy usually resolves if the bone disease can be brought under control.

Myoglobinuria

Myoglobinuria is one of the many important causes of acute renal failure. It has numerous etiologies that can be broadly grouped into genetic and metabolic defects of muscle; excessive heat and exercise; extreme cold; a wide variety of systemic infections; crush and ischemia of muscle; drugs and toxins, including alcohol; and electrolyte and water disturbances, particularly severe hypokalemia (Penn, 1986). The main clinical picture is largely determined by the underlying cause. The renal threshold for myoglobin is often low, so this substance is cleared rapidly by the kidney. Thus, while the urine is burgundy red in color, the serum may simply be amber to tan in color, but never pinkish as in hemolysis. Heme proteins can be detected in the urine by testing

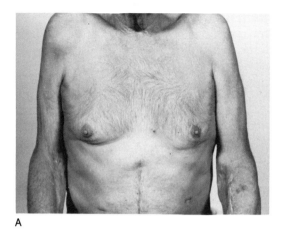

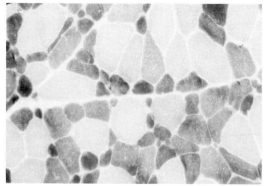

Figure 6.3. Selective atrophy of type II fibers (stained dark). Angulated, rounded, and polygonal shapes are seen. Adenosine triphosphatase pH 9.4 (original magnification, ×80). (Reprinted with permission from Bautista et al., 1983.)

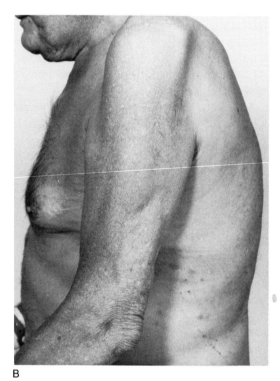

Figure 6.2 A and B. Severe muscle wasting in a 67-year-old man receiving chronic hemodialysis for seven years. It was associated with underlying pain secondary to progressive bone disease. He also had a progressive dementia, but aluminum intoxication was never proven. While he had a mild uremic polyneuropathy, needle electromyography of shoulder girdle muscles revealed only an increased proportion of polyphasic units, consistent with a primary myopathy.

with peroxidase-sensitive chromagens. Myoglobin can be specifically identified by an immunochemical method. In addition to the abnormal color of the urine, it will characteristically lack red blood cells but may contain golden brown pigmented casts. The muscles have been traditionally described as weak, swollen, and painful, but they may be surprisingly normal on examination. The creatine phosphokinase level is invariably elevated.

The ultimate prognosis largely depends on the nature of the underlying disease, but the degree of recovery of muscle strength is often good. The major complication is acute renal failure. The precise mechanism by which this occurs is not well understood, although precipitation of protein with blockage of renal tubules is still the favored mechanism. This complication developed in 19 of 44 patients with myoglobinuria at the Hospital of the University of Pennsylvania (Grossman et al., 1974). The renal disorder is characterized by oliguria, orthotolidine-positive urine, pigmented granular casts in the urinary sediment, very high serum urate and creatinine concentrations, and a resulting low ratio of blood urea nitrogen to creatinine. Hyperkalemia may be high enough to threaten cardiac arrest. Hypocalcemia may occur at the same time, but it is later followed by hypercalcemia as calcium is released from necrotic muscle. These patients should be promptly hydrated with alkaline fluids and diuresis instituted with mannitol or other osmotic diuretics. If the renal failure is severe, some form of dialysis will be required. Penn (1986) has suggested that plasmapheresis might theoretically be of value.

Acquired Immune Deficiency Syndrome

There is increasing awareness of the association of renal failure with acquired immune deficiency syndrome (AIDS). Rao et al. (1987) reported 78 cases of renal failure in 750 patients with AIDS (10.8 percent) attending two hospitals in New York City. Renal syndromes with AIDS can be divided into four groups (Rao et al., 1987):

> Group 1 contains patients with acute reversible renal failure probably secondary to allergic, toxic and ischemic factors. This group has the best prognosis, with survival for 10–24 months after recovery. Short term dialysis, if warranted by the severity of the renal failure, appears to be beneficial.
>
> Group 2 with AIDS-related nephropathy constitutes the largest group. Patients present with massive proteinuria, azotemia, or both and most develop irreversible renal failure. Such patients develop severe, progressive, refractory cachexia and show a median survival of only 1.4 months whether dialysis is used or not.
>
> Group 3 patients are found to have AIDS while they are being treated with maintenance hemodialysis for chronic renal failure. It is unlikely these patients acquired AIDS as a result of nosocomial infection. Survival in this group was also very short, with a median of 1.0 months, despite intensive nutritional support and continued hemodialysis.
>
> Group 4 patients constitute a poorly defined population with glomerular lesions suggestive of immune-complex glomerulonephritis. This group is small and needs further study to determine prognosis.

These observations raise important considerations regarding management. In Group 1 patients, intensive medical support, including hemodialysis, appears to be beneficial, while in Groups II and III, such measures are of

Table 6.6. Neurological Complications of Human Immunodeficiency Virus

	Incidence
Central Nervous System	
Encephalopathy	
Aids dementia complex	63%
Cerebral toxoplasmosis	5%
Cryptococcal meningitis	5%
Lymphoma—primary or secondary	2%
Progressive multifocal leukoencephalopathy	2%
Cytomegalovirus infections	?
Herpes simplex encephalitis	—
Varicella—Zoster virus	—
Epstein-Barr virus	—
Cerebrovascular disease	12%
Meningovascular syphilis	—
Other infection	
Myelopathy	22%
Peripheral Nervous System	
Distal symmetrical peripheral neuropathy	
Inflammatory demyelinating polyradiculoneuropathy	
Mononeuropathy multiplex	
Progressive polyradiculopathy	

dubious value. Rao et al. (1987) use the analogy of offering hemodialysis and vigorous support to individuals with terminal malignancies. Such decisions clearly must be individualized. The nervous system is involved in approximately 40 percent of patients with AIDS (Bredesen et al., 1989). It is outside the scope of this book to discuss such involvement, but we have included a table (Table 6.6) to illustrate the type and relative incidence. The subject has been recently reviewed by Bredesen et al. (1989). It will be noted that the CNS is involved approximately 60 percent of the time, and the peripheral nervous system 15 percent (Miller et al., 1988). See Chapter 8 for a brief discussion of AIDS in relationship to renal transplantation.

References

Adachi M, Rosenblum WI, Feigin I. Hypertensive and cerebral edema. J Neurol Neurosurg Psychiatry 1966;29:451–455.

Adams RD, Cammermeyer J, Fitzgerald PJ. The neuropathological aspects of thrombocytic acroangiothrombosis. J Neurol Neurosurg Psychiatry 1948;11:27–43.

Adams RD. Case records of the Massachusetts General Hospital (case 3). N Engl J Med 1973;288:150–156.

Adams RD. Diseases of muscle. 3rd ed. Hagerstown, MD: Harper & Row, 1975.

Adams HP, Dawson G, Coffman TJ, Corry RJ. Stroke in renal transplant recipients. Arch Neurol 1986;43:113–115.

Albers JW. Inflammatory demyelinating polyradiculopathy. In: Brown WF, Bolton CF, eds. Clinical electromyography. Boston: Butterworths, 1987:209–244.

Amair P, Khanna R, Leibel B, et al. Continuous ambulatory peritoneal dialysis in diabetics with end-stage renal disease. N Engl J Med 1982;306:625–630.

Anderson JM, Jamieson DG, Jefferson JM. Non-healing granuloma and the nervous system. Q J Med 1975;174:309–323.

Andrianakos AA, Duffy J, Suzuki M, Sharp JT. Transverse myelopathy in systemic lupus erythematosus: report of three cases and review of the literature. Ann Intern Med 1975;83:616–624.

Arieff AI, Kleeman CR. Cerebral edema in diabetic comas. II. Effects of hyperosmolality, hyperglycemia and insulin in diabetic rabbits. J Clin Endocrinol Metab 1974;38:1057–1067.

Arkin A. A clinical and pathological study of periarteritis nodosa: a report of five cases, one histologically healed. Am J Pathol 1930;6:401–420.

Asbury AK. Focal and multifocal neuropathies of diabetes. In: Dyck PJ, Thomas PK, Asbury AK, et al., eds. Diabetic neuropathy. Philadelphia: WB Saunders, 1987:45–55.

Avram MM, Wolf RE, Gan A, et al. Uremic hypoglycemia: a preventable life-threatening complication. NY Stat J Med 1984;84:593–596.

Bacon PA. Evolving concepts in vasculitis. Q J Med [New Ser] 1985;57:609–610.

Badran RHA, Weir RJ, McGuiness JB. Hypertension and headache. Scott Med J 1970;15:48–51.

Bagdade JD, Porte D, Bierman EI. Hypertriglyceridemia: a metabolic consequence of chronic renal failure. N Engl J Med 1968;279:181–185.

Bale JF, Brasher C, Siegler L. CNS manifestations of the hemolytic-uremic syndrome. Am J Dis Child 1980;134:869–872.

Banker BQ, Engel AG. Basic reactions of muscle. In: Engel AG, Banker BQ, eds. Myology. Vol 1. New York: McGraw-Hill, 1986:851.

Barnett HJM, Mohr JP, Stein BM, Yatsu FM. Stroke: pathophysiology, diagnosis and management. New York: Churchill-Livingstone, 1986:767,1092–1093, 1096.

Bautista J, Gil-Necija E, Castilla J, et al. Dialysis myopathy: report of 13 cases. Acta Neuropathol (Berl) 1983;61:71–75.

Bazzato G, Mezzina C, Ciman M, Guarnieri G. Myasthenialike syndrome associated with carnitine in patients on long-term hemodialysis. Lancet 1979;1:1041–1042.

Behrman RE, Vaughan VC. Nelson's textbook of pediatrics. 13th ed. Philadelphia: WB Saunders, 1987:1124–1125.

Beisswenger PJ. Neuropathic and vascular complications occurring in diabetes. Postgrad Med 1976; 59:169–174.

Bernardi D, Ferreri A, Moretti P, et al. Carotid artery atherosclerotic disease assessed by flow velocity wave form analysis in hemodialyzed normotensive and hypertensive patients. Nephron 1986;44:180–185.

Bihari D, Smithies M, Gimson A, Tinker J. The effects of vasodilation with prostacyclin on oxygen delivery and uptake in critically ill patients. N Engl J Med 1987;317:397–402.

Binder H, Gerstenbrand F. Scleroderma. In: Vinken PJ, Bruyn GW, eds. Handbook of clinical neurology. Vol 39, Part 2. Neurological manifestations of systemic diseases. Amsterdam: North-Holland, 1980: 355–378.

Binswanger O. Die Abgrenzung der allgemeinen progressiven Paralyse. Klin Wochenschr 1894;31:1180–1186.

Bitter T. Systemic lupus erythematosus. Rheumatology 1974;5:49–243.

Block MB, Rubenstein AH. Spontaneous hypoglycemia in diabetic patients with renal insufficiency. JAMA 1970;213:1863–1866.

Blohme I, Ahlmen J. Late complications after successful renal transplantation. Scand J Urol Nephrol [Suppl] 1977;42:173–175.

Bluestein HG, Zvaifler NJ. Brain-reactive lymphocytotoxic antibodies in the serum of patients with systemic lupus erythematosus. J Clin Invest 1976;57:509–516.

Bolton CF, Gilbert JJ, Hahn AF, Sibbald WJ. Polyneuropathy in critically ill patients. J Neurol Neurosurg Psychiatry 1984;47:1223–1231.

Bolton CF, Laverty DA, Brown JD, et al. Critically ill polyneuropathy: electrophysiological studies and differentiation from Guillain-Barré syndrome. J Neurol Neurosurg Psychiatry 1986;49:563–573.

Borzotta AP, Polk HC. Multiple system organ failure. Surg Clin North Am 1983;63:315–336.

Bredesen DE, Levy RM, Rosenblum ML. Human immunodeficiency virus-related neurological dysfunction. In: Aminoff MJ, ed. Neurology and General Medicine. The Neurological Aspects of Medical Disorders, Chapter 37, 1989. Churchill-Livingstone, New York;pp.673–689.

Bresnihan B. CNS lupus. Clin Rheum Dis 1982;8:183–195.

Bronte-Stewart B, Heptinstall RH. The relationship between experimental hypertension and cholesterol-induced atheroma in rabbits. J Pathol Bacteriol 1954;68:407–417.

Brunner FP, Brynger H. Chantler C, et al. Combined report on regular dialysis and transplantation in Europe. Proc Eur Dial Transplant Assoc 1979;16:3–73.

Byrom FB. The pathogenesis of hypertensive encephalopathy and its relation to the malignant phase of hypertension. Experimental evidence from the hypertensive rat. Lancet 1954;2:201–211.

Cameron JS. Acute renal failure—the continuing challenge. Q J Med 1986;59:228,337–343.

Caplan LP, Schoene WC. Clinical features of subcortical arteriosclerotic encephalopathy (Binswanger's disease). Neurology 1978;28:1206–1215.

Cassaretto AA, Marchiuro JC, Bagdade JD. Hyperlipidemia following renal transplant. Trans Am Soc Artif Intern Organs 1973;19:154.

Castaigne P, Cathala H-P, Beaussart-Boulengé L, Petrover M. Effect of ischaemia on peripheral nerve function in patients with chronic renal failure undergoing dialysis treatment. J Neurol Neurosurg Psychiatry 1972;35:631–637.

Castaigne P, Lhermitte F, Gautier J-C, et al. Internal carotid artery occlusion. A study of 61 instances in 50 patients with post-mortem data. Brain 1970;93:231–258.

Cavanagh JB. Liver bypass and the glia. In: Plum F, ed. Brain dysfunction in metabolic disorders. Res Publ Assoc Res Nerve Ment Dis 1974;53:13–38.

Chaudry IH, Schleck S, Clemens MG, et al. Altered hepatocellular active transport: an early change in peritonitis. Arch Surg 1982;117:151–157.

Cheson BD, Bluming AZ, Alroy J. Cogan's syndrome: asystemic vasculitis. Am J Med 1976;60:549–555.

Chester EM, Agamanolis DP, Banker BQ, Victor M. Hypertensive encephalopathy: a clinicopathological study of 20 cases. Neurology 1978;28:928–939.

Chiappa K, Young R. The EEG as a definitive diagnostic tool in the course of Creutzfeldt-Jakob disease. Electroencephalogr Clin Neurophysiol 1978;45:26.

Clarke E. Spinal cord involvement in multiple myelomatosis. Brain 1956;79:332–348.

Clarke E, Murphy EA. Neurological manifestations resulting from malignant hypertension. Br Med J 1956;2:1319–1326.

Clyne N, Lins L-E, Pehrsson SK. Occurrence and significance of heart disease in uremia: an autopsy study. Scand J Urol Nephrol 1986;20:307–311.

Cogan DG, Kubik CS, Smith WL. Unilateral internuclear ophthalmoplegia: report of eight cases with one post-mortem study. Arch Ophthalmol 1950;44:783–796.

Conn DL, Dyck PJ. Angiopathic neuropathy in connective tissue diseases. In: Dyck PJ, Thomas PK, Lambert EH, Bunge R, eds. Peripheral neuropathy. Philadelphia: WB Saunders, 1984:2039.

Cooper RA, Bunn HF. Hemolytic anemias. In: Braunwald E, Isselbacher KJ, Petersdorf RG, et al., eds. Harrison's principles of internal medicine. 11th ed. New York: McGraw-Hill, 1987:1506–1518.

De Fronzo RA, Andres R, Edgar P, Walker WG. Carbohydrate metabolism in uremia: a review. Medicine 1973;52:469–481.

Delgado-Escueta AV, Wasterlain C, Treiman DM, Porter RJ. Status epilepticus: mechanisms of brain damage and treatment, New York: Raven Press, 1883:539.

De Reuck J, Crevits L, de Coster W, et al. Pathogenesis of Binswanger's chronic progressive subcortical encephalopathy. Neurology (Minneap) 1980;30:920–928.

Devinsky O, Petito CK, Alonso DR. Clinical and neuropathological findings in systemic lupus erythematosus: the role of vasculitis, heart emboli and thrombocytopenic purpura. Ann Neurol 1988;23:380–384.

Dintenfass L, Ibels LS. Blood viscosity factors and occlusive arterial disease in renal transplant recipients. Nephron 1975;15:456–465.

Dolin S, Dewar JP. Extramedullary plasmacytoma. Am J Pathol 1956;32:83–103.

Drachman D. Neurological complications of Wegener's granulomatosis. Arch Neurol 1963;8:145–155.

Dubois EL, Tuffanelli D. Clinical manifestation of systemic lupus erythematosus. JAMA 1964;190:104–111.

Dyck PJ, Hansen S, Karnes J, et al. Capillary number and percentage closed in human diabetic sural nerve. Proc Natl Acad Sci USA 1985;82:2513–2517.

Earnest M, Fahn S, Karp J, et al. Normal pressure hydrocephalus and hypertensive cerebrovascular disease. Arch Neurol 1974;31:262–266.

Editorial. Uraemic hypoglycemia. Lancet 1986;1:660–661.

Evans WE, Manninen DL, Garrison LP, et al. The quality of life of patients with end-stage renal disease. N Engl J Med 1985;312:553–558.

Fagerburg SE. Diabetic neuropathy: a clinical and histologic study on the significance of vascular affections. Acta Med Scand 1959;164(Suppl 345):1–80.

Feigin I, Popoff N. Neuropathological observations on cerebral edema. Arch Neurol 1962;6:151–160.

Feigin I, Popoff N. Neuropathological observations on cerebral edema: the relation to trauma, hypertensive disease and Binswanger's encephalopathy. J Neuropathol Exp Neurol 1963;22:500–511.

Felig P, Owen OE, Wahren J, Cahill GC Jr. Amino acid metabolism during prolonged starvation. J Clin Invest 1969;48:584–594.

Ferrendelli JA. Cerebral utilization of nonglucose substrates and their effect in hypoglycemia. In: Plum F, ed. Brain dysfunction in metabolic disorders. Res Publ Assoc Res Nerv Ment Dis 1974;53:113–123.

Fischer JE. False neurotransmitters and hepatic coma. In: Plum F, ed. Brain dysfunction in metabolic disorders. Res Publ Assoc Res Nerve Ment Dis 1974;53:53–73.

Fischer KF, Lees JA, Newman JH. Hypoglycemia in hospitalized patients: causes and outcomes. N Engl J Med 1986;315:1245–1250.

Fisher CM. The pathological and clinical aspects of thalamic hemorrhage. Trans Am Neurol Assoc 1959;84:56–59.

Fisher CM, Cole M. Homolateral ataxia and crural paresis: a vascular syndrome. J Neurol Neurosurg Psychiatry 1965;12:48–55.

Fisher CM. A lacunar stroke: the dysarthria–clumsy hand syndrome. Neurology 1967;17:614–617.

Fisher CM. Capsular infarcts: the underlying vascular lesion. Arch Neurol 1979;36:65–73.

Ford RG, Siekert RG. Central nervous system manifestations of periarteritis nodosa. Neurology 1965;15:114–122.

Foster DB, Malamud N. Periarteritis nodosa: a clinicopathological reference to the central nervous system, a preliminary report. Univ Hosp Bull Ann Arbor 1941;7:102–124.

Foster DW. Diabetes mellitus. In: Braunwald E, Isselbacher KJ, Petersdorf RG, et al., eds. Harrison's principles of internal medicine. 11th ed. New York: McGrow-Hill, 1987:1778–1797.

Freund H, Atamian S, Holroyde J, Fischer JE. Plasma amino acids as predictors of the severity and outcome of sepsis. Ann Surg 1979;190:571–576.

Garber AJ, Bier DM, Cryer PE, Pagliara AS. Hypoglycemia in compensated renal insufficiency: substrate limitations of gluconeogenesis. Diabetes 1974;23:982–986.

Garraway WM, Whisnant JP, Kurland LT, O'Fallen WM. Changing pattern of cerebral infarction: 1947–1974. Stroke 1979;10:657–663.

Gianantonio CA, Vitacco M, Mendilarzu F, et al. Hemolytic-uremic syndrome. Nephron 1973;11:174–192.

Gilliland BC. Progressive systemic sclerosis (diffuse scleroderma). In: Braunwald E, Isselbacher KJ, Petersdorf RG, et al., eds. Harrison's principles of internal medicine. 11th ed. New York: McGraw-Hill, 1987:1428–1432.

Glaser GH. Collagen diseases and the nervous system. Med Clin North Am 1963;41:1475–1495.

Gloor P, Kalabay O, Giard N. The electroencephalogram in diffuse encephalopathies: EEG correlates of gray and white matter lesions. Brain 1968;91:779–802.

Goetz CG. Polyarteritis nodosa. In: Vinken PJ, Bruyn GW, eds. Handbook of clinical neurology. Vol 39, Part 2. Neurological manifestations of systemic diseases. Amsterdam: North-Holland, 1980:295–311.

Gordon RM, Silverstein A. Neurologic manifestations of progressive systemic sclerosis. Arch Neurol 1970;22:126–134.

Green RN. The unconscious diabetic. Can Fam Physician 1976;22:47–49.

Grenfell A. Acute renal failure in diabetics. Intensive Care Med 1986;12:6–12.

Griffith JG Jr. Involvement of the facial nerve in malignant hypertension. Arch Neurol Psychiatry 1933;29:1195–1202.

Grigor R, Edmonds J, Lewkonia R, et al. Systemic lupus erythematosus: a prospective analysis. Ann Rheum Dis 1978;37:121–128.

Grossman RA, Hamilton RW, Morse BM, et al. Nontraumatic rhabdomyolysis and acute renal failure. N Engl J Med 1974;291:807–811.

Haas LF. Stroke as an early manifestation of systemic lupus erythematosus. J Neurol Neurosurg Psychiatry 1982;45:554–556.

Hachinski VC, Lassen NA, Marshall J. Multi-infarct dementia: a cause of mental deterioration in the elderly. Lancet 1974;2:207–210.

Hachinski VC, Norris JW. The acute stroke. Philadelphia: FA Davis, 1985:141–163.

Hansen S, Ballantyne JP. A quantitative electrophysiological study of uremic neuropathy. Diabetic and renal neuropathies compared. J Neurol Neurosurg Psychiatry 1978;41:128–134.

Harris EN, Boey MI, Mackworth-Young CG, et al. Anticardiolipin antibodies: detection by radioimmunoassay and association with thrombosis in systemic lupus erythematosus. Lancet 1983;2:1211–1214.

Harris EN, Hughes GRV. Cerebral infarction in systemic lupus erythematosus. Clin Exp Rheumatol 1984;2:47–51.

Haust MD. The morphogenesis and date of potential and early atherosclerotic lesions in man. Hum Pathol 1971;2:1–29.

Haynes BF, Fishman ML, Fauci AS, Wolff WM. The ocular manifestations of Wegener's granulomatosis. Am J Med 1977;63:131–141.

Higgins MR, Grace M, Dossetor JB. Survival of patients treated for end-stage renal disease by dialysis and transplantation. Can Med Assoc J 1977;117:880–883.

Hollenberg NK. Vascular injury to the kidney. In: Braunwald E, Isselbacher KJ, Petersdorf RG, et al., eds. Harrison's principles of internal medicine. 11th ed. New York: McGraw-Hill, 1987:1200–1205.

Holman RC, Herron CA, Sinnock P. Epidemiologic characteristics of mortality from diabetes with acidosis or coma, United States, 1970–78. Am J Public Health 1983;73:1169–1173.

Hudson AJ, Hyland HH. Hypertensive cerebrovascular disease: a clinical and pathologic review of 100 cases. Arch Intern Med 1958;49:1049–1072.

Hughes W, Dodson MCH, MacLennan DC. Chronic cerebral hypertensive disease. Lancet 1954;2:770–774.

Ibels LS, Stewart JH, Mahony JF, et al. Deaths from occlusive arterial disease in renal allograft recipients. Br Med J 1974;3:552–554.

Ibels LS, Simons LA, King JO, et al. Studies on the nature and causes of hyperlipidemia in uremia, maintenance hemodialysis and renal transplantation. Q J Med [New Ser 44] 1975;176:601–614.

Ingelfinger JR, Grupe WE, Levey RH. Post-transplant hypertension in the absence of rejection or recurrent disease. Clin Nephrol 1981;15:235–239.

Jablecki CK. Myopathies. In: Brown WF, Bolton CF, eds. Clinical electromyography. Boston: Butterworths, 1987:385–416.

Jackson AJ, Gilbert JJ, Young GB, Bolton CF. The encephalopathy of sepsis. Can J Neurol Sci 1985;12:303–307.

Jefferson A. Hypertensive cerebral vascular disease and intracranial tumor. Q J Med 1955;24:245–268.

Jellinek EH, Painter M, Prineas J, Russell RR. Hypertensive encephalopathy with cortical disorders of vision. Q J Med 1964;33:239–256.

Jennekins FGI. Disuse, cachexia and aging. In: Mastaglia FL, Walton J, eds. Skeletal muscle pathology. London: Churchill-Livingstone, 1982:605.

Johnson RT, Richardson EP Jr. The neurological manifestations of systemic lupus erythematosus: a clinical-pathological study of 24 cases and review of the literature. Medicine 1968;47:337–369.

Kaladelfos G, Edwards KDG. Increased prevalence of coronary heart disease in analgesic nephropathy: relations to hypertension, hypertriglyceridemia and combined hyperlipidemia. Nephron 1976;162:388–400.

Kannel WB. Epidemiology of cerebrovascular disease. In: Ross Russell RW, ed. Cerebral arterial disease. London: Churchill-Livingstone, 1976:1–23.

Keller V, Berger W, Troug P. Course and prognosis of 86 episodes of diabetic coma: a five year experience with a uniform schedule of treatment. Diabetologia 1975;11:93–100.

Kelly JJ. Polyneuropathies associated with malignancies and plasma cell dyscrasias. In: Brown WF, Bolton CF, eds. Clinical electromyography. Boston: Butterworths, 1987:314–317.

Kernohan JW, Woltman HW. Periarteritis nodosa: a clinicopathologic study with special reference to the nervous system. Arch Neurol 1938;7:655–686.

Khauli RB, Novick AC, Steinmuller DR, et al. Comparison of renal transplantation and dialysis in rehabilitation of diabetic end-stage renal disease patients. Urology 1986;27:521–525.

Kimmelstein P, Wilson C. Intercapillary lesions in the glomeruli of the kidney. Am J Pathol 1936;12:83–98.

Kinkaid-Smith PJ, McMichael J, Murphy EA. The clinical course and pathology of hypertension with papilloedema (malignant hypertension). Q J Med 1958;27:117–153.

Kinkel WR, Jacobs L. Computerized axial transverse tomography in cerebrovascular disease. Neurology 1976;26:924–930.

Kjellstrand CM, Shideman JR, Simmons RL, et al. Renal transplantation in insulin-dependent diabetic patients. Kidney Int 1974;6(Suppl 1):S21–S22.

Konishi T, Hiroshi N, Motomura S. Single fiber electromyography in chronic renal failure. Muscle Nerve 1982;5:458–461.

Krane EJ, Roackoff MA, Wallman JD, Wolfsldorf JI. Subclinical brain swelling in children during treatment of diabetic ketoacidosis. N Engl J Med 1985;312:1147–1151.

Krolewski AS, Warram JH, Christlieb AR, et al. The changing natural history of nephropathy in type I diabetes. Am J Med 1985;78:785–794.

Kubisz P, Parizek M, Seghier F, et al. Relationship between platelet aggregation and plasma β-thromboglobulin levels in arteriovascular and renal diseases. Atherosclerosis 1985;55:363–368.

Lacombe M. Arterial stenosis complicating allotransplantation in man. A study of 38 cases. Ann Surg 1975;181:283–288.

Lampert PW, Oldstone MBA. Host immunoglobulin G and complement deposits in the choroid plexus during spontaneous immune complex disease. Science 1973;180:408–410.

Lane RJM, Mastaglia FL. Drug-induced myopathies in man. Lancet 1978;1:562–566.

Leavitt RY, Fauci AS. Polyangiitis overlap syndrome. Classification and prospective clinical experience. Am J Med 1986;81:79–85.

Lee JE, Haynes JM. Carotid arteritis and cerebral infarction due to scleroderma. Neurology 1967;17:18–22.

Levitt MF, Altchek A. Hypertension and toxemia of pregnancy. In: Rovinsky JJ, Guttmacher AF, eds. Medical, surgical and gynecological complications of pregnancy. Baltimore: Williams & Wilkins, 1965;76–110.

Lewis BI, Sinton DW, Nott JR. Central nervous system involvement in disorders of collagen. Arch Intern Med 1954;93:315–327.

Lhermitte F, Gautier JC, Derouesné C, Guiraud B. Ischemic accidents in middle cerebral artery territory. Arch Neurol 1968;19:248–256.

Lim L, Ron MA, Ormerod IEC, et al. Psychiatric and neurological manifestations in systemic lupus erythematosus. Q J Med 1988;66:27–38.

Lindner A, Charra B, Sherrard DJ, Scribner BH. Accelerated atherosclerosis in prolonged maintenance hemodialysis. N Engl J Med 1974;290:697–701.

Lindstrom BJ. Late complications after primary renal transplantation. Scand J Urol Nephrol 1977;42 (Suppl):165.

Loizou LA, Jefferson JM, Smith WT. Subcortical arteriosclerotic encephalopathy (Binswanger's type) and cortical infarcts in a young, normotensive patient. J Neurol Neurosurg Psychiatry 1982;45:409–417.

Lovshin LL, Kernohan JW. Peripheral neuritis in periarteritis nodosa. Arch Intern Med 1948;82:321–328.

Low PA, Tuck RR, Takeuchi M. Nerve microenvironment in diabetic neuropathy. In: Dyck PJ, Thomas PK, Asbury, et al., eds. Diabetic neuropathy. Philadelphia: WB Saunders, 1987:266–278.

Lowitzsch K, Göhring U, Hecking E, Köhler H. Refractory period, sensory conduction velocity and vibration before and after haemodialysis. Acta Neurol Scand 1979;60(Suppl 73):133.

Lucas CE. Renal response to acute injury and sepsis. Surg Clin North Am 1976;56:953–975.

Lundin AP, Friedman EA. Vascular consequences of maintenance hemodialysis—an unproven case. Nephron 1978;21:177–180.

Mackenzie ET, Strandgaard S, Graham DI, et al. Effects of acutely induced hypertension in cats on pial arteriolar caliber, local cerebral blood flow, and the blood-brain barrier. Circ Res 1976;39:33–41.

Maher ER, Smyth-Walsh B, Pugh S, et al. Aortic and mitral valve calcification in patients with end-stage renal disease. Lancet 1987;2:875–877.

Mahony JF, Sheil AGR, Etheridge SB, et al. Delayed complications of renal transplantation and their prevention. Med J Aust 1982;2:426–429.

Makovi C, Williams CL, Roman J. Polycythemia of renal transplantation. NC Med J 1980;41:23–25.

Mannik M, Gilliland BC. Systemic lupus erythematosus. In: Petersdorf RG, Adams RD, Braunwald E, et al., eds. Harrison's principles of internal medicine. 10th ed. New York: McGraw-Hill, 1983:387–391.

McCurdy DK. Hyperosmolar hyperglycaemic non-ketotic diabetic coma. Med Clin North Am 1970;54:683–699.

McGonigle RJS, Trafford JAP, Bewick M, Parsons V. Hypertensive encephalopathy complicating renal artery stenosis. Postgrad Med J 1984;60:356–358.

Medeiros LJ, Schotte D, Gersib B. Reliability and significance of increased kinase MB iso-enzyme in the serum of uremic patients. Am J Clin Pathol 1987;87:103–108.

Mela L. Direct and indirect effects of endotoxin on mitochondrial function. Prog Clin Biol Res 1981;62:15–21.

Mendelsohn DB, Hertzanu Y, Chaitowitz B, Cartwright JD. Cranial CT in the haemolytic uraemic syndrome. J Neurol Neurosurg Psychiatry 1984;47:876–878.

Meyer JS, Rogers RL, Mortel KF, Judd BW. Hyperlipidemia is a risk factor for decreased cerebral perfusion and stroke. Arch Neurol 1987;44:418–422.

Miller RG, Parry GJ, Pfaeffl W, Lang W, Lippert R, Kiprov D. The spectrum of peripheral neuropathy associated with ARC and AIDS. Muscle Nerve 1988;11:857–863.

Miller SI, Wallace RJ, Musher DM, et al. Hypoglycemia as a manifestation of sepsis. Am J Med 1980;68:649–654.

Mitchell JRA, Schwartz CJ. Arterial disease. Oxford: Blackwell Scientific, 1965.

Mitz M. Benedetto MD, Klingbeil GE, et al. Neuropathy in end-stage renal disease secondary to primary renal disease and diabetes. Arch Phys Med Rehabil 1984;65:235–238.

Mohr JP. Lacunes. Neurol Clin 1983;1:201–221.

Mohri H, Noguchi T, Kodama F, et al. Acquired von Willebrand disease due to inhibitor of human myeloma protein specific for von Willebrand factor. Am J Clin Pathol 1987;87:663–668.

Monier-Vinard R, Puech P. Nephrite chronique et paralysie faciale. Bull Mem Soc Hop Paris 1930;4:977–980.

Moore S. Atheroma. In: Harrison MJG, Dyken ML, eds. Cerebral vascular disease. Boston: Butterworths 1983:3–26.

Moschowitz E. An acute febrile pleiochromic anemia with hyaline thrombosis of the terminal arterioles and capillaries. An undescribed disease. Arch Intern Med 1925;36:89–93.

Nag S, Robertson DM, Dinsdale HB. Cerebral cortical changes in acute experimental hypertension. An ultrastructural study. Lab Invest 1977;36:105–161.

Najarian JS, Sutherland DER, Simmons RL, et al. Ten year experience with renal transplantation in juvenile onset diabetes. Ann Surg 1979;190:487–500.

Nordoy A. The interaction of lipids, platelets and endothelial cells in thrombogenesis. Acta Med Scand 1980;208(Suppl):208–220.

Nossel H. Disorders of blood coagulation factors. In: Petersdorf RG, Adams RD, Braunwald E, et al., eds. Harrison's principles of internal medicine. 10th ed. New York: McGraw-Hill, 1983:1905–1908.

O'Connor JF. Psychoses associated with systemic lupus erythematosus. Ann Intern Med 1959;51:526–530.

Onoyama K, Kumagai H, Miischima T, et al. Incidence

of strokes and its prognosis in patients on maintenance hemodialysis. Jpn Heart J 1986;27:685–691.

Oppenheimer BS, Fishberg AM. Hypertensive encephalopathy. Arch Intern Med 1928;41:264–278.

Oppenheimer S, Hoffbrand BI. Optic neuritis and myelopathy in systemic lupus erythematosus. Can J Neurol Sci 1986;13:129–132.

Patten GM, Bilezikian JP, Mallette LE. Neuromuscular disease in primary hyperparathyroidism. Ann Intern Med 1974;80:182–193.

Peitaman SJ, Agarwal BN. Spontaneous hypoglycemia in end-stage renal failure. Nephron 1977;19:131–139.

Penn AS. Myoglobinuria. In: Engel AG, Banker BQ, eds. Myology. 1st ed. New York: McGraw-Hill, 1986.

Pickering GW. High blood pressure. 2nd ed. London: Churchill, 1968.

Piper WN, Helwig EB. Progressive systemic sclerosis. Arch Dermatol 1955;72:535–546.

Plum F, Posner JB. The diagnosis of stupor and coma. 3rd ed. Philadelphia: FA Davis, 1980:198–200.

Podolsky S. Hyperosmolar non-ketotic coma in the elderly diabetic. Med Clin North Am 1978;62:815–828.

Polk HC, Shields CL. Remote organ failure: a valid sign of intra-abdominal infection. Surgery 1977;81:310–313.

Potter DJ. Death as a result of hyperglycemia without ketosis—a complication of hemodialysis. Ann Intern Med 1966;64:399–401.

Pulsinelli WA, Waldman S, Rawlinson D, Plum F. Moderate hyperglycemia augments ischemic brain damage: a neuropathologic study in the rat. Neurology 1982;32:1239–1246.

Pun KK, Yeung CK, Ho PWM, et al. Effects of propranolol and haemodialysis on the response of glucose, insulin, C-peptide and cyclic AMP to glucagon challenge. Clin Nephrol 1984;21:235–240.

Pun KK, Yeung CK, Yeung RTT. Effects of propranolol and metoprolol on glucose, cyclic AMP and insulin responses during pharmacologic hyperglucagonemia in hemodialysis patients. Nephron 1985; 39:175–178.

Rao KV, Smith EJ, Alexander JW, et al. Thromboembolic disease in renal allograft recipients. Arch Surg 1976;111:1086–1092.

Rao TK, Friedman EA, Nicastri AD. The types of renal disease in acquired immune deficiency syndrome. N Engl J Med 1987;316:1062–1068.

Richardson EP Jr. Systemic lupus erythematosus. In: Vinken PJ, Bruyn GW, eds. Handbook of clinical neurology. Vol 30, Part 2, Neurological manifestations of systemic diseases. Amsterdam: North-Holland, 1980:273–294.

Rigg GA, Bergu BA. Hypoglycemia—a complication of hemodialysis. N Engl J Med 1967;277:1139–1140.

Rimmer JM, Sussman M, Foster R, Gennari J. Renal transplantation in diabetes mellitus: influence of pre-existing vascular disease on outcome. Nephron 1986;42:304–310.

Ritsky EA, McDaniel HG, Thorpe DL, et al. Spontaneous hypoglycemia in chronic renal failure. Arch Intern Med 1978;138:1364–1368.

Robertson WB, Strong JP. Atherosclerosis in persons with hypertension and diabetes mellitus. Lab Invest 1968;18:538–551.

Robins M. Baum HM. Incidence. Stroke 1981;12(Suppl I):I45–I55.

Rooney JR, Anderson RM, Hopkins IJ. Clinical and pathological aspects of the central nervous system involvement in the haemolytic-uremic syndrome. Aust Paediatr J 1971;17:28–33.

Ross R, Glomset J, Harker L. Response to injury and atherogenesis. Am J Pathol 1977;86:675–684.

Rothenberg RJ. Isolated angiitis of the brain. Am J Med 1985;79:629–632.

Rotter W, Roettger P. Comparative pathologic-anatomic study of cases of chronic global renal insufficiency with and without preceding hemodialysis. Clin Nephrol 1973;1:257–265.

Russell RWR. Observations on intracerebral aneurysms. Brain 1963;86:425–442.

Sanford JP. Epidemiology and root of the problem. In: Root RK, Sande MA, eds. Septic shock. New York: Churchill-Livingstone, 1985:1–11.

Schoenberg BS, Schoenberg DG, Pritchard DA, et al. Differential risk factors for completed stroke and transient ischemic attacks (TIA): study of vascular diseases (hypertension, cardiac disease, peripheral vascular disease) and diabetes mellitus. Trans Am Neurol Assoc 1980:105:165–167.

Sheehan B, Harriman DGF, Bradshaw JPP. Polyarteritis nodosa with ophthalmologic and neurological complications. Arch Ophthalmol 1958;60:537–547.

Siebold JR, Buckingham RB, Medsger TA Jr, Kelly RH. Cerebrospinal fluid immune complexes in systemic lupus erythematosus involving the central nervous system. Semin Arthritis Rheum 1982;12:68–76.

Siegl H, Ruffel B, Petric R, et al. Cyclosporine, the renin-angiotensin-aldosterone system and renal adverse reactions. Transplant Proc 1983;15:2719–2725.

Silberstein LE, Abrahm J, Shattil SJ. The efficacy of intensive plasma exchange in acquired von Willebrand's disease. Transfusion 1987;27:234–237.

Silverstein A, Doniger DE. Neurological complications of myelomatosis. Arch Neurol 1963;9:534–544.

Solders G, Wilczek H, Gunnarsson R, et al. Effects of combined pancreatic and renal transplantation on diabetic neuropathy; a two-year follow-up study. Lancet 1987;2:1232–1235.

Solomon A. Neurological manifestations of macroglobulinemia. In: Brain WR, Norris F, eds. The remote effects of cancer on the nervous system. New York: Grune & Stratton, 1965:12–15.

Someren A, Osgood CP, Brylski J. Solitary posterior fossa plasmacytoma. J Neurosurg 1971;35:223–228.

Spaar FW. Paraproteinaemias and multiple myeloma. In: Vinken PJ, Bruyn GW, eds. Handbook of clinical neurology. Vol 39. Amsterdam: North-Holland, 1980:131–179.

Stehbens WE. Pathology of the cerebral blood vessels. St. Louis: CV Mosby, 1972.

Steinberg A, Ish-Horowitz M, El-Peleg O, et al. Stroke in a patient with hemolytic-uremic syndrome and a good outcome. Brain Dev 1986;8:70–72.

Still JL, Cottom D. Severe hypertension in childhood. Arch Dis Child 1967;42:34–39.

Swift TR. Weakness from magnesium containing cathartics: electrophysiologic studies. Muscle Nerve 1979;2:295–298.

Swift TR. Disorders of neuromuscular transmission other than myasthenia gravis. Muscle Nerve 1981;4:334–353.

Tackmann W, Ullerich D, Cremer W, Lehmann HJ. Nerve conduction studies during the relative refractory period in sural nerves of patients with uremia. Eur Neurol 1974;12:331–339.

Tackmann W. Ullerich D, Lehmann HJ. Impulse series neurography and paired stimuli in early stages of human polyneuropathy. In: Kunze K, Desmedt JE, eds. Studies on neuromuscular diseases. Basel: S Karger, 1975:251–257.

Takahashi K, Yamamura F, Motoyama H. IgM myeloma—its distinction from Waldenström's macroglobulinemia. Acta Neuropathol Jpn 1986;36:1553–1563.

Tan EM, Cohen AS, Fries JF, et al. The 1982 revised criteria for the diagnosis of systemic lupus erythematosus. Arthritis Rheum 1982;25:1271–1277.

Tanaka H. Udea Y, Hayashi M, et al. Risk factors for cerebral hemorrhage and cerebral infarction in a Japanese rural community. Stroke 1982;13:62–73.

Taylor RD, Corcoran AC, Page IH. Increased cerebrospinal fluid pressure and papilledema in malignant hypertension. Arch Intern Med 1954;93:818–824.

Tegnér R. The effect of skin temperature on vibratory sensitivity in polyneuropathy. J Neurol Neurosurg Psychiatry 1985;48:176–178.

Thiele B, Stålberg E. Single fibre EMG findings in polyneuropathies of different aetiology. J Neurol Neurosurg Psychiatry 1975;38:881–887.

Thomas FT, Lee HM. Factors in the differential rate of arteriosclerosis between long surviving renal transplant recipients and dialysis patients. Ann Surg 1976;84:342–351.

Thomas PK. Classification and electrodiagnosis of hereditary neuropathies. In: Brown WF, Bolton CF, eds. Clinical electromyography. Boston: Butterworths, 1987:184–185.

Thomsen AC. The kidney in diabetes mellitus. Copenhagen: Munksgaard, 1965.

Tornheim P. Regional localization of cerebral edema following fluid and insulin therapy in streptozotocin-diabetic rats. Diabetes 1981;30:762–766.

Tvedegaard E, Falk E, Nielsen M. Uremic arterial disease in rabbits with special reference to the coronary arteries. Acta Pathol Microbiol Immunol Scand 1985;93:81–88.

Ueda K, Omae T, Hirota Y, et al. Decreasing trend in incidence and mortality from stroke in Hisayama residents, Japan. Stroke 1981;12:154–160.

Walsh TD. Hypoglycemia and septicemia. Postgrad Med J 1984;60:431–432.

Walton EW. Giant-cell granuloma of the respiratory tract (Wegener's granulomatosis). Br Med J 1958;2:265–270.

Weiner LP, Anderson RN, Allen JC. Cerebral plasmacytoma with myeloma protein in the cerebrospinal fluid. Neurology 1966;16:616–618.

Wetzels JFM, Hoitsma AJ, Berden JHM, Koene RAP. The changing natural history of nephropathy in type I diabetes. Am J Med 1986;80:A63.

White JC. Periodic EEG activity in subcortical arteriosclerotic encephalopathy (Binswanger's type). Arch Neurol 1979;36:485–489.

White MG, Kurtzman NA. Hypoglycemia in diabetes with renal insufficiency. JAMA 1971;15:117.

Wieloch T. Hypoglycemia-induced neuronal damage prevented by an N-methyl-D-aspartate antagonist. Science 1985;230:681–683.

Williams GH, Braunwald E. Hypertensive encephalopathy. In: Braunwald E, Isselbacher KJ, Petersdorf RG, et al., eds. Harrison's principles of internal medicine. 11th ed. New York: McGraw-Hill 1987:1024–1037.

Wolff SM. Wegener's granulomatosis and midline granuloma. In: Petersdorf RG, Adams RD, Braunwald E, et al., eds. Harrison's principles of internal medicine. 11th ed. New York: McGraw-Hill, 1987:1255–1257.

Young GB, Bolton CF, Austin TW, Archibald YM. The electroencephalography (EEG) in sepsis. Can J Neurol Sci 1986;13:164.

Young GB, Bolton CF, Austin TW, Archibald YM. Encephalopathy in sepsis: a clinical prospective study. In press.

Ziegler DK, Zosa A, Zileli T. Hypertensive encephalopathy. Arch Neurol (Chicago) 1965;12:472–478.

Zeumer H, Schonsky B, Strum KW. Predominant white matter involvement in subcortical arteriosclerotic encephalopathy (Binswanger disease). J Comput Assist Tomogr 1980;4:14–19.

Zochodne DW, Bolton CF, Wells GA, et al. Polyneuropathy associated with critical illness: a complication of sepsis and multiple organ failure. Brain 1987;110:819–842.

PART THREE

Neurological Complications of Treatment

Chapter 7

Neurological Complications of Dialysis

Contents

Acronyms

ATP   adenosine triphosphate
CJD   Creutzfeldt-Jakob disease
CNS   central nervous system
CSF   cerebrospinal fluid
DDS   dialysis dysequilibrium syndrome
DE   dialytic encephalopathy
DFO   deferoxamine
DNA   deoxyribonucleic acid
EEG   electroencephalogram

FIRDA frontal intermittent rhythmic delta
        activity
GABA   γ-aminobutyric acid
HU   Hounsfield unit
IPD   intermittent peritoneal dialysis
RNA   ribonucleic acid
SDAT   senile dementia of the Alzheimer
        type

In this chapter, we shall discuss the complications of peritoneal and hemodialysis therapy for the treatment of renal failure. These range from the relatively minor dialysis headache to the often fatal dialytic encephalopathy.

With modern dialysis techniques, vitamin deficiencies and dialysis dysequilibrium are infrequent. Hyperglycemia or hypoglycemia associated with dialysis are now rarely encountered. Better understanding of dialytic encephalopathy has allowed preventive measures; early recognition of the entity may permit the arrest or reversal of the condition.

The object of this chapter is to acquaint the reader with the preventable and treatable neurological complications of dialysis. In some respects, the chapter serves as a review of recent history. It is hoped that the lessons learned will allow such future reviews to be purely historical in nature.

Dialytic Encephalopathy

Dialytic encephalopathy is a syndrome with specific neurological signs and associated electroencephalographic (EEG) abnormalities found in association with the treatment of chronic renal failure. The condition is progressive and fatal unless treated early. There is good evidence that DE is due to chronic toxicity from aluminum accumulation in the brain. Alternate terms include dialysis encephalopathy, dialysis dementia, progressive myoclonic dialysis encephalopathy, progressive dialysis encephalopathy, progressive dialytic encephalopathy, progressive uremic encephalopathy, and hemodialysis encephalopathy. The first three names are the most commonly used. There are some problems with these labels, in that not all patients are on hemodialysis; some are on peritoneal dialysis (Smith et al., 1980) and some may not have been dialyzed at all. Furthermore, since the disease is reversible in its early stages, it is not always progressive. However, some terms have been used so often that we shall not suggest yet another appellation. We shall use the term dialytic encephalopathy (DE) throughout this book.

The section on dialytic encephalopathy was written in collaboration with Anthony B. Hodsman, M.B., F.R.C.P.(C.), Associate Professor, Department of Medicine, University of Western Ontario, and Director of the Dialysis Unit, St. Joseph's Health Centre, London, Ontario, Canada.

Clinical Features and Population Studies

The first clear description of DE as a recognized entity was by Alfrey et al. (1972). The authors described five patients who had each been treated with hemodialysis for more than three years. The dialysis regimens in each case were adequate, yet the patients showed a progressive neurological syndrome. Four had died by the time of publication, two from incapacity due to the neurological illness and a third from aspiration of toilet paper during an organic psychosis.

Since that time, DE has been reported from numerous centers, and the clinical features have shown a remarkable similarity. In Europe for 1976 and 1977, the two-year prevalence of DE was 600 per 100,000 dialysis patients (Wing et al., 1980). There was considerable variation from center to center (Figure 7.1). Dewberry et al. (1980) in Tennessee found 14 cases among 320 patients over five years, an annual incidence of about one percent. In the United States, the overall attack rate among several dialysis centers was four percent and varied from 2.2 to 14.7 percent (Schreeder et al., 1983). The latter study likely reflects selection bias, with inclusion of centers experiencing a higher than average incidence of DE.

Recent progress in understanding the pathogenesis and resultant preventive and early therapy have reduced these figures (Pierides et al., 1980). Although "epidemics" of DE, or

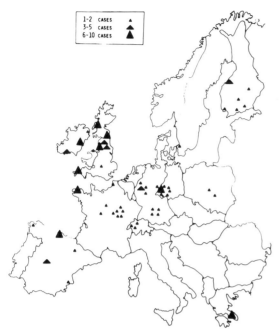

Figure 7.1. Geographic distribution of 150 cases of dialysis dementia in Europe, 1976–1977. Centers that reported numerous cases are shown with larger triangles (see key). Note that many areas of high population density—e.g., Thames valley, the Ruhr, and Italy—did not report many cases, despite large numbers of patients on treatment. (Reprinted with permission from Wing et al., 1980.)

high occurrences in certain centers are less common, La Greca et al. (1985) point out that sporadic cases still occur.

It is likely that individual patient factors also play a role in DE. Overall, males outnumber females about 1.4 to 1 (Dewberry et al., 1980). The age range for disease onset is reportedly from 21 to 68 years (Jack et al., 1983–1984), although this is skewed towards older patients, as the mean age was 50 years. Probably no age is exempt; there is a report of a similar syndrome in five children (Foley et al., 1981).

The time of DE symptoms from onset of dialysis can range from 0.5 to 112 months, with a mean of 35 months (Jack et al., 1983–1984). In fatal cases, the duration of disease from onset till death has ranged from 0.5 to 57 months, with a mean of 6 months (Jack et al., 1983–1984).

Signs and Symptoms

The manifestations of DE include an initial speech disturbance, involuntary motor phenomena (myoclonus, tremulousness, asterixis, and seizures), gait disturbance, and other mental and neurological changes. DE is commonly associated with vitamin D–resistant osteomalacia, with a propensity for fractures (Platts et al., 1977), proximal myopathy in the lower limbs, and a severe, refractory, non-iron-deficient, microcytic, hypochromic anemia (O'Hare and Murnahagan, 1982; O'Hare et al., 1983). All of these have been linked to increased aluminum in the body (Wills and Savory, 1983).

The various neurological components of the syndrome will be discussed separately, although it should be realized that they occur and progress together in the advanced phase of the syndrome. There are often striking fluctuations early in the course of the illness, even with brief periods of complete remission of symptoms. Further, there is considerable variation in the tempo of the illness. In clusters of DE cases, in which a significant percentage of dialysis unit patients are simultaneously affected, the disease usually progresses more quickly than in sporadic cases (La Greca et al., 1985).

Speech Disturbance

A disturbance in speech is commonly, but not invariably, among the first signs of DE (Alfrey et al., 1972; Chokroverty et al., 1976). It is not a feature of other metabolic encephalopathies and is therefore a helpful diagnostic sign. It is found during the course of illness in 93 percent of patients (Jack et al., 1983–1984). In the early part of the illness, the speech disturbance most frequently comes on just after hemodialysis and then may clear, only to return again and again, becoming more persistent (Alfrey, 1986).

Case studies have revealed a variety of speech abnormalities. In some patients, the initial speech problem is articulatory, in the form of dysarthria and stuttering (Canter, 1971;

Rosenbek et al., 1975; Madison et al., 1977; Baratz and Herzog, 1980; Parkinson et al., 1981). Some patients sound as if they are "gagging on their words" (Madison et al., 1977). A breakdown of articulation occurs; speech becomes effortful. Some authors use the term "apraxia of speech" (Rosenbek et al., 1975) in reference to the inconsistent sound substitutions, omissions or repetitions of sounds and syllables, and labored speech. This may relate, in part, to the manner in which the vocal apparatus works in order to produce certain phonemes. Sometimes there is faulty contact between the tongue and the alveolar ridge of the hard palate (Baratz and Herzog, 1980). Speech may be slowed in some cases in a deliberate attempt to correct mispronounced words, and in others, because of impaired concentration (O'Hare et al., 1983).

Another type of nonfluent speech disorder is Broca's aphasia, a language disorder due to dysfunction of the inferior frontal region of the dominant hemisphere. It is characterized by effortful, low-output speech, word-finding difficulties, and agrammatisms, associated with insight into the deficit and frustration. Fluency may be reduced to the point of complete muteness. Although sometimes mistaken for a stroke when it appears suddenly as the initial speech disorder, muteness usually occurs later in the disease.

Word-finding difficulties are often associated with circumlocution, in which the object is described but not named (e.g., one patient, who could not find the word "cups," described the objects as "little bowls with handles").

Prosody refers to the rhythm, melody and intonation of speech. It is affected in various ways: it may take the form of a slow "scanning" speech similar to that found in patients with cerebellar disease; other cases may show a staccato quality, in which each syllable has pronounced loudness and stress (Baratz and Herzog, 1980).

Thus, some patients have true Broca's aphasia, while others show apraxia of speech and dysarthria. Aphasia and dysarthria are often found in the same patient (Chokroverty et al., 1976; O'Hare et al., 1983; Lederman and Henry, 1978).

Comprehension of oral speech is relatively preserved, but it may be impaired, as may other functions of the "posterior speech center," impairment of which is manifested by perseveration, neologisms, and paraphasic errors.

Dysgraphia is common (see illustrative Case 2 later in this chapter). The writing is slow and laborious, with misspellings, inappropriate omissions and substitutions, and frequent attempts at correcting errors (Baratz and Herzog, 1980; O'Hare et al., 1983).

The time course of the speech disturbance is worthy of comment. Reduced fluency and fluctuations are early features; beyond this, the course and features show considerable variability from patient to patient. Some patients may show more comprehension problems. Others may even become hyperfluent in later stages, while still others may again become mute. Some may show striking hallucinations and perseveration. The patients may show variable degrees of confusion, and in advanced cases, there is always an associated decline in other aspects of intellect besides language functions. The type of dysarthria or aphasia may change during the course of the illness, e.g., dysarthria typical of cerebellar dysfunction may be replaced by spastic dysphonia.

Mental Changes

Behavioral changes appear early, sometimes preceding the speech disturbance, but they are less specific and often insidious in onset and progression. Apathy, inappropriate behavior and attitude alterations are among the first manifestations. The main affective change is depression (Jack et al., 1983–1984), which is commonly accompanied by lethargy and apathy. Personality change, paranoia, and suicidal tendencies have been described (Mayor and Burnatowska-Hiedin, 1986). Daytime somnolence is common, and directional disorientation may also occur. Although such features are not uncommon in the general dialysis population (Abram et al., 1971), such a mental *change* may be the clue that an organic brain syndrome has occurred.

English et al. (1978) carried out a prospective study on the mental status of home dialysis patients. They found that some individuals showed inability to acquire new information. They also found that results of digit-symbol, block design, and picture arrangement tests were abnormal, but not the full-scale intelligence quotient. The authors argue that these features may be the earliest cognitive changes in DE, and that such psychological tests could be used to screen dialysis patients. This would be a great asset, as it would (1) allow recognition of patients at an early, and hopefully reversible, phase of DE and (2) detect those patients who might soon lose abilities to perform self-dialysis. Unfortunately, results of follow-up were not reported.

Memory failure, inattention, poor concentration, and disorientation are common and may fluctuate. They may be difficult to assess if speech problems predominate early in the illness. Confusional states may come and go and are sometimes more dramatic. Frank delirium, or an agitated confusional state, is not uncommon after initial mental changes or speech problems have appeared (Chokroverty et al., 1976). Sometimes, visual or auditory hallucinations, paranoid delusions, or even manic behavior occurs (Chokroverty et al., 1976; Jack et al., 1983; 1983–1984). These psychotic features usually occur later in the illness, but they can be the presenting symptom and cause diagnostic problems (Jack et al., 1983).

Apraxia is the inability of the patient to perform a task in the absence of basic motor deficit and despite understanding the command. Although myoclonus and incoordination can interfere with motor activity, many patients with DE show an intellectual inability to execute tasks such as writing and drawing. This may progress to the point where patients can no longer feed themselves, comb their hair, or do other activities of daily living. In some patients, the initiation of movement is the most difficult part; this can affect even walking (apraxia of gait).

Other intellectual dysfunctions such as dyscalculia may be prominent, but more typically there is a general reduction in mental status, or dementia. This is progressive in later stages of the disease and may progress to incontinence, incapacity, and dependence; the patient may become immobile and die of pneumonia (Bates et al., 1985; Alfrey, 1986).

Motor Phenomena

Myoclonus, or brief, involuntary jerking movements of groups of muscles, occurred in 78 percent of DE cases pooled from the literature (Jack et al., 1983–1984). It is less common than the speech disturbance and usually appears later. Myoclonus may be regional in early stages, especially in the upper limbs (Bakir et al., 1986), but it then becomes more generalized, usually as multifocal myoclonus (Mahurkar, 1978). Myoclonus is often found in conjunction with asterixis (see next paragraph) (Bates et al., 1985). The face may be involved. In some patients, the myoclonus is stimulus sensitive, brought on by movement or by external stimuli (Bates et al., 1985). In one patient, the sensitivity to light, sound, and startle was such that the condition resembled Creutzfeldt-Jakob disease (Chokroverty et al., 1976). Bates et al. (1985) describe the myoclonus beginning distally in the extremities and ultimately involving more proximal limb muscles and even the trunk. The jerking movements may persist in sleep. Occasionally, the myoclonus may be severe enough to cause the patient to fall (Chokroverty et al., 1976). The transition from myoclonus to seizures is sometimes blurred.

Asterixis is a brief loss of postural tone, causing an extended wrist or limb to transiently drop. Like postural action tremor, it is commonly associated with metabolic encephalopathies, including uremic encephalopathy. In DE, asterixis and/or tremor occur principally in advanced disease (Alfrey, 1986).

Grimacing has occasionally been reported (Chokroverty et al., 1976), as have athetotic movements (Mahurkar et al., 1973), raising the likelihood of striatal dysfunction in these patients.

Gait disturbance, a common and often early symptom and sign, may take the form of a wide-based ataxia or apraxia of gait (see description of gait under Subdural Hematoma, Chapter 7C). Proximal muscle weakness, and pelvic girdle osteomalacia and fractures often cause difficulty in sorting out the mechanism.

Upper limb ataxia may also be present. Along with apraxia, this may be disabling (Bates et al., 1985).

Focal motor signs are rare. In one case described by Bakir et al. (1986), focal weakness may have been due to hypertensive vascular disease.

Seizures

Seizures occur in about 60 percent of patients with DE (Jack et al., 1983–1984). They tend to occur in the advanced phase of the disease (Jack et al., 1983–1984), although they may be the first manifestation in a small proportion of cases (Bates et al., 1985). Attacks are usually generalized tonic-clonic in type, although generalized myoclonic (Chui and Damasio, 1980) and simple or complex partial seizures have been noted (Bates et al., 1985). Convulsive status epilepticus is sometimes the terminal event (Jack et al., 1983–1984).

Although diazepam may temporarily help the speech disorder, myoclonus, and other early symptoms, it is not especially effective in preventing recurrent epileptic seizures in DE. Bates et al. (1985) have noted that phenytoin or carbamazepine is often effective. However, control tends to fall off with progression of the disease, and higher drug doses may be necessary.

Apnea

Garcia-Bunuel et al. (1980) described apneic spells in a 53-year-old man who was considered to have DE. After hemodialysis for four years, he presented with episodes of light-headedness and dysarthria, then with 20-second episodes of difficulty concentrating or muteness. He later developed episodes of apnea and unresponsiveness in association with paroxysms of bilaterally synchronous, high-voltage slow waves on the EEG. Such episodes began and ended abruptly and lasted from 5 to 50 seconds. For a time, the apneic spells and the

paroxysmal EEG abnormality were helped by diazepam therapy. The patient later became more obtunded, developed status epilepticus, and died. The postmortem examination showed multiple small vascular lesions in cerebral white matter. The cerebral cortex and brainstem were normal.

The explanation for the apneic episodes is uncertain. One possibility is that they represented an unusual form of central sleep apnea. However, this would not be expected to respond to diazepam. Alternatively, the apneic spells may have been epileptic seizures. Nonconvulsive seizures may produce apnea if they involve the limbic system (Jackson, 1899; Nelson and Ray, 1968). It is difficult to fully substantiate either hypothesis. Other explanations of episodic dysfunction of the brainstem reticular formation and respiratory centers may be necessary.

Infants and Children

Aluminum-induced encephalopathy in infants and children is likely a special form of DE. Young children appear to be especially susceptible to aluminum intoxication, which has been reported in uremic infants before maintenance dialysis therapy was initiated. Foley et al. (1981) reported five children, aged 2 to 5 years, with chronic renal failure who developed a progressive encephalopathy consisting of ataxia, loss of motor abilities, myoclonus, seizures, dementia, and bulbar dysfunction. The latter consisted of dysphagia and decreased facial and palatal movements. Two children had died at the time of publication, at 10 months and 4 years from disease onset. The "survivors," who were followed for two to four years, were incapacitated.

At autopsy in one case, the brain was atrophic and showed severe neuronal loss, spongiform change in the cortex, and gliosis.

The only possible etiological feature that was common to all the patients was the ingestion of large amounts of aluminum hydroxide gel.

Freundlich et al. (1985) described two infants with congenital uremia who died at 1 and

3 months of age. The deterioration was abrupt, consisting mainly of impaired consciousness. Autopsy of one patient showed neuronal degeneration in basal ganglia, diencephalon, pontine nuclei, and deeper layers of the cerebral cortex. The white matter showed diffuse gliosis, edema, and axonal swelling. The other autopsy showed "reduced brain tissue." Aluminum content of the brain was increased to 60 times normal in gray matter and four times normal in white matter. Bone aluminum was only slightly increased.

Neither baby had been dialyzed. The apparent source of aluminum was infant formulas, most of which contain between 120 and 390 ng/ml of aluminum.

Illustrative Cases

The following cases illustrate many of the above features. The first case is a progressive disorder, terminating in death as a complication of dementia. In the second case, the disease was halted and partly reversed.

Case 1

In 1972, at age 51 years, this man was diagnosed as having chronic renal failure due to glomerulonephritis. Two years later, he was treated with hemodialysis, and aluminum hydroxide (Amphojel, 180 mL/day) by mouth as a phosphate binder. He was stable until, on June 1, 1979, he had a transient episode of hesitant speech just after dialysis. Speech problems recurred after subsequent dialysis treatments, consisting mainly of word-finding difficulty and hesitancy; episodes lasted about two hours. He also showed intermittent episodes of disorientation and inappropriate activity: he would awaken in the middle of the night and clean the sink or take a shower. His upper limbs sometimes seemed uncoordinated; he also tended to drop things, sometimes breaking glasses when drinking.

By July 1979, the speech disorder was persistent and consisted of stuttering and apraxic elements and increased effort in speaking. By early August, he showed multifocal myoclonus affecting all limbs. He was then tried on diazepam, 5 mg t.i.d., which produced a significant improvement in myoclonus, speech, and writing (Figure 7.2). He was able to converse and write normally for approximately 10 days. Despite the diazepam, he slipped back to his impaired state in a few days and remained impaired thereafter.

When formally assessed on August 20, 1979, his speech showed hesitancy, difficulty initiating phonation, and blocking on the first syllable. Speech was telegraphic, with frequent pauses. He tended to repeat single phonemes and whole words and showed increased underlying vocal tension. There was mild dysarthria and general slowing of speech. Auditory comprehension, reading, and writing were moderately impaired. Neuropsychological testing showed an IQ (Wechsler Adult Intelligence Scale) of 82, with performance and verbal IQs of 78 and 87, respectively. Memory quotient (Wechlser Memory) was 86. These were decreased, it was estimated, at least 15 points from premorbid values. He showed distortions on the Rey figure and mild constructional apraxia. He showed right-left confusion on testing mirror image, but not for self.

Intellectual deterioration continued. He required hospital admission in August 1979. He was closely supervised, but early on September 10, 1979, went to the bathroom, turned on only the hot water in the bath, and got in the tub. He was found two minutes later, but suffered 30 percent surface area second- and third-degree burns. Despite careful fluid replacement, he developed hypotension and died on September 12, 1979.

The brain was normal on gross and microscopic examination.

Case 2

This woman required hemodialysis for chronic renal failure since 1981 at age 65. In the fall of 1986, she seemed more frail. By December, she would get up at night and wander about the house. In mid-December a transient aphasia with naming errors occurred after hemodialysis. Over a week, this worsened until she had a moderate Wernicke's aphasia, with fluent (although less fluent than her usual) speech and impaired comprehension, repetition, and naming. She was perseverative and showed occasional paraphasic errors. Attention and idiomotor praxis were mildly impaired. Over that same week, she developed multifocal myoclonus, upper-limb ataxia, intention tremor, and an ataxic gait. She tended to drop things placed in either hand. She was markedly dysgraphic (see Figure 7.3A). Dialysis treatment caused no noticeable deterioration in central nervous system (CNS) symptoms. Her EEG showed frequent generalized bursts of rhythmic delta activity and triphasic waves (Figure 7.3B), confirming a clinical diagnosis of DE.

By that time she had undergone hemodialysis for 54 months. Routine management included standard

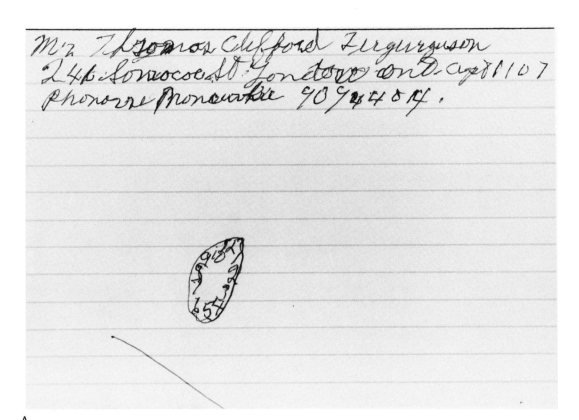

A

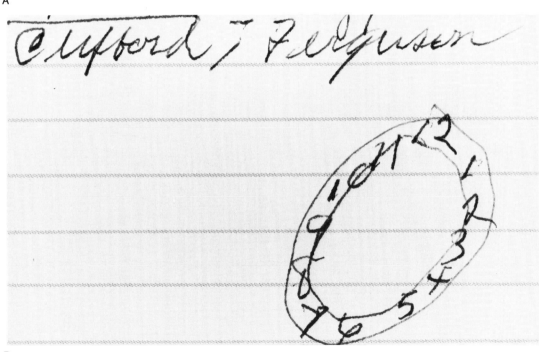

B

Figure 7.2. Evaluation of a patient with dialysis dementia (case 1). (A) The patient attempted writing his name, address, and telephone number. He was also asked to draw a clock. Note the spelling errors with perseveration, shaky handwriting, and errors on drawing a clock (omitted 11, poorly aligned numbers). (B) Several days later, the patient transiently improved on diazepam. Writing his name and drawing the clock have both improved. (Reproduced with permission of the family.)

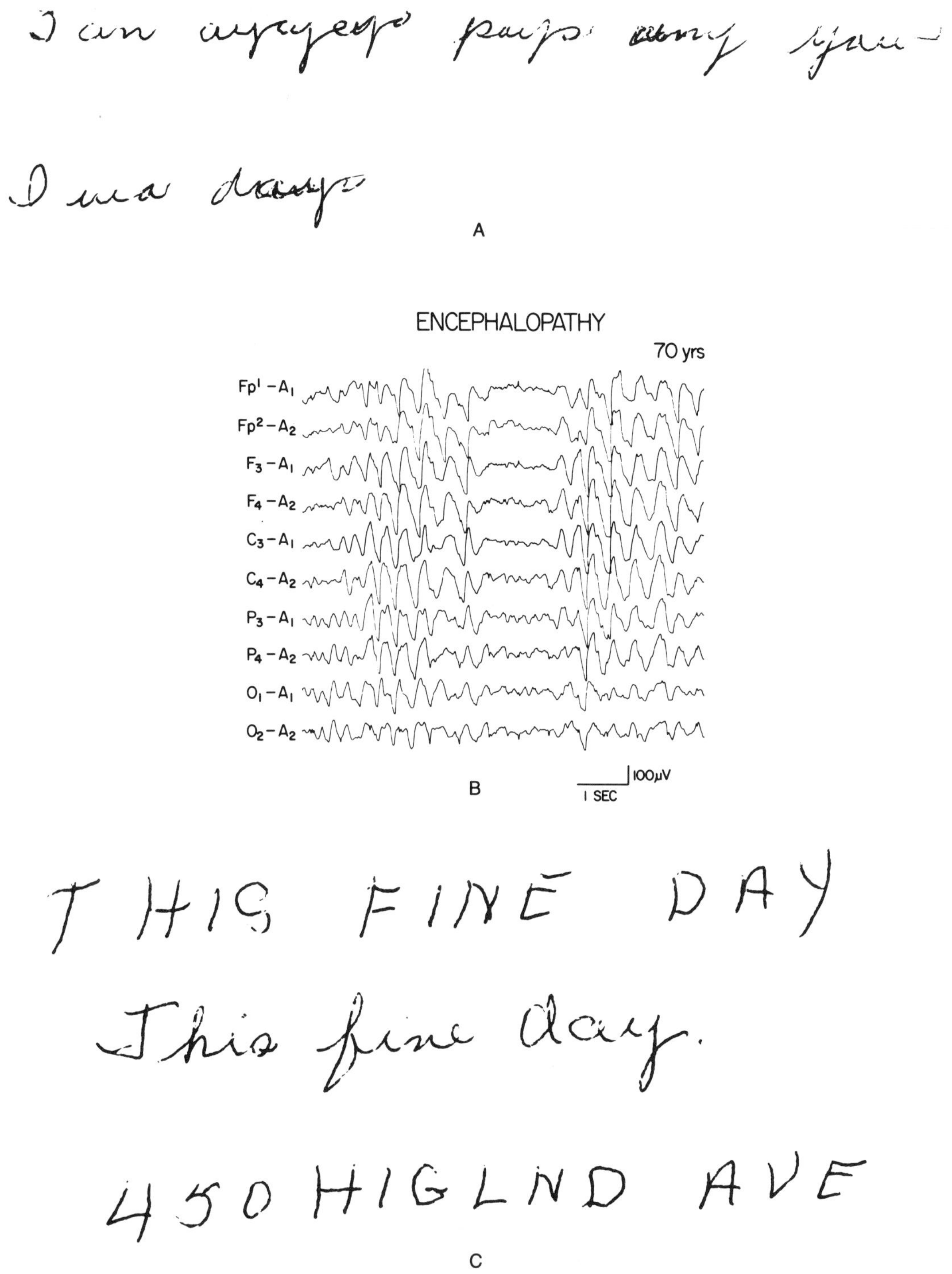

Figure 7.3. Case 2 (A) Handwriting in December 1986. She was asked to write "This is a fine day." (B) EEG performed at the same time as handwriting sample in Figure 7.3A. The background is abnormally slow, and there are frequent bisynchronous bursts of high voltage delta mixed with triphasic waves. (C) Writing in April, 1987. She was asked to write "This is a fine day" and her address, 450 Highland Ave. Note the omitted words and letters.

treatment with Al(OH)$_3$ for controlling dietary phosphate absorption in doses averaging 4.5 g/day. However, it should be noted that routine measurements of serum aluminum averaged 206 µg/L (7,630 nmol/L). At the time the diagnosis of DE was established, serum aluminum was 284 µg/L (10,300 nmol/L).

She began therapy with the chelating agent, deferoxamine, in late December, receiving 4 g intravenously once a week for a period of one year. Over the next three months, her speech improved to a mild nominal aphasia. The myoclonus and tremor subsided, and her gait improved. By the end of 12 months of chelation therapy, she was fully independent at home, with only minimal functional impairment to speech.

When reassessed in April of 1987, four months after presentation, she had difficulty repeating "no ifs, ands, or buts" and was still not as fluent as prior to December 1986. Her writing had improved, but she left out verbs, articles, and even some letters (Figure 7.3C). At this time, the EEG showed only a mild generalized abnormality with excessive diffuse, low-voltage, 2 to 6-Hz waves, which were more prominent in both frontal and the left temporal regions.

Differential Diagnosis

When the presentation is classic, particularly when, at the onset, a speech disorder occurs in a transient manner related to dialysis and is combined with the other features and EEG findings, the diagnosis is not difficult. When the speech disorder does not play a prominent initial role and the course is steadily progressive, DE can sometimes be difficult to differentiate from a number of conditions.

Other Complications of Dialysis and Toxic/Metabolic Conditions

Uremic encephalopathy and complications of dialysis (dialysis dysequilibrium, subdural hematoma, Wernicke's encephalopathy, and abnormalities related to fluid, electrolyte, and mineral balance) have to be considered. These various considerations are easily differentiated from DE using clinical evaluation, appropriate laboratory tests, and sometimes, a therapeutic change such as correcting a fluid or mineral imbalance or reducing or withdrawing a medication.

Drug effects, altered drug handling in uremia, drug intoxication, and idiosyncratic or hypersensitivity reactions should always be considered. Benzodiazapine intoxication has been reported to occasionally cause confusion with DE (Taclob and Needle, 1976), but drowsiness dominates the picture with such drug accumulation. The EEG in barbiturate intoxication is also vastly different from that of DE. In the former, a mixture of beta (fast-frequency waves) and slower frequencies (theta and delta) is characteristic.

Occasionally, acute hypercalcemia in patients on hemodialysis may cause an encephalopathy with dysarthria, myoclonus, seizures, hallucinations, and behavioral changes (Rivera-Vasquez et al., 1980). The acuteness of presentation, clinical course, reversibility with correction of serum calcium, and the EEG are again helpful in differentiating the two conditions.

Depressive Psychosis

Depression is common in dialysis patients; the associated psychomotor retardation can mimic dementia. Occasionally, a functional psychosis can occur, just as it can in any population. Aphasia, dysarthria, myoclonus, and gait disturbance are not features of depression or functional psychosis. Speech output in depression may be reduced, but aphasic errors are not expected.

Psychotic features with hallucinations, delusions, or manic behavior may be difficult to differentiate from delirium sometimes found in DE or uremic encephalopathy. However, gross tremor, multifocal myoclonus, asterixis, or seizures are indicative of a metabolic encephalopathy, rather than a functional psychosis. Fortunately, agitated behavior is not long-lasting, and it is eventually possible to sort out the problem after the patient has been treated symptomatically.

The EEG can be helpful in differentiating functional from organic mental conditions such as depression, in which case the EEG is normal. However, the EEG may not be feasible if the patient is agitated or poorly cooperative.

Degenerative Conditions

Senile dementia of the Alzheimer type (SDAT) is the most common cause of dementia in our population. The uremic population is not exempt from this "quiet epidemic." The onset is often subtle, as it may be with DE. The patient becomes more withdrawn, abandons hobbies and interests, and neglects routine tasks. Forgetfulness is also often an early feature. Although aphasia is not a prominent feature, patients often develop word-finding difficulties, similar to anomic aphasia, and later, a gradual reduction in more complex language functions. Impaired cognition and incompetence in dealing with financial or work-related responsibilities become more apparent with time. The patient may get lost and may become unreasonably preoccupied with a trivial matter. Failure of judgment, decreased control of temper, and accentuation of previous personality traits are seen. All intellectual faculties may be impaired; in advanced stages more well-defined aphasic, apraxic, and agnostic syndromes may appear.

The patient with SDAT does not have the hesitancy, stuttering, muteness, and dysarthria commonly found in early phases of DE. Patients with SDAT do not show the marked fluctuations that characterize the intermittent speech disturbance of early DE. Myoclonus, asterixis, tremor, and ataxia are not found in SDAT, although such patients occasionally show some apraxia of gait.

The EEG in SDAT usually exhibits slowing of the occipital background rhythm and variable amounts of diffuse slow waves (Letemendia and Pampiglione, 1958; Rae-Grant and Blume, 1987). Single sharp waves are more likely than spikes in SDAT (Letemendia and Pampiglione, 1958). Usually, the distinction between early SDAT and DE is not difficult on EEG, but in severe cases of SDAT there may be more slowing and paroxysmal activity resembling that of DE (Rae-Grant and Blume, 1987). The EEG findings in SDAT are not specific for that condition; several metabolic abnormalities, including those with hypothyroidism and pernicious anemia, can resemble SDAT electrographically. Sundaram and Blume (1987) noted triphasic waves in some patients with SDAT; this may cause some difficulty in the EEG differentiation between SDAT and metabolic encephalopathies.

SDAT is *consistently* associated with neurofibrillary degeneration and senile plaques. Such findings are *extremely rare* in DE (see Pathology, below). Granulovacuolar degeneration occurs in SDAT but never in DE.

There are other, less common, neurodegenerative disorders associated with dementia and a variety of neurological signs and symptoms. Most of these do not include the speech problems and myoclonus which are characteristic of DE. Also, many contain other features, such as predominant parkinsonism, amyotrophy, or appendicular ataxia, which are not features of DE.

Creutzfeldt-Jakob Disease

Creutzfeldt-Jakob disease (CJD) is a slow virus infection of the CNS. Characteristically, it is a subacute illness characterized by dementia and myoclonus. In early phases, focal features may occur, depending on the topography of the cerebral cortical and subcortical involvement. Patients may present with a dominant hemisphere syndrome, including aphasia (Zochodne et al., 1988). Gait disturbance is common, related to cerebellar, basal ganglia, or bifrontal disease. The disease progresses to a vegetative state. Survival is usually a matter of months, although cases of long duration are well described (Brown et al., 1984).

CJD, unlike DE, does not show fluctuations in the early phases. It tends to be steadily progressive. Parkinsonian features, muscular wasting and fasciculations, cortical blindness, and Balint's syndrome sometimes occur in CJD but not in DE.

The EEG in the two conditions is quite different. In CJD, the EEG typically shows periodic sharp-wave complexes, which are usually generalized but may be lateralized in the early stages (Levy et al., 1986). Occasionally, periodic sharp-wave complexes fail to occur (Zochodne et al., 1988), but even then, the EEG does not resemble that of DE. Pathologically, CJD and DE are distinctive. A spongiform encephalopathy, accompanied by neuronal loss and gliosis affecting cortical and subcortical gray matter, is the hallmark of CJD. In DE, there are no consistent findings, although spongiform change has been described in some infants with aluminum-induced encephalopathy (Foley et al., 1981).

Focal Brain Lesions

Ischemic, neoplastic, inflammatory, or traumatic lesions and spontaneous subdural hematoma (see Chapter 7C) could cause similar speech disturbance, apraxia, etc. These would cause problems in diagnosis, especially if they affected the dominant (usually left) cerebral hemisphere, but multifocal lesions could even more closely mimic the mental status profile of DE. With extra-axial lesions, e.g., subdural hematomas or meningiomas, the neurological disorder may fluctuate considerably, similar to the transient speech disturbance that may follow dialysis in early DE.

Investigative Tests

The Electroencephalogram in Dialytic Encephalopathy

The EEG is the principal investigative test for the diagnosis of DE. As noted in the original description by Alfrey et al. (1972), the EEG abnormalities constitute an important component of the disease entity. The combination of the clinical and EEG features in the appropriate setting, especially in the presence of an adequate dialysis program, establishes the diagnosis.

Table 7.1 shows data from three series, those of Lederman and Henry (1978), Hughes and Schreeder (1980), and Chokroverty and Gandhi (1982). Although the studies are not identical, there is agreement on a number of aspects.

Chokroverty and Gandhi (1982) found that intermittent bursts of frontally predominant delta (less than 3 Hz) activity, especially more than 50 bursts per routine recording, was a reliable feature of DE. The other series did not differentiate *intermittent* slow waves from persistent slowing; the latter did not reliably differentiate DE from uremic encephalopathy. Care should be exercised in attributing frontal intermittent delta activity to DE: such bursts are common in patients immediately after dialysis and in healthy elderly individuals in drowsiness.

All studies are in agreement with respect to the specificity and sensitivity of paroxysmal generalized bursts of spike-and-wave activity. The paroxysms lacked the stereotypy and consistent symmetry of the 3/s spike and wave seen in absence epilepsy. Instead, they were irregular (Figure 7.4). Hughes and Schreeder (1980) correctly classified 77 percent of their DE patients and 85 percent of their records using this criterion alone. Several of their patients showed generalized spike-and-wave activity *before* clinical signs of DE developed, indicating the potential usefulness of the EEG as a screening test for the risk of early DE. It should be remembered that generalized spike-and-wave activity is not 100 percent specific for DE and that it does not occur in all records on patients with DE (see Table 7.1). Such a spike-and-wave pattern may occur in uremic encephalopathy, either spontaneously or with photic stimulation, although DE patients more commonly show such activation (Chokroverty and Gandhi, 1982).

The occurrence of triphasic waves, especially in association with frontal intermittent delta activity, or generalized epileptiform activity supports the diagnosis of DE (Noriega-Sanchez et al., 1978). Their mere presence, however, is not helpful in differentiating DE from uremic encephalopathy.

To summarize, the EEG can help in the diagnosis of DE when the characteristic features are present in a patient without an acute metabolic derangement who has received adequate dialysis.

Table 7.1. EEG Abnormalities in Dialytic Encephalopathy and Chronic Renal Failure

EEG Finding	DE (% EEGs)	CRF (% EEGs)
FIRDA		
Lederman and Henry[a]	—	—
Hughes and Schreeder[b]	—	—
Chokroverty and Gandhi[c]	94	12
Spike and wave		
Lederman and Henry	nearly all	—
Hughes and Schreeder	81	1
Chokroverty and Gandhi	76	6
Diffuse slowing		
Lederman and Henry	—	—
Hughes and Schreeder	96	91
Chokroverty and Gandhi	82	47
Focal spikes		
Lederman and Henry	—	—
Hughes and Schreeder	5	8
Chokroverty and Gandhi	6	6
Reactivity		
Lederman and Henry	—	—
Hughes and Schreeder	—	—
Chokroverty and Gandhi	0	12
Triphasic waves		
Lederman and Henry	33[d]	—
Hughes and Schreeder	3	7
Chokroverty and Gandhi	0	0
Normal		
Lederman and Henry	3	—
Hughes and Schreeder	3	7
Chokroverty and Gandhi	0	53

Note: EEG = electroencephalogram; DE = dialysis encephalopathy; CRF = chronic renal failure; FIRDA = frontal intermittent rhythmic delta activity.
[a]Lederman and Henry (1978): DE only—17 patients, 28 EEGs.
[b]Hughes and Schreeder (1980): DE—26 patients, 80 EEGs; CRF—51 patients, 76 EEGs.
[c]Chokroverty and Gandhi (1982): DE—17 patients, 17 EEGs; CRF—17 patients, 17 EEGs.
[d]Percent of patients.

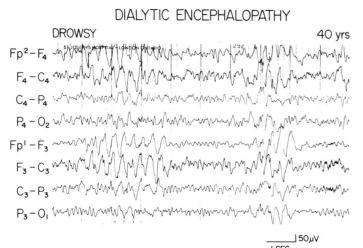

DIALYTIC ENCEPHALOPATHY

DROWSY   40 yrs

Fp2–F4
F4–C4
C4–P4
P4–O2
Fp1–F3
F3–C3
C3–P3
P3–O1

50μV
I SEC

Figure 7.4. EEG from a 40-year-old man with early DE. Bursts of poorly stereotyped spike-and-wave activity mixed with low-frequency waves are accentuated in the anterior head.

Improvement in the EEG may not always parallel clinical improvement. O'Hare et al. (1983) reported a patient whose EEG abnormalities persisted after signs of DE cleared following renal transplantation. Although clinical features of DE and the EEG abnormalities may quickly improve after diazepam, this effect is transient (Nadel and Wilson, 1976). Transient worsening in the EEG may occur with deferoxamine therapy, possibly as a result of increased release of aluminum from bone (Luda 1983).

Serum Aluminum Levels and the Deferoxamine Infusion Test

These tests are less specific and less sensitive than EEG studies. They are discussed under Clinical Management later in this chapter.

Pathology

The neuropathology of DE has not shown consistent abnormalities (Cartier et al., 1981). Brain weight is normal or slightly reduced, even though some cases show edema. Usually the brain is macroscopically and microscopically normal or similar to that of a patient with chronic renal failure. One finding that is, perhaps, more consistently found in DE is a reduction in Purkinje cells of the cerebellum.

Neurofibrillary degeneration and/or senile plaques, somewhat similar to those found in Alzheimer's disease or SDAT, have been described in seven patients with DE (Brun and Dictor, 1981; Kogeorgos and Scholtz, 1982; Scholtz et al., 1987). The age at death ranged from 34 to 67 years. This finding does not appear to be merely the coincidental occurrence of Alzheimer's disease in these patients for the following reasons: (1) the patients had clinical and EEG features of DE; (2) neurofibrillary degeneration in DE was more marked in the cingulate gyrus and motor cortex than in the hippocampus, in contrast to Alzheimer's disease or SDAT in which the hippocampus shows maximal involvement; (3) the neurofibrillary material in patients with DE more

closely resembled that produced by experimental toxicity with aluminum than that found in Alzheimer's disease or SDAT: it was not doubly refractile with polarized light, did not stain with Congo red, and reacted with antibody against the 210-kilodalton portion of neurofilament polypeptide (Scholtz et al., 1987); and (4) the aluminum in DE was intracytoplasmic rather than intranuclear as in Alzheimer's disease or SDAT (Scholtz et al., 1987). It should be emphasized that neurofibrillary degeneration is rare in DE, but it gives support to the etiological role of aluminum.

Electron microscopy in DE shows numerous lysosomes in cerebral neurons (Galle et al., 1979). On further analysis, these were found to contain aluminum phosphate. Further neurochemistry is discussed under Neurotoxicology of Aluminum, and Role of GABA and the Benzodiazepine Receptor, in the next section.

Etiology of Dialytic Encephalopathy

Role of Aluminum Toxicity

The exact cause of DE is unknown. Neuropathological examination of brain tissue obtained from patients dying of DE has yielded few clues; moreover, there is no animal model for the disease. The evidence for aluminum as the responsible toxin is compelling but circumstantial. Aluminum likely facilitates or accelerates a neurodegenerative process in susceptible uremic patients. As such, its association with DE may be analogous to that seen in other neurodegenerative disorders such as Alzheimer's disease and Guamian amyotrophic lateral sclerosis. The evidence incriminating aluminum in the genesis of DE may be summarized as follows:

Brain Accumulation of Aluminum

When Alfrey et al. first described DE in 1972, they suspected the presence of a water-borne toxin that contaminated the dialysate, probably a trace metal. Subsequently, the same group reported three- to fourfold elevations of aluminum levels in brain, bone, and other tissues obtained from dialysis patients dying from DE, compared with control uremic subjects (Alfrey et al., 1976). Unfortunately, there are relatively few studies of brain aluminum content in dialysis patients. Arieff has pointed out that there is some overlap in aluminum content between brain tissue from patients with and those without DE, while brain aluminum levels are significantly elevated in other diseases with quite different neurological manifestations (Arieff et al., 1979; Fraser and Arieff, 1988). Nonetheless, brain aluminum content is significantly higher in patients dying from DE than in those dying from any other condition in which it has been measured. This is illustrated in Figure 7.5. However, brain aluminum levels in DE are about one-tenth the value of bone aluminum from patients with dialysis osteomalacia associated with aluminum toxicity (see Association of Dialytic Encephalopathy with Dialysis Osteomalacia, below). This implies that the blood-brain barrier is relatively effective in controlling aluminum entry into the brain.

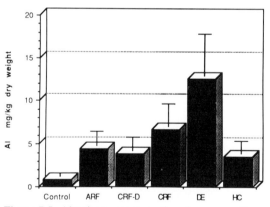

Brain Aluminum Concentration

Figure 7.5. Aluminum concentrations in gray matter of control patients, those with acute renal failure (ARF), patients with chronic renal failure on hemodialysis (CRF-D), patients with chronic renal failure not treated with dialysis (CRF), patients with dialytic encephalopathy (DE), and patients with hepatic coma (HC). (Modified from Sideman and Manor, 1982).

Epidemiological Association

Further implications of aluminum as the causative agent were provided by epidemiological studies. Platts et al. (1977) in the Trent Region of England and Elliot et al. (1978) in the west of Scotland, correlated the geographic distribution of DE with elevated water aluminum levels in those areas. These initial findings were corroborated in large-scale surveys of dialysis patients in England and Europe (Parkinson et al., 1979) (see Figure 7.1) and subsequently in epidemic outbreaks of DE in individual dialysis units where abrupt failures occurred in the dialysate water purification systems (Flendrig et al., 1976; Berkseth and Shapiro, 1980; Dunea et al., 1978). It is now clear that epidemics of DE are no longer seen, provided that adequate purification of dialysate water by reverse osmosis maintains dialysate aluminum levels below the recommended acceptable limits of 10 μg/L (270 nmol/L) (Savory et al., 1983; Davison et al., 1982; Parkinson et al., 1979).

However, DE is still seen in sporadic instances. The prevalence of this endemic form is unknown but is certainly very low; it has been variably reported between 0.6 and 1.0 percent (Wing et al., 1980; Dewberry et al., 1980). In this instance, the source of aluminum must be via the oral ingestion of $Al(OH)_3$ used to control dietary phosphate absorption (Dewberry et al., 1980). Since most dialysis patients have been treated with large amounts of $Al(OH)_3$, the very low prevalence of DE probably indicates that factors other than aluminum operate to select those patients who ultimately develop DE.

*Association of Dialytic
Encephalopathy with Dialysis
Osteomalacia*

The association between DE and fracturing dialysis osteodystrophy, or dialysis osteomalacia, was noted very early in dialysis units using dialysates contaminated with high aluminum levels (Ward et al., 1976; Parkinson et al., 1979; Platts et al., 1977). In its most severe form, dialysis osteomalacia is a crippling syndrome associated with severe bone pain and fractures. Bone biopsy reveals severe osteomalacia, without concurrent evidence of secondary hyperparathyroidism (Hodsman et al., 1981). The epidemiological evidence linking the osteomalacia to accumulation of aluminum salts in bone is similar to that outlined previously for DE. However, the availability of bone biopsy material allows comparisons between this syndrome and other forms of renal osteodystrophy; similar comparisons cannot be made in encephalopathic patients. Thus, bone aluminum content is significantly higher in dialysis patients with osteomalacia than in those with other forms of uremic bone disease (Hodsman et al., 1982).

Aluminum can be detected by light microscopy using a specific histochemical stain (Marcus et al., 1984). Aluminum deposition is found predominantly at the osteoid–mineralized bone interface, the site at which mineralization of osteoid matrix begins. Stainable aluminum can be quantitated histomorphometrically and is found to have a strong positive correlation with extractable bone aluminum content as measured by flameless atomic absorption spectrophotometry and with the amount of unmineralized osteoid matrix found in the biopsy (Maloney et al., 1982). These correlations between aluminum and osteoid tissue imply that aluminum is preferentially deposited in osteoid matrix and that this deposition may, in some way, inhibit normal mineralization of the matrix by calcium and phosphate ions. Patients with other forms of renal osteodystrophy do not have positive staining for aluminum and have much lower levels of extractable bone aluminum content (Hodsman et al., 1982; Maloney et al., 1982).*

Just as there are epidemics of DE in addition to an endemic form with a much lower prevalence, similar differences have been found for dialysis osteomalacia. In North America, the severe, symptomatic form of osteomalacia has an endemic prevalence of around two to four percent (Hodsman et al., 1981). However, in endemic cases of osteomalacia, the concurrent existence of DE is low, with less than 20 percent of aluminum-associated osteomalacic patients becoming demented (Hodsman et al., 1981) (Hodsman, et al. unpublished observations of the regional dialysis population in southwestern Ontario, Canada, 1988). Similarly, not all cases of endemic DE have histological evidence of aluminum-associated osteomalacia (A.B. Hodson, personal communication, 1988). Clearly, the interrelationship between aluminum, DE, and dialysis osteomalacia is not straightforward.

Nature of Brain Dysfunction in Toxic Dialytic Encephalopathy

The fluctuation, asterixis, multifocal myoclonus, EEG features, and reversibility found in early DE are characteristic of a metabolic encephalopathy. It could be argued that the characteristic speech disturbance sets DE apart from typical metabolic encephalopathies. This is true, but focal features can occur in metabolic encephalopathies. Chédru and Geschwind (1972) found that writing disturbances are common in toxic encephalopathies. It could be that language-related operations, by virtue of their complexity, are especially vulnerable in metabolic or toxic disorders.

Nadel and Wilson (1976) proposed that DE is a seizure disorder. They based their argument on the epileptiform activity on the EEG and the clinical and EEG response to diazepam. They propose that the seizure arises in the diencephalon and involves corticoreticular and thalamoreticular systems. Three features of DE argue against this simple explanation. First, although bursts of epileptiform activity are found, no patient has been reported to have continuous epileptiform activity or status epilepticus, which would be required to explain the prolonged episodes of altered function. Second, although cerebral

---

Osteomalacic bone in patients with aluminum-associated osteomalacia contains 175 ± 22 mg aluminum per kg dry weight of tissue compared with 60 ± 10 mg/kg in renal osteodystrophy not related to aluminum intoxication. The difference between bone and brain is striking (Hodsman et al., 1982).

cortical benzodiazepine binding sites are slightly reduced in DE, binding sites for γ-aminobutyric acid (GABA), the principal inhibitory neurotransmitter in the brain, are not reduced (Kish et al., 1985). This is in contradistinction to temporal lobe epilepsy in humans, in which GABA receptor binding is reduced (Lloyd et al., 1983). Finally, diazepam is helpful for seizures when given intravenously for acute seizures, but it is not a very effective antiepileptic drug for maintenance use, because of rapid development of tolerance and uncertain serum and brain levels (Schmidt, 1982). It seems, therefore, unlikely that diazepam would be the only antiepileptic drug effective against DE if the mechanism involved continuous epileptic seizures. Other mechanisms, perhaps involving the benzodiazepine receptor, seem a more likely explanation for diazepam's effect.

The advanced, apparently irreversible phase of DE suggests that some structural change has taken place in the brain. Even though there is no consistent macroscopic or microscopic lesion, an irreversible biochemical effect (e.g., on nucleic acid transcription) seems likely. The derangement passes the point of no return beyond which the brain cannot repair itself, and progressive deterioration occurs.

Neurotoxicology of Aluminum

One of the earliest reports of aluminum toxicity (Spofforth, 1921) was in a metal worker who suffered memory disturbances, tremor, myoclonus, and incoordination. McLaughlin et al. (1962) later described a ball-mill worker who developed a similar encephalopathy, as well as pulmonary fibrosis, from the inhalation of aluminum dust.

In experimental animals, mental and motor deficits, similar to those described in DE, have been produced by systemic or intracerebral injection of aluminum (Scherp and Church, 1937; Crapper and Dalton, 1973a; 1973b; Petit et al., 1980). Learning and short-term memory defects, delayed response and avoidance tasks, and incoordination were followed by apathy and convulsions. Alumina cream applied directly onto the cerebral cortex produces a sta-

ble epileptic focus with loss of neuronal dendritic spines and reduced branching of dendrites (Westrum et al., 1964). Neurofibrillary tangles have been produced by aluminum in intact animals, as well as in human neuronal cell culture (Crapper and Dalton, 1973a; 1973b; De Boni et al., 1980).

There are both ontogenetic and phylogenetic factors in the development of experimental aluminum-induced neurotoxicity. Younger animals are more resistant than adults, and primates take longer than cats and rabbits to develop the behavioral and motor abnormalities (Petit, 1985). Monkeys develop neurofibrillary tangles after only 180 days (Petit, 1985). Humans are likely to be more resistant to aluminum than other mammals.

There are several possible mechanisms by which aluminum may produce encephalopathy in uremic patients (Sarkander et al., 1983; Ganrot, 1986). These include: binding with adenosine triphosphate (ATP) and interfering with phosphate transfer involving various enzymes and membrane transport systems; interference with calcium uptake and utilization; altered function of various neurotransmitters and neuromodulators; effects on membrane lipid attachment to deoxyribonucleic acid (DNA) and ribonucleic acid (RNA), resulting in reduced RNA synthesis; and a colchicine-like effect on microtubular function, causing reduced axoplasmic transport. These may not be mutually exclusive. It is unclear whether there is any pathophysiological explanation for the reversible and irreversible phases of DE based on the different toxic actions of aluminum or whether the point of no return reflects a brain and body burden of aluminum that cannot be adequately removed. The dying back of dendrites and neurofibrillary changes found in experimental animals, as well as the effects on DNA represent irreversible toxicity. However, the brain levels of aluminum in DE are very high (see the earlier section, Role of Aluminum Toxicity), and the mechanisms for transfer of aluminum out of the brain are likely inadequate (Ganrot, 1986); the cytosol, nucleic acids, and cellular proteins may be chronically poisoned.

Aluminum has been shown to form stable

complexes with ATP (Solheim and Fromm, 1980); this creates the potential for inhibition of a large number of reactions in neurons and glia that are mediated by enzymes including hexokinase (Solheim and Fromm, 1980), adenylate cyclase (Mansour et al., 1983), 3,5-nucleotide phosphodiesterase (Ganrot, 1986), sodium-potassium adenosine triphosphatase (Staurnes et al., 1984), acetylcholinesterase (Patoka, 1971), catechol-O-methyltransferase (Mason and Weinkove, 1983) and dihydropteridine reductase (Mayor and Burnatowska-Hiedin, 1986). The inhibition of phosphodiesterase is likely due to interaction between the aluminum ion and calmodulin (Siegal and Haug, 1983). Interference with calmodulin activity could also affect other cell activity by reducing calcium entry into the cell. It should be understood that all of these actions have been shown using *in vitro* model systems; it remains to be shown that aluminum can exist in a free (unbound) state in sufficient concentration in the brain to produce these effects.

Aluminum has been reported to interfere with the uptake of several putative neurotransmitters in synaptosomes (isolated nerve terminals) *in vitro*. These include GABA, glutamic acid (Wong et al., 1981), choline (Lai et al., 1980), norepinephrine, and serotonin (Lai et al., 1982). This could alter the activity of these chemicals at receptor sites in the brain. Furthermore, aluminum was shown to form complexes with leu-enkephalin, a neuromodular endorphin (Mazarguil et al., 1982).

Aluminum can inhibit the incorporation of inositol into phospholipids and the hydrolysis of phosphoinositides (Johnson and Jope, 1986). This system serves as the second messenger system in those neurons not using cyclic adenosine monophosphate for this purpose. Thus, the receptor physiology may be seriously compromised in cholinergic and other systems. The "turning off" of these receptors is also altered, and calcium overstimulation may cause eventual neuronal death (Birchall and Chappell, 1988).

Aluminum has affinity for DNA, RNA, and a number of nucleotides (Ganrot, 1986) in the nuclei of both in neurons and glia (De Boni et al., 1974). With DNA, the binding is much greater to heterochromatin, which makes it less harmful than if it were bound to the metabolically active euchromatin. The degree and type of aluminum reaction with DNA is dependent on pH and whether or not aluminum is associated with the hydroxyl ion (Karlik et al., 1980). Cross-linking and other interactions may prevent information transfer from DNA. Aluminum inhibits RNA synthesis in isolated rat brain nuclei in a concentration of 0.5 mmol/L (Sarkander et al., 1983). If such concentrations are achieved in brain nucleic acid proteins, this could alter protein synthesis.

Although neurofibrillary degeneration is rare in DE, it is possible that a physiological reduction in dendritic physiology and neurotubular axoplasmic transport may occur without frank neurofibrillary change (Bizzi et al., 1984). Farnell et al. (1982), using a hippocampal slice preparation, provide evidence that this can occur. The hippocampal preparations were taken from animals at various stages of aluminum-induced encephalopathy. Neurons in the CA 1 region of the hippocampus showed reduced orthodromic spike generation in response to stimulation of the stratum radiatum, a region from which these neurons receive synaptic input. In addition, the authors demonstrated reduced long-term potentiation, thought to be the neurophysiological basis of memory, in this *in vitro* system. These electrophysiological events occurred before any histological or electron microscopical evidence of neurofibrillary degeneration in the pyramidal neurons under study. There is no definitive explanation for these observations.

Modifying Factors in Aluminum Intoxication

Uremic patients have diminished ability to clear aluminum once it enters the body. Since aluminum becomes highly protein bound, there is a gradient of free (unbound) aluminum ions between the dialysis fluid and the plasma. This favors transfer of aluminum from the dialysate across the dialysis membrane into the blood. Aluminum ionization is pH dependent: less than 40 percent is in ionic form at pH 6, but nearly 100 percent is ionized at pH 4 and pH

9 (Parkinson et al. 1981). Thus, the aluminum concentration and pH of the dialysate as well as the aluminum concentration and protein concentration of the plasma determine the net transfer of aluminum from dialysate to blood in hemodialysis. Notwithstanding these considerations, it is possible that net transfer of aluminum occurs from dialysate to blood at any level of dialysate aluminum in excess of 10 μg/L (370 nmol/L) (Kaehny et al., 1977). Transfer across the peritoneal membrane depends on the same factors.

It has been proposed that abnormalities in the blood-brain barrier facilitate entry of aluminum into brain in DE (Fraser and Arieff, 1988). This has not been established, however.

Role of GABA and the Benzodiazepine Receptor

Special mention should be made of GABA, which has been shown by Perry et al. (1985) to be deficient in the cerebral cortex taken postmortem from 10 repeatedly dialyzed uremic patients, eight of whom probably had DE. It is unclear if aluminum toxicity played a role, but it may have. The authors also found a deficiency of pyridoxal phosphate, a cofactor in the synthesis of GABA by the enzyme glutamic acid decarboxylase.

A deficiency of GABA, along with the above-mentioned reduction in benzodiazepine binding sites (Kish et al., 1985), which are linked to the GABA ionophore, may account for the temporary benefit from diazepam. However, since this is only a temporary benefit, it appears unlikely that GABA and the benzodiazepine receptor play a major role in the development and progression of DE. Pathophysiologically, some of the early features of the reversible phase of the disease may relate to these neurochemical derangements, however.

Other Factors

Although the importance of aluminum in the production of DE seems incontrovertible, the role of other factors, which may be important in individual susceptibility, should still be considered. These include: level of parathyroid hormone, vitamin D administration, imbalance of other trace elements and minerals, variations in amino acid transport into and out of the brain and CSF, damage to the blood-brain barrier, and missing or depleted substances.

Clinical Management

Prevention

The diagnosis of DE is made on clinical grounds, in association with a characteristic EEG. However, arrest or reversal of the encephalopathy once it becomes clinically apparent may not be possible. Therefore, some consideration should be given to prevention of the syndrome. From the foregoing sections, it is likely that aluminum toxicity is one of the major, if not *the* major, etiological agents responsible for the development of DE. Some general measures should be taken in all patients entering a dialysis program, to monitor the development of aluminum accumulation.

Monitoring Dialysate Aluminum Levels

Over 90 percent of circulating aluminum is bound to plasma proteins, particularly transferrin (Martin, 1986). For this reason, there is a net transfer of aluminum from dialysate to blood unless the dialysate aluminum can be reduced to extremely low levels. There is a general consensus that the "safe" dialysate aluminum concentration should be no higher than 10 μg/L (370 nmol/L) (Savory et al., 1983); in practice, this is reliably achieved only by reverse osmosis purification of the water used to reconstitute dialysate. Since inadvertent contamination of concentrates used to make hemodialysate or peritoneal dialysate theoretically can occur during the manufacturing process, it would seem prudent to monitor hemo- and peritoneal dialysate solutions on a regular basis. Values in excess of 10 μg/L should prompt a full evaluation of the tap water purification system within the dialysis unit and, if this seems to be functioning properly, of the manufacturing process of the dialysate.

Predictive Value of Serum Aluminum Levels

Serum aluminum levels are conveniently measured by flameless atomic absorption spectrophotometry; with modern instrumentation, the assay is both precise and accurate. In nonuremic patients, serum aluminum levels are less than 15 μg/L (550 nmol/L). Among patients who are dialyzed against aluminum-free dialysate, serum aluminum levels increase with time in all patients treated with aluminum-based phosphate binders; in general, the increased serum aluminum reflects the total dose of $Al(OH)_3$ consumed during the previous uremic history (Salusky et al., 1984; McCarthy et al., 1986). Cross-sectional studies of serum aluminum in dialysis patients treated with $Al(OH)_3$ reveal average values of 50 to 70 μg/L (Hodsman et al., 1985; vonHerrath et al., 1986). However, clinical features of aluminum toxicity can be seen at any level of serum aluminum; thus, there is no safe range.

For dialysis osteomalacia, whether or not there are symptoms of bone pain, baseline levels of serum aluminum in excess of 150 μg/L are strongly associated with bone histological evidence of aluminum poisoning (Hodsman et al., 1985; Milliner et al., 1984; Roodhooft et al., 1987); in our experience, serum aluminum levels in excess of this value have an 80 percent positive predictive value for histological evidence of aluminum-associated osteomalacia (Hodsman, AB et al., unpublished observations, 1988). The evidence is less clear regarding serum aluminum levels in DE patients dialyzed against low dialysate aluminum levels. Dialysis encephalopathy has been described in patients with serum aluminum levels ranging from 15 to over 1,000 μg/L (McKinney et al., 1982; Adhemar et al., 1980) (the higher levels due to severe aluminum contamination of dialysate). In a large cross-sectional study reported by Rovelli et al. (1988), DE was found only in patients with serum aluminum levels in excess of 50 μg/L; serum aluminum concentration averaged 150 μg/L in patients with DE. This accords well with our own unpublished observations in a five-year follow-up of over 300 dialysis patients in southwest Ontario. However, while serum aluminum levels of below 50 μg/L are less likely to be associated with aluminum toxicity, they do not exclude it. It is likely that serum aluminum levels have less predictive value for DE than they do for dialysis osteomalacia.

Deferoxamine Infusion Test

In attempts to enhance the specificity and sensitivity of serum aluminum in predicting the total body aluminum burden, changes in serum aluminum after deferoxamine (DFO) administration have been evaluated. This chelating agent removes aluminum from tissue binding sites, resulting in a significant rise in total circulating aluminum. Since the drug is primarily cleared by dialysis and is distributed in the extracellular fluid space, total serum aluminum levels rise progressively after DFO infusion, reaching a plateau at 24 to 36 hours. Milliner et al. (1984) found that using the criterion of an increment in serum aluminum in excess of 200 μg/L 48 hours after a standardized DFO infusion (40 mg/kg) greatly increased the sensitivity of the serum aluminum measurement to predict underlying aluminum-associated osteomalacia, compared to measuring baseline serum aluminum concentrations. However, it must be pointed out that the *specificity* of the serum aluminum measurement after the DFO infusion test is greatly reduced, since patients with other forms of renal osteodystrophy may have comparable changes (Milliner et al., 1984). Other workers have not found the DFO infusion test to be any more valuable in managing renal osteodystrophy than a simple baseline serum aluminum level (Hodsman et al., 1985; Roodhooft et al., 1987). When applying the DFO infusion test to patients with DE, Rovelli et al. (1988) also found little additional value of the DFO infusion test over the baseline serum aluminum measurement.

Dialysis, Diet, and Phosphate Binders

Sustained hyperphosphatemia from dietary phosphate is an inevitable accompaniment of progressive renal failure, and is usually seen when the glomerular filtration rate has fallen to less than 30 mL/min. Because hyperphosphatemia results in a reduction in serum ionized calcium, it is a potent trigger for the development of progressive hyperparathyroidism, which is almost universally seen in patients entering a dialysis program. In the early days of clinical dialysis programs, severe hyperparathyroidism was responsible for the development of renal osteodystrophy (particularly the bone lesion known as osteitis fibrosa) and was strongly associated with vascular calcification. For this reason, control of hyperphosphatemia remains a vigorously adhered-to goal in most dialysis units. The major determinants of phosphate absorption are the absolute dietary intake of phosphate and the limitation of phosphate absorption by the administration of phosphate-binding agents, conventionally in the form of aluminum-containing antacid gels. Because of the ubiquity of phosphorus in most meat and dairy products, it is unrealistic to expect the average patient with advanced renal failure to accept a diet containing less than 600 to 900 mg of phosphorus per day (about a 25 percent reduction from normal) (Fournier et al., 1971a). Thus, aluminum-based phosphate-binding agents have become the mainstay of dietary phosphate control (Fournier et al., 1971b). At the same time, it must be recognized that the administration of aluminum-containing phosphate binders will lead to increasing whole body aluminum burdens. Although it is poorly absorbed, some degree of aluminum absorption occurs with the most commonly used preparation, $Al(OH)_3$, and this appears to be responsible for the sporadic or endemic cases of DE and dialysis osteomalacia (discussed under Role of Aluminum Toxicity, above). Many nephrologists now believe that the long-term risks of aluminum toxicity offset the benefits of controlling dietary phosphate absorption in preventing renal osteodystrophy (Hercz and Coburn, 1986; Savory et al., 1983).

Although $Al(OH)_3$ has so far proven to be the most effective phosphate binder, the most widely used alternative is calcium carbonate.

Calcium carbonate ($CaCO_3$) has been shown to be an effective dietary binder (Meyrier et al., 1973), in addition to its proven ability to augment calcium absorption. Besides the obvious advantage of minimizing the total body aluminum burden, additional benefits include suppression of secondary hyperparathyroidism in both children and adults (Alon et al., 1986; Mak et al., 1985). However, there are significant disadvantages to therapy with $CaCO_3$: (1) with current dialysate calcium concentrations (1.5 to 1.75 mmol/L), many patients develop postdialysis hypercalcemia; (2) in general, serum phosphate levels are not as easily controlled as with $Al(OH)_3$; and (3) the dose of $CaCO_3$ required to achieve control of serum phosphate levels averages 8 g/day (about 16 to 32 tablets per day) (Hercz and Coburn, 1987). Moreover, simultaneous use of 1-hydroxylated vitamin D metabolites and $CaCO_3$ should be avoided because of the risks of vitamin D–induced hypercalcemia.

Although dietary measures and antacids lead to acceptable control of serum phosphate in most patients, it may be necessary to increase the duration of dialysis treatment beyond that needed to maintain acceptable levels of blood urea and creatinine in a small minority of patients. However, it must be appreciated that even with the introduction of newer, more permeable dialysis membranes during the past decade, the unit removal of phosphate per hour of dialysis has not improved to any clinically significant degree (Hercz and Coburn, 1987).

As a general recommendation, dialysis patients who remain well and free of any symptoms suggesting the development of aluminum toxicity can probably be continued on $Al(OH)_3$ treatment, provided serum aluminum levels remain below 100 μg/L. The risk of developing symptomatic aluminum toxicity is considerably increased if serum aluminum levels remain in excess of 150 μg/L. It may be prudent to switch such patients to a non–aluminum-based phosphate binding agent such as $CaCO_3$.

Treatment of Established Dialytic Encephalopathy

Withdrawal from Sources of Aluminum

The development of symptoms suggestive of DE should prompt a full evaluation of the likely underlying tissue aluminum burden. This should include measurement of serum and dialysate aluminum levels, and perhaps the performance of the DFO infusion test (see Prevention, above). Even if serum aluminum levels are less than 150 μg/L, or the patient is developing a dementia with none of the attendant clinical or EEG hallmarks of DE, it should be mandatory to discontinue $Al(OH)_3$ as a dietary phosphate binder. Such patients should continue phosphate binding management with $CaCO_3$.

It is now widely recognized that the epidemic incidence of DE falls after adequate steps are taken to guarantee the use of aluminum-free dialysate. Indeed, this measure alone may lead to improvement in symptomatic DE (Davison et al., 1982; O'Hare et al., 1983). Furthermore, there are a number of reports suggesting amelioration of encephalopathic symptoms following the discontinuation of oral aluminum-containing phosphate binders (Masselot et al., 1978; Poisson et al., 1978; Dewberry et al., 1980; McKinney et al., 1982). In this context, it should be noted that children may be at special risk for aluminum intoxication from the use of $Al(OH)_3$ (Nathan and Pedersen, 1980; Griswold et al., 1983; Andreoli et al., 1984; Freundlich et al., 1985). While withdrawal of aluminum alone may result in arrest or regression of encephalopathy, significant reduction in the total tissue aluminum burden is unlikely. Aluminum is so tightly bound (at least 90 percent) to circulation plasma proteins and other tissues, that the very small amount of free circulating aluminum is inefficiently dialyzed (Kaehny et al., 1977); the average clearance during a standard dialysis treatment may amount to only 0.3 mg (Nebecker and Coburn, 1986).

Deferoxamine in the Management of Aluminum Toxicity

The demonstration that aluminum is probably the major etiological agent responsible for the development of DE and dialysis osteomalacia has led to the concept that chelation therapy might be able to reverse these syndromes. Initial results using the chelating agent DFO have been very encouraging in light of the almost universal failure of other therapeutic measures.

DFO has been used for many years as a chelating agent to accelerate removal of excessive iron stores in nonuremic subjects. DFO was first used to enhance the clearance of aluminum from a dialysis patient with DE on an empirical basis, leading to striking resolution of his symptoms (Ackrill et al., 1980).

In subsequent reports, it has become clear that chronic DFO therapy may lead to substantial clinical improvement in up to 70 percent of patients with DE, occasionally to the point where no residual neurological deficit is detectable; unfortunately, failure to respond or a fatal outcome was seen in the remaining patients (Ackrill et al., 1980; Arze et al., 1981; Milne et al., 1983; deGencarelli et al., 1986). It is very possible that the unreported failure rate is even higher. Symptoms of bone pain and myopathy usually respond dramatically in aluminum-intoxicated patients with dialysis osteomalacia treated with DFO chelation (Brown et al., 1982; Hood et al., 1984; Andress et al., 1987).

In the presence of DFO, the dialyzable fraction of the total serum aluminum, circulating as aluminoxamine, increases to more than 75 percent as a major result of the increased chelator-bound aluminum. Thus, whole body aluminum removal (usually less than 0.3 mg during standard dialysis treatment) may increase to 4 to 8 mg after DFO infusion, depending on the total body aluminum burden (Nebecker and Coburn, 1986). However, the biliary/fecal clearance of aluminoxamine may be five to 10 times more efficient than dialysis (McCarthy et al., 1987).

Given that total body aluminum burdens typically exceed 1.5 g in aluminum-poisoned patients (Williams et al., 1980), aluminum removal during DFO therapy is still rather slow (perhaps 70 to 80 mg/month). Since the clinical response to DFO therapy is usually observed within three to six months of starting such therapy, the benefits of DFO therapy may be the result of depleting a small but selected pool of tissue aluminum.

DFO therapy can be given safely and on a long-term basis. The simplest therapeutic regimens have used doses of 30 to 40 mg DFO/kg body weight (to a maximum dose of 4 g) given intravenously over the last two hours of a dialysis treatment, once weekly. Doses of 1 to 2 g/week may be just as effective. Less data is available for chronic ambulatory peritoneal dialysis patients; however, DFO can be given by weekly intravenous infusion or by weekly addition to the overnight dialysate exchange with comparable efficacy (Molitoris et al., 1987). Although symptomatic improvement in the encephalopathy may be seen within three months, the optimum duration of DFO therapy has not been established. As an empirical guide, we have followed the total serum aluminum levels pre- and 48 hours post-DFO infusion; provided there are significant increments of serum aluminum post-DFO, it is likely that the tissue-bound aluminum is still available for chelation and continued depletion of total body aluminum stores will be maintained. Total treatment periods of six to 12 months should be anticipated.

Although the long-term side effects of prolonged parenteral DFO therapy have largely been observed in nondialysis patients, they have occurred in dialysis patients as well. These include an ill-defined flulike syndrome for 48 hours or so after receiving the weekly dose of DFO, visual and auditory neurotoxicity (Olivieri et al., 1986; Davies et al., 1983) and an increased risk of contracting atypical infections, including *Yersinia enterocolitica* and mucormycosis, both of which thrive in an iron-depleted environment (Molitoris et al., 1987). Iron stores are often low in dialysis patients; regular DFO therapy will, of course, exacerbate underlying iron deficiency. However, the development of iron deficiency can be followed in the usual way by regular assessment of serum ferritin levels, and concurrent iron therapy can be instituted as necessary.

A word of caution should also be added. A recent report by Sherrard et al. (1988) described five patients with very high serum aluminum levels and severe aluminum-associated dialysis osteomalacia who were treated with standard doses of DFO (1 to 2 g parenterally every week). This appeared to precipitate DE in all five patients, which was fatal in three. There are other sporadic reports documenting a worsening of CNS symptoms when patients with DE have been treated with DFO (Ackrill and Day, 1984; Luda et al., 1983). The pathophysiology of DFO-induced dialysis dementia is unclear. Direct CNS toxicity seems unlikely, as this has not been described in extensive experience with the use of DFO to treat iron overload. Since the DFO-aluminum complex has a relatively low molecular weight (less than 600 daltons), it may cross the blood-brain barrier more readily than the normally circulating aluminum that is largely bound to protein. Unfortunately, the limited available data does not indicate the lowest safe dose of DFO that might successfully avoid the exacerbation of DE symptoms during chelation therapy.

Symptomatic Management of Neurological Dysfunction

Although seizures may respond initially to diazepam, phenytoin and carbamazepine are more effective in long-term management. Hospitalization is usually necessary with confusional states, seizures, or ataxia, as well as for initial specific therapy. Diazepam therapy, as mentioned, is only of temporary benefit. We have not found it of practical value in therapy.

Intellectual Impairment in Dialysis Patients

Whether there is a syndrome of chronic intellectual impairment in uremic patients treated by dialysis, which is separate from DE, is controversial. Some psychological surveys suggest a reduction in information processing capabilities (McDaniel, 1971; Osberg et al., 1982). Other studies, even on patients hemodialyzed for more than 10 years fail to show any significant cognitive dysfunction (Treischmann and Sand, 1971; Brancaccio et al., 1981). A subpopulation of hemodialyzed patients shows a significant slowing of EEG frequencies, but most patients have normal recordings or minimal to no deterioration (Teschan et al., 1981). The specific factors involved in cerebral dysfunction in the affected subpopulation are uncertain.

References

Abram HS, Moore GL, Westervelt FB. Suicidal behavior in chronic dialysis patients. Am J Psychiatry 1971;127:1119–1204.

Ackrill P, Day JP. Therapy of aluminum overload II. Contrib Nephrol 1984;38:78–80.

Ackrill P, Ralston AJ, Day JP, Hodge KC. Successful removal of aluminum from patients with dialytic encephalopathy. Lancet 1980;2:692–693.

Adhemar JP, Laederich J, Jaudon MC, et al. Dialysis encephalopathy. Diagnostic and prognostic value of clinical and EEG signs, and aluminum levels in serum and cerebrospinal fluid. Proc Eur Dial Transplant Assoc 1980;17:234–239.

Alfrey A. Dialysis encephalopathy. Kidney Int 1986; 29:S53–S57.

Alfrey AC, LeGendre GR, Kaehny WD. The dialysis encephalopathy syndrome. Possible aluminum intoxication. N Engl J Med 1976;294:184–188.

Alfrey AC, Mishell JM, Burks J, et al. Syndrome of dyspraxia and multifocal seizures associated with chronic hemodialysis. Trans Am Soc Artif Intern Organs 1972;18:257–261.

Alon U, Davidai G, Bentur L, et al. Oral calcium carbonate as phosphate-binder in infants and children with chronic renal failure. Miner Electrolyte Metab 1986;12:320–325.

Andreoli SP, Bergstein JM, Sherrard DJ. Aluminum intoxication from aluminum-containing phosphate binders in children with azotemia not undergoing dialysis. N Engl J Med 1984;310:1079–1084.

Andress DL, Nebeker HG, Ott SM, et al. Bone histologic response to deferoxamine in aluminum-related bone disease. Kidney Int 1987;31:1344–1350.

Arieff AI, Cooper JD, Armstrong D, Lazarowitz VC. Dementia, renal failure and brain aluminum. Ann Intern Med 1979;90:741–747.

Arze RS, Parkinson IS, Cartlidge NE, et al. Reversal of aluminum dialysis encephalopathy after desferrioxamine treatment. Lancet 1981;2:1116.

Bakir AA, Hryhorczuk O, Berman E, Dunea G. Acute fatal hyperaluminemic encephalopathy in undialyzed

and recently dialyzed uremic patients. Trans Am Soc Artif Intern Organs 1986;32:171–176.

Baratz R, Herzog AG. The communication disorders of dialysis dementia. Brain Lang 1980;10:378–389.

Bates D, Parkinson IMS, Ward MK, Kerr DNS. Aluminum encephalopathy. Contrib Nephrol 1985;45:29–41.

Berkseth RO, Shapiro FL. An epidemic of dialysis encephalopathy and exposure to high aluminum dialysate. In: Scheiner GE, Winchester JF, eds. Controversies in nephrology. 2nd ed. Washington, DC: Georgetown University Press, 1980:42–51.

Birchall JD, Chappell JS. Aluminum chemical physiology and Alzheimer's disease. Lancet 1988;2:1008–1010.

Bizzi A, Crane RC, Autilo-Gambetti L, Gambetti P. Aluminum effect on slow axoplasmic transport: a novel impairment of neurofilament transport. J Neurosci 1984;4:722–731.

Brancaccio D, Damasso R, Spinnler R, et al. Neuropsychological performances of patients dialyzed for more than 10 years. In: Giordano C, Friedman EI, eds. Uremia: pathobiology of patients treated for 10 years or more. Milan: Wichtig Editore, 1981;46:126–129.

Brown DJ, Dawborn JK, Ham KN, Xipell JM. Treatment of dialysis osteomalacia with desferrioxamine. Lancet 1982;2:343–345.

Brown P, Rodgers-Johnson P, Cathala F, et al. Creutzfeldt-Jakob disease of long duration: clinico-pathological characteristics, transmissibility and differential diagnosis. Ann Neurol 1984;16:295–304.

Brun A, Dictor M. Senile plaques and tangles in dialysis dementia. Acta Pathol Microbiol Scand [A] 1981;89:193–198.

Canter GJ. Observations in neurogenic stuttering: a contribution and differential diagnosis. Br J Commun Dis 1971;6:139–143.

Cartier F, Chatel M, Allain P. Aluminum toxicity in renal failure. In: Zurukzoglu W, Papadimitriou M, Pyrpasapoulos M, et al., eds. Proceedings of the Eighth International Congress of Nephrology. Basel: Karger, 1981:1022–1029.

Chédru F, Geschwind N. Writing disturbances in acute confusional states. Neuropsychologia 1972;10:343–353.

Chokroverty S, Bruetman ME, Berger V, Reyes MG. Progressive dialytic encephalopathy. J Neurol Neurosurg Psychiatry 1976;39:411–419.

Chokroverty S, Gandhi V. Electroencephalograms in patients with progressive dialytic encephalopathy. Clin Electroencephalogr 1982;13:122–127.

Chui HC, Damasio AR. Progressive dialysis encephalopathy (dialysis dementia). J Neurol 1980;222:145–157.

Crapper DR, Dalton AJ. Alterations in short-term retention conditioned avoidance response acquisition and motivation following aluminum-induced neurofibrillary degeneration. Physiol Behav 1973a; 10:925–933.

Crapper DR, Dalton AJ. Aluminum-induced neurofibrillary degeneration, brain electrical activity and alterations in acquisition and retention. Physiol Behav 1973b;10:935–945.

Davies SC, Hungerford JL, Arden GB, et al. Ocular toxicity of high-dose intravenous desferrioxamine. Lancet 1983;2:181–184.

Davison AM, Oli H, Walter GS, Lewins AM. Water supply, aluminum concentration, dialysis dementia and effect of reverse-osmosis water treatment. Lancet 1982;2:785–786.

De Boni U, Scott JW, Crapper DR. Intranuclear aluminum binding: a histochemical study. Histochemistry 1974;40:31–37.

De Boni U, Seger M, Crapper McLachlan DR. Functional consequences of chromatin bound aluminum in cultured human cells. Neurotoxicology 1980;1:65–81.

DeGencarelli NC, Cournot-Witmer G, Zingraff J, Drueke T. The role of parathyroid function and parathyroidectomy in the outcome of aluminum-related dialysis encephalopathy. Nephrol Dial Transplant 1986;1:192–198.

Dewberry FL, McKinney TD, Stone WJ. The dialysis dementia syndrome: report of fourteen cases and review of the literature. Trans Am Soc Artif Intern Organs 1980;3:102–108.

Dunea G, Mahurkar SD, Mamdani B, Smith EC. Role of aluminum in dialysis dementia. Ann Intern Med 1978;88:502–504.

Elliot HL, MacDougall AI, Dryburgh F, et al. Aluminum toxicity during regular haemodialysis. Br Med J 1978;1:1101–1103.

English A, Savage RD, Britton PG, et al. Intellectual impairment in chronic renal failure. Br Med J 1978;1:888–889.

Farnell BJ, De Boni U, Crapper McLachlan DR. Aluminum neurotoxicity in the absence of neurofibrillary degeneration in CA 1 hippocampal pyramidal neurons in vitro. Exp Neurol 1982;78:241–258.

Flendrig JA, Kruis H, Das HA. Aluminum and dialysis dementia. Lancet 1976;1:1235.

Foley CM, Polinsky MS, Gruskin AB, et al. Encephalopathy in infants and children with chronic renal disease. Arch Neurol 1981;38:656–658.

Fournier AE, Arnaud CD, Johnson WJ, et al. Etiology of hyperparathyroidism and bone disease during chronic hemodialysis. II. Factors affecting serum immunoreactive parathyroid hormone. J Clin Invest 1971a;50:599–605.

Fournier AE, Johnson WJ, Taves DR, et al. Etiology of hyperparathyroidism and bone disease during chronic hemodialysis. Association of bone disease with potentially etiologic factors. J Clin Invest 1971b;50:592–598.

Fraser CL, Arieff AI. Nervous system complications in uremia. Ann Intern Med 1988;109:143–153.

Freundlich M, Abitol C, Zilleruelo G, Strauss J. Infant formula as a cause of aluminum toxicity in neonatal uremia. Lancet 1985;2:527–529.

Galle P, Chatel M, Berry JP, Menault F. Encéphalopathie myoclonique progressive des dialysés: présence d'aluminum en forte concentration dans les lysosomes des cellules cérébrales. Nouv Presse Med 1979;8:4091–4094.

Ganrot PO. Metabolism and possible health hazards of aluminum. Environ Health Perspect 1986;65:363–441.

Garcia-Bunuel L, Elliott DC, Blank NK. Apneic spells in progressive dialysis encephalopathy. Arch Neurol 1980;37:594–596.

Griswold WR, Reznik V, Mendoza SA, et al. Accumulation of aluminum in a nondialyzed uremic child receiving aluminum hydroxide. Pediatrics 1983;71:56–58.

Hercz G, Coburn JW. Prevention of phosphate retention and hyperphosphatemia in uremia. Kidney Int 1987;32(Suppl):S215–S220.

Hodsman AB, Hood SA, Brown P, Cordy PE. Do serum aluminum levels reflect underlying skeletal accumulation and bone histology before or after chelation by desferrioxamine? J Lab Clin Med 1985; 106:674–681.

Hodsman AB, Sherrard EJ, Alfrey AC, et al. Bone aluminum and histomorphometric features of renal osteodystrophy. J Clin Endocrinol Metab 1982; 54:539–546.

Hodsman AB, Sherrard DJ, Wong EG, et al. Vitamin-D resistant osteomalacia in hemodialysis patients lacking secondary hyperparathyroidism. Ann Intern Med 1981;94:629–637.

Hood SA, Clark WF, Hodsman AB, et al. Successful treatment of dialysis osteomalacia and dementia, using desferrioxamine infusions and oral 1-alpha hydroxycholecalciferol. Am J Nephrol 1984;4:369–374.

Hughes JR, Schreeder MT. EEG in dialysis encephalopathy. Neurology 1980;30:1148–1154.

Jack R, Rabin PL, McKinney TW. Dialysis encephalopathy: a review. Int J Psychiatry Med 1983–1984;13:309–326.

Jack RA, Ribers-Buckeley NT, Rabin PL. Secondary mania as a presentation of progressive dialysis encephalopathy. J Nerv Ment Dis 1983;171:193–195.

Jackson JH. On asphyxia in slight epileptic paroxysms: on the symptomatology of slight epileptic fits supposed to depend on discharges of the uncinate gyrus. Lancet 1899;1:199–207.

Johnson GVW, Jope RS. Aluminum impairs glucose utilization and cholinergic activity in rat brain in vitro. Toxicology 1986;40:93–102.

Kaehny WD, Alfrey AC, Holman RE, Shorr WJ. Aluminum transfer during hemodialysis. Kidney Int 1977;12:361–365.

Karlik SJ, Eichhorn GL, Crapper McLachlan DR. Molecular interactions of aluminum with DNA. Neurotoxicology 1980;1:83–88.

Kish SJ, Perry TL, Sweeney VP, Hornykiewicz O. Brain γ-aminobutyric acid and benzodiazepine receptor binding in dialysis encephalopathy. Neurosci Lett 1985;58:241–244.

Kogeorgos J, Scholtz C. Neurofibrillary tangles in aluminum encephalopathy: a new finding. Neuropathol Appl Neurobiol 1982;8:246.

La Greca G, Biasioli S, Borin D, et al. Dialytic encephalopathy. Contrib Nephrol 1985;45:9–28.

Lai JCK, Guest JF, Leung TKC, et al. The effects of cadmium, manganese and aluminum on sodium-potassium-activated and magnesium-activated adenosine triphosphate activity and choline uptake in rat brain synaptosomes. Biochem Pharmacol 1980; 29:141–146.

Lai JCK, Lim L, Davison AN. Effects of Cd^{2+}, Mn^{2+} and Al^{3+} on brain synaptosomal uptake of noradrenalin and serotonin. J Inorg Biochem 1982;17:215–225.

Lederman RJ, Henry CE. Progressive dialysis encephalopathy. Ann Neurol 1978;4:199–204.

Letemendia F, Pampiglione G. Clinical and electroencephalographic observations in Alzheimer disease. J Neurol Neurosurg Psychiatry 1958;21:167–172.

Levy SR, Chiappa KH, Burke CJ, Young RR. Early evolution and incidence of electrographic abnormalities in Creutzfeldt-Jakob disease. J Clin Neurophysiol 1986;3:1–21.

Lloyd KG, Murani C, Bossi L, Morselli PL. Status of GABA-ergic neurons in human epileptic foci, as defined by neurochemistry. J Neurochem 1983; 41(Suppl):S1010.

Luda E. EEG study on progressive dialytic encephalopathy in treatment with desferrioxamine. Int J Artif Intern Organs 1983;6:215–216.

Madison DP, Baehr ET, Bazell M, et al. Communicative and cognitive deterioration in dialysis dementia: two case studies. J Speech Hear Disord 1977; 42:238–246.

Mahurkar SD, Salta R, Smith EC, et al. Dialysis dementia. Lancet 1973;1:1412–1415.

Mahurkar SD, Smith EC, Mandani BH, Dunea G. Dialysis dementia: the Chicago experience. J Dial 1978;2:447–458.

Mason L, Weinkove C. Radioenzymic assay of catecholamines: reversal of aluminum inhibition of enzymatic o-methylation by desferrioxamine. Ann Clin Biochem 1983;20:105–111.

Mak RHK, Turner C, Thompson T, et al. Suppression of secondary hyperparathyroidism in children with chronic renal failure by high dose phosphate binders: calcium carbonate versus aluminum hydroxide. Br Med J 1985;291:623–627.

Maloney NA, Ott SM, Alfrey AC, et al. Histological

quantitation of aluminum in iliac bone from patients with renal failure. J Lab Clin Med 1982;99:206–216.

Mansour JM, Ehrlich A, Mansour TE. The dual effect of aluminum as activator and inhibitor of adenylate cyclase in the liver fluke Fasciola hepatica. Biochem Biophys Res Commun 1983;112:911–918.

Marcus R, Madvig P, Young G. Age-related changes in parathyroid hormone action in normal humans. J Clin Endocrinol Metab 1984;58:223–230.

Martin RB. The chemistry of aluminum as related to biology and medicine. Clin Chem 1986;32:1797–1806.

Masselot JP, Adhemar JP, Jandon MC, et al. Reversible dialysis encephalopathy: role for aluminum-containing gels. Lancet 1978;2:1386–1387.

Mayor GH, Burnatowska-Hiedin M. The metabolism of aluminum and aluminum-related encephalopathy. Semin Nephrol 1986;4(Suppl 1):1–4.

Mazarguil N, Haran R, Laussac J-B. The binding of aluminum to (Leu^5)-enkephalin. An investigation using ^1H, ^{13}C and ^{27}Al NMR spectroscopy. Biochim Biophys Acta 1982;717:465–472.

McCarthy JT, Kurtz SB, Mussman GV. Deferoxamine-enhanced fecal losses of aluminum and iron in a patient undergoing continuous ambulatory peritoneal dialysis. Am J Med 1987;82:367–370.

McCarthy JT, Milliner DS, Kurtz SB, et al. Interpretation of serum aluminum values in dialysis patients. Am J Clin Pathol 1986;86:629–636.

McDaniel JW. Metabolic and central nervous system correlates of cognitive dysfunction with renal failure. Psychophysiology 1971;8:704–713.

McKinney TD, Basinger M, Dawson E, Jones MM. Serum aluminum levels in dialysis dementia. Nephron 1982;32:53–56.

McLaughlin AIG, Kazantzis G, King E, et al. Pulmonary fibrosis and encephalopathy associated with inhalation of aluminum dust. Br J Ind Med 1962;19:253–263.

Meyrier A, Marsac J, Richet G. The influence of high calcium carbonate intake on bone disease in patients undergoing hemodialysis. Kidney Int 1973;4:146–153.

Milliner DS, Nebeker HG, Ott SM, et al. Use of the deferoxamine infusion test in the diagnosis of aluminum-related osteodystrophy. Ann Intern Med 1984;101:775–780.

Milne FJ, Sharf B, Bell P, Meyers AM. The effect of low aluminum water and desferrioxamine on the outcome of dialysis encephalopathy. Clin Nephrol 1983;20:202–207.

Molitoris BA, Alfrey PS, Miller NL, et al. Efficacy of intramuscular and intraperitoneal deferoxamine for aluminum chelation. Kidney Int 1987;31:986–991.

Nadel AM, Wilson WP. Dialysis encephalopathy: a possible seizure disorder. Neurology 1976;26:1130–1134.

Nathan E, Pedersen SE. Dialysis encephalopathy in a nondialysed uraemic boy treated with aluminum hydroxide orally. Acta Paediatr Scand 1980;69:793–796.

Nebecker HG, Coburn JW. Aluminum and renal osteodystrophy. Annu Rev Med 1986;37:79–95.

Nelson DA, Ray CD. Respiratory arrest from seizure discharges in the limbic system. Arch Neurol 1968; 19:199–207.

Noriega-Sanchez A, Martinez-Maldonado M, Haiffe RM. Clinical and electroencephalographic changes in progressive uremic encephalopathy. Neurology 1978;28:667–669.

O'Hare JA, Callaghan NM, Murnaghan DJ. Dialysis encephalopathy: clinical, electroencephalographic and interventional aspects. Medicine 1983;62:129–141.

Olivieri NF, Buncic JR, Chew E, et al. Visual and auditory neurotoxicity in patients receiving subcutaneous deferoxamine infusions. N Engl J Med 1986;314:869–873.

Osberg JW, Meares GJ, McKee DC, Burnett GB. Intellectual functioning in renal failure and chronic dialysis. J Chronic Dis 1982;35:445–457.

Parkinson IS, Feest TG, Ward MK, et al. Fracturing dialysis osteodystrophy and dialysis encephalopathy: an epidemiological survey. Lancet 1979;1:406–409.

Parkinson IS, Ward MK, Kerr DNS. Dialysis encephalopathy, bone disease and anemia: the aluminum syndrome during regular hemodialysis. J Clin Pathol 1981;34:1285–1294.

Patoka J. The influence of Al^{3+} on cholinesterase and acetylcholinesterase activity. Acta Biol Med Ger 1971;26:845–846.

Perry TL, Yong VW, Kish SJ, et al. Neurochemical abnormalities in brains of renal failure patients treated by repeated hemodialysis. J Neurochem 1985; 45:1043–1048.

Petit TL. Aluminum in human dementia. Am J Kidney Dis 1985;6:313–316.

Petit TL, Biederman GB, McMullen PA. Neurofibrillary degeneration, dendritic dying back and learning-memory deficiencies after aluminum administration: implications for brain aging. Exp Neurol 1980;67:152–162.

Pierides AM, Edwards WG, Cullum UX Jr, et al. Hemodialysis encephalopathy with osteomalacic fractures and muscle weakness. Kidney Int 1980; 1:115–124.

Platts MM, Goode GC, Hislop JS. Composition of the domestic water supply and the incidence of fractures and encephalopathy in patients on home dialysis. Br Med J 1977;2:657–660.

Poisson M, Mashally R, Lebkiri B. Dialysis encephalopathy: recovery after interruption of aluminum intake. Br Med J 1978;2:1610–1611.

Rae-Grant A, Blume WT. The electroencephalogram in Alzheimer-type dementia: a sequential study correlating the electroencephalogram with psychometric and quantitative pathologic data. Arch Neurol 1987;44:50–54.

Rivera-Vasquez AB, Noriega-Sanchez A, Ramirez-Gonzazel R, Martinez-Maldonado M. Acute hypercalcaemia in haemodialysis patients: distinction from "dialysis dementia." Nephron 1980;25:243–246.

Roodhooft AM, VandeVyver FL, D'Haese PC, et al. Aluminum accumulation in children on chronic dialysis: predictive value of serum aluminum levels and desferrioxamine infusion test. Clin Nephrol 1987; 28:125–129.

Rosenbek JC, McNeil MR, Lemme ML, et al. Speech and language findings in a chronic hemodialysis patient: a case report. J Speech Hear Disord 1975; 40:245–252.

Rovelli E, Luciani L, Pagani I, et al. Correlation between serum aluminum concentration and signs of encephalopathy in a large population of patients dialysed with aluminum-free fluids. Clin Nephrol 1988;29:294–298.

Salusky B, Coburn JW, Paunier L, et al. Role of aluminum hydroxide in raising serum aluminum levels in children undergoing continuous ambulatory peritoneal dialysis. J Pediatr 1984;105:715–720.

Sarkander H-I, Balss G, Schlosser R, et al. Blockade of neuronal brain RNA initiation sites by aluminum: a primary molecular mechanism of aluminum-induced neurofibrillary changes. In: Cervos-Navarro J, Sarkander H-I, eds. Brain aging: neuropathology and neuropharmacology. New York: Raven Press, 1983:259–274.

Savory J, Merlin A, Courtoux C, et al. Summary report of an international workshop on "The role of biological monitoring in the prevention of aluminum toxicity in man: aluminum analysis in biological fluids." Ann Clin Lab Sci 1983;13:1983–1990.

Scherp HW, Church CF. Neurotoxic action of aluminum salts. Proc Soc Exp Biol Med 1937;36:851–853.

Schmidt D. Diazepam. In: Woodbury DM, Penry JK, Pippinger DE, eds. Antiepileptic drugs. New York: Raven Press, 1982:711–735.

Scholtz C, Swash M, Gray A, et al. Neurofibrillary neuronal degeneration in dialysis dementia: a feature of aluminum toxicity. Clin Neuropathol 1987;6:93–97.

Schreeder MT, Favero MS, Hughes JR, et al. Dialysis encephalopathy and aluminum exposure: an epidemiologic analysis. J Chronic Dis 1983;36:581–593.

Sherrard DJ, Walker JV, Boykin JL. Precipitation of dialysis dementia by deferoxamine treatment of aluminum-related bone disease. Am J Kidney Dis 1988;12:126–130.

Sideman S, Manor D. The dialysis dementia syndrome and aluminum intoxication. Nephron 1982;31:1–10.

Siegal N, Haug A. Aluminum interaction with calmodulin: evidence for altered structure and function from optical and enzymatic studies. Biochim Biophys Acta 1983;744:36–45.

Smith DB, Lewis JA, Burks JS, Alfrey AC. Dialysis

encephalopathy in peritoneal dialysis. JAMA 1980; 244:365–366.

Solheim LP, Fromm HJ. A simple method for removing aluminum from adenosine-5'-triphosphate. Anal Biochem 1980;109:266–269.

Spofforth J. Case of aluminum poisoning. Lancet 1921;1:1301.

Staurnes M, Sigholt T, Reite OB. Reduced carbonic anhydrase and Na-K-ATPase activity in gills of salmonids exposed to aluminum-containing acid water. Experientia 1984;40:226–227.

Sundaram M, Blume WT. Triphasic waves: clinical correlates and morphology. Can J Neurol Sci 1987; 14:136–140.

Taclob L, Needle M. Drug induced encephalopathy in patients on maintenance hemodialysis. Lancet 1976;2:704–705.

Teschan PE, Ginn HE, Bourne JR, et al. Neurobehavior in long-term hemodialyzed patients. In: Giordano C, Friedman EA, eds. Uremia: pathobiology of patients treated for 10 years or more. Milan: Wichtig Editore, 1981:117–125.

Treischmann RB, Sand PL. WAIS and MMPI correlates of increasing renal failure in adult medical patients. Psychol Rep 1971;29:1251–1262.

VonHerrath D, Asmus G, Pauls A, et al. Renal osteodystrophy in asymptomatic hemodialysis patients: evidence of a sex-dependent distribution and predictive value of serum aluminum measurements. Am J Kidney Dis 1986;8:430–435.

Ward MK, Pierides AM, Fawcett P, et al. Dialysis encephalopathy syndrome. Proc Eur Dial Transplant Assoc 1976;13:348–354.

Westrum LE, White LE, Ward AA Jr. Morphology of the experimental epileptic focus. J Neurosurg 1964;1:1033–1044.

Williams ED, Elliott HL, Boddy K, et al. Whole body aluminum in chronic renal failure and dialysis encephalopathy. Clin Nephrol 1980;14:198–200.

Wills MR, Savory J. Aluminum poisoning: dialysis encephalopathy, osteomalacia, and anaemia. Lancet 1983;2:29–33.

Wing AJ, Brunner FP, Brynger H, et al. Dialysis dementia in Europe. Lancet 1980;2:190–192.

Wong PCK, Lai JCK, Lim L, Davison AN. Selective inhibition of L-glutamate and gamma aminobutyrate transport in nerve ending particles by aluminum, manganese and cadmium chloride. J Inorg Biochem 1981;14:253–260.

Zochodne DW, Young GB, McLachlan RS, et al. Creutzfeldt-Jakob disease without periodic sharp wave complexes: a clinical, electroencephalographic and pathologic study. Neurology 1988;38:1056–1060.

B

Dialysis Dysequilibrium Syndrome

Dialysis dysequilibrium syndrome (DDS) is a term used for a set of signs and symptoms that come on during or just following a dialysis procedure. The syndrome, in its mildest form, consists of headache, nausea, vomiting, restlessness or drowsiness, and muscle cramps. Moderate cases show asterixis, myoclonus, disorientation, and somnolence. In severe cases, the patient may develop an organic psychosis, generalized convulsive seizures, stupor, or coma (Port et al., 1973). All ages are affected, but the very young and very old may be more susceptible (Port et al., 1973). In some severe cases, the condition is fatal (Peterson and Swanson, 1964), either from the neurological problems or from the associated cardiac arrhythmias (Wakim, 1969).

EEG Findings

Port et al. (1973) found that nine of 13 patients showed a deterioration in their EEGs during or immediately following routine hemodialysis. The first changes are insidious, but encephalopathic patients ultimately (usually by two to three hours after the start of dialysis) show bursts of symmetrical, bisynchronous, rhythmic waves of medium or high voltage, mainly in the delta frequency range (less than 3 Hz) (Kennedy et al., 1963). Sometimes a mixture of rhythmic theta (3 to 8 Hz) and delta frequencies are present. The background, or ongoing continuous rhythm, is variably normal, mildly abnormal, or markedly dysrhythmic with more continuous polymorphic wave forms. In general, the severity of EEG change reflects the severity of the clinical encephalopathy. In most cases, the EEG returns to normal shortly after the procedure, unless complications such as severe cerebral edema or altered mental status persist.

Arieff et al. (1978) used a manual counting method to quantitate the percent of waves less than 5 Hz in the particular EEG channel's record. This technique is of some value, as is power spectral analysis. The main problem is that criteria for selection of the strip to be analyzed are not stated. It is very difficult to control for drowsiness; this could be at least partly corrected by sampling just following hyperventilation or some other task requiring concentration. Another problem with manual or automated frequency analysis is that paroxysmal abnormalities can be entirely missed; these sometimes constitute the main abnormality.

Neuroimaging Findings

Using computed tomographic (CT) x-ray scans, La Greca et al. (1982) measured the density of the brain in healthy persons and uremic

198

patients. They found that nonuremic individuals showed densitometric values ranging from 25 to 35 Hounsfield units (HU). In uremic subjects studied before dialysis, the values range from 35 to 45 HU. During and after hemodialysis or intermittent peritoneal dialysis (IPD), there was a consistent reduction in brain parenchymal density. These changes began during hemodialysis and persisted for at least 10 hours after the onset of dialysis. The reduction in brain density values for hemodialysis and IPD averaged between 20 and 30 percent of predialysis values. Density fell more rapidly in those patients on conventional hemodialysis with polyacrylonitrile membranes and standard dialysis solutions, reaching a plateau at the end of the four-hour dialysis procedure. The density fell less rapidly in hemodialysis patients treated similarly but using a Cuprophan membrane, reaching a plateau 10 hours after dialysis onset. In those on IPD, densities fell at an intermediate rate. The brain density measurements essentially returned to normal in these patients. Values remained constant and close to normal in continuous ambulatory peritoneal dialysis patients.

Although the density changed, presumably due to a combination of imbibition of water and some loss of osmotic particles, there was little evidence of significant brain swelling, as evidenced by change in ventricular size or compression of subarachnoid space.

Pathophysiology

The initial hypothesis was that DDS is due to a "reverse urea effect" (Peterson and Swanson, 1964). Urea crosses the blood-brain barrier and equilibrates between the plasma and brain or plasma and cerebrospinal fluid (CSF) compartments. With dialysis, the urea concentration in the plasma compartment is rapidly lowered. Because of the time lag for diffusion of urea from brain and CSF compartments back into the plasma compartment, there is an osmotic gradient, resulting in a net diffusion of water from plasma into brain and CSF. Rosen et al. (1964) found that the magnitude of the urea gradient between the plasma and the CSF was proportional to the predialysis plasma urea concentration. Further, they showed that the gradient persisted for about 24 hours from the onset of dialysis. Gilliland and Hegstrom (1963a; 1963b) found that a rise in CSF pressure occurred as part of DDS and that it could be prevented by adding isotonic urea to the dialysate.

Pappius et al. (1966), using an acutely uremic dog model, showed that the osmotic gradient between cerebral tissues and plasma was not maintained. The concentration gradient was most marked 30 to 60 minutes after the onset of rapid hemodialysis. Following dialysis, plasma urea levels increased, probably from urea diffusing back into the blood compartment from the tissues. The equilibration time for urea between cerebral gray matter and plasma (on the order of 1 to 3 hours) was shorter than that for white matter and plasma and much longer than that for CSF and plasma. There was a consistent rise in CSF fluid pressure in all cases. Brain tissue was sampled at intervals for up to four hours from onset of dialysis. Swelling (increased water content) was found in the gray matter in 50 percent, and in white matter in 75 percent, of dialyzed uremic animals. The significance of the observed lowering of cortical potassium concentration is unclear, particularly since the animals did not show a metabolic acidosis.

Arieff et al. (1973) showed that with rapid hemodialysis in the acute uremic dog model an intracellular acidosis occurs in the brain in association with an increase in brain "idiogenic osmols," osmotic particles of unknown chemical composition. The latter, rather than urea, may largely account for the increased water content of gray and white matter as part of DDS. Arieff et al. (1978), using the same model, also found a decrease in the pH of CSF, as well as reduced sodium and increased calcium concentrations in the brain. The acidosis in the brain is of uncertain pathogenesis. In steady state uremia, without or between dialyses, the brain does not show an acidosis, despite the presence of a systemic metabolic acidosis (Posner, 1965). With rapid hemodialysis, even when PCO_2 levels in arterial blood are controlled, the intracellular acidosis still occurs (Arieff et al., 1978). It may be that there is a formation of organic acids in the CNS. In any case, the intracellular acidosis may play a role as great or greater than that of swelling in the production of the EEG slowing and the signs and symptoms of DDS.

Treatment and Prevention

It appears that preventing a rapid osmotic shift of water into brain is the essential element in preventing DDS. This can be at least partly accomplished by using slower blood flow rates in dialysis (Arieff et al., 1973) and by increasing osmolality in the dialysate by addition of urea (Gilliland and Hegstrom, 1963b), sodium (Port et al., 1973), mannitol, or glycerol (Arieff et al., 1978). Glycerol is the most successful of these in preventing all of the changes found in experimental DDS (Arieff et al., 1978).

Arieff et al. (1978) propose that glycerol increases glycolysis and the availability of dihydroxyacetone phosphate. Lactate rather than lactic acid is produced, and each mole of lactate utilizes one mole of hydrogen ions, thus creating bicarbonate and prompting a rise rather than a fall of intracellular pH in the brain. Glycerol is also a well-known osmotic diuretic.

References

Arieff AI, Lazarowitz VC, Guisado R. Experimental dialysis dysequilibrium syndrome: prevention with glycerol. Kidney Int 1978;14:270–278.

Arieff AI, Massry SG, Barrientos A, Kleeman CR. Brain, water and electrolyte metabolism in uremia: effects of slow and rapid hemodialysis. Kidney Int 1973;4:177–187.

Gilliland KG, Hegstrom RM. Effect of hemodialysis on cerebrospinal fluid pressure in dogs. Clin Res 1963a;11:120.

Gilliland KG, Hegstrom RM. The effect of hemodialysis on cerebrospinal pressure in uremic dogs. Trans Am Soc Artif Intern Organs 1963b;9:44–48.

Kennedy AC, Linton AL, Luke RG, Renfrew S. Electroencephalographic changes during haemodialysis. Lancet 1963;1:408–411.

La Greca G, Biasioli S, Chiaramonte S, et al. Studies of brain density in hemodialysis and peritoneal dialysis. Nephron 1982;31:146–150.

Pappius HM, Oh JH, Dossetor JB. The effects of rapid hemodialysis on brain tissues and cerebrospinal fluid of dogs. Can J Physiol Pharmacol 1966;45:129–147.

Peterson H deC, Swanson AG. Acute encephalopathy occurring during hemodialysis. Arch Intern Med 1964;113:877–880.

Port FK, Johnson WJ, Klass DW. Prevention of dialysis dysequilibrium syndrome by the use of high sodium concentration in the dialysate. Kidney Int 1973;3:327–333.

Posner JB. Acid-base balance in cerebrospinal fluid. Arch Neurol 1965;12:479–496.

Rosen SM, O'Connor K, Shaldon S. Haemodialysis disequilibrium. Br Med J 1964;2:672–675.

Wakim KG. The pathophysiology of the dialysis dysequilibrium syndrome. Mayo Clin Proc 1969;44:406–429.

C

Subdural Hematoma

Clinical Features

Subdural hematomas are collections of blood trapped between the dura and arachnoid membranes. They are commonly produced by tearing of veins draining into the superior sagittal sinus. In most cases, the collection of blood lies over the frontal and parietal lobes. An outer wall forms over the hematoma, composed of highly vascularized granulation tissue that is prone to rebleeding, causing the hematoma to grow in size.

Chronic subdural hematomas are a well-recognized complication in 1 to 3.3 percent of uremic patients receiving hemodialysis and anticoagulation therapy (Talalla et al., 1970; Leonard et al., 1969; Leonard and Shapiro, 1975; Adams and Victor, 1985; Meyer and Barron, 1960). Rotter and Roettger (1973) found nontraumatic subdural hematomas at autopsy in 2.7 percent of routinely dialyzed uremic patients. The hemorrhage was large in only one of the nine patients with subdural hematomas. Most cases were fresh, but some were older with evidence of rebleeding. Undoubtedly, the coagulation problems that occur as part of the uremic syndrome play a major role in the pathogenesis of subdural hematomas in uremic patients. Prolongation of bleeding time, decreased platelet factor III activity, reduced platelet aggregation and adhesiveness, and impaired prothrombin utilization constitute the coagulopathy. The use of anticoagulants, such as heparin for dialysis purposes, adds to the risk. The exact mechanism, however, is still uncertain (Rotter and Roettger, 1973).

There may not be a history of injury. Although in the general population, older individuals are more likely to develop chronic subdural hematomas with or without a history of trauma, young uremic adults are susceptible, as are young persons with hematological disorders (Talalla et al., 1970). The clinical presentation is highly variable. Whatever features are present may show considerable fluctuation, sometimes so markedly as to stimulate transient ischemic attacks or threatened stroke. Headache is commonly present, and percussion of the head may be painful. The patient may show general decrease in alertness and cognition, mimicking a dementing or depressive illness. Alternatively, focal signs and symptoms such as language disturbance or hemiparesis may predominate. Sensory complaints and hemianopsia are not common, possibly because of difficulty testing sensation in the presence of impaired mental status; also, the deeper optic radiations may not be as subject to compressive symptoms as is the motor pathway.

Gait disturbance is sometimes striking, usually as a gait apraxia or ataxia or as a hemiparetic gait (McLachlan et al., 1981). Most patients are over 60 years of age (McLachlan et al., 1981). With gait apraxia, the patient may have difficulty initiating walking, and appears glued to the floor, or may walk with small steps (marcher à petits pas) (Meyer and Barron, 1960). Gait apraxia is more likely when the subdural collections are bilateral, as they are in up to 20 percent of all cases of subdural hematomas (McKissock et al., 1960; Grant, 1928). With gait ataxia, such patients complain of poor balance. They stagger and fall and have a typical wide-based gait. In such individuals, the subdural collection was found to be invariably unilateral by McLachlan et al. (1981), but the hematoma did not predominate over one hemisphere or over one particular lobe. Apraxia may be due to a dysfunction in the frontal lobe regulation of initiation of gait or to a physiological disruption in the parietal lobe connections with the frontal lobes (McKissock et al., 1960). The ataxia could result from a dysfunction of the reciprocal connections of the frontal lobe(s) and cerebellum or to a transmission of diffuse increases in intracranial pressure to the posterior fossa structures (McLachlan et al., 1981; Grant, 1928).

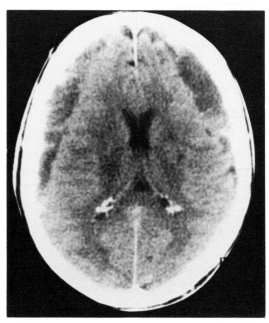

Figure 7.6. Computed tomographic head scan of a 63-year-old man on chronic hemodialysis. Fluid collections are external to the brain parenchyma bilaterally. These are hypodense and, therefore, likely chronic, but the brighter regions within them probably represent small recent hemorrhages.

Management

Because subdural hematomas are treatable and highly variable in presentation, the condition should be considered in any dialysis patient who shows focal or generalized central nervous system dysfunction. Subdural hematomas may easily be confused with uremic encephalopathy, dialysis dysequilibrium, dialytic encephalopathy, drug intoxication, or stroke. The condition is easily diagnosed with computed tomography (Figure 7.6) or magnetic resonance imaging scans. Magnetic resonance imaging has some advantage over computed tomography in not being affected by the hematoma becoming isodense with brain or showing volume averaging effect with bone. Prior to the advent of CT and MRI, cerebral angiography was the most sensitive and definitive diagnostic test. Radioisotope brain scans can detect significant supratentorial subdural hematomas. The EEG is almost always abnormal with supratentorial subdural hematomas, but cannot be reliably differentiated from other conditions (Figure 7.7).

Treatment is surgical. Drainage or evacuation of the clot is curative, providing the patient has not suffered irreversible damage from compression and brain herniation. Because of coagulation problems, uremic patients are at higher risk for rebleeding. With close monitoring, however, it should be possible to successfully manage such patients, even with the need for ongoing dialysis in the recovery period. If the patient is treated before severe brain compression or herniation occurs, recovery is often complete.

References

Adams RD, Victor M. Principles of neurology. 3rd ed. New York: McGraw-Hill, 1985:798.

Grant FC. Cerebellar symptoms produced by supratentorial tumors: further report. Arch Neurol Psychiatry 1928;20:292–308.

Leonard A, Shapiro FL. Subdural hematoma in regularly hemodialyzed patients. Ann Intern Med 1975;82:650–658.

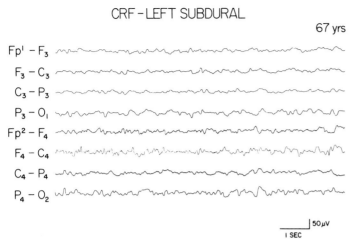

CRF – LEFT SUBDURAL

67 yrs

Fp¹ – F₃

F₃ – C₃

C₃ – P₃

P₃ – O₁

Fp² – F₄

F₄ – C₄

C₄ – P₄

P₄ – O₂

50 μV

I SEC

Figure 7.7. This 67-year-old man with chronic renal failure was on hemodialysis for several years. One day after hemodialysis, he was aphasic. Dialytic encephalopathy was suspected but the EEG showed suppression of faster frequencies from the left cerebral hemisphere, along with generalized slowing. The CT scan showed a left-sided chronic subdural hematoma.

Leonard CD, Weil E, Scribner BH. Subdural haematomas in patients undergoing haemodialysis. Lancet 1969;2:239–240.

McKissock W, Richardson A, Bloom WH. Subdural hematoma: a review of 389 cases. Lancet 1960;1:1365–1369.

McLachlan RS, Bolton CF, Coates RK, Barnett HJM. Gait disturbance in chronic subdural hematoma. Can Med Assoc J 1981;125:865–868.

Meyer JS, Barron DW. Apraxia of gait: a clinicopathological study. Brain 1960;83:261–284.

Rotter W, Roettger P. Comparative pathologic-anatomic study of cases of chronic global renal insufficiency with and without preceding dialysis. Clin Nephrol 1973;1:257–265.

Talalla A, Halbrook H, Barbour BH, et al. Subdural hematoma associated with long-term hemodialysis for chronic renal disease. JAMA 1970;212:1847–1849.

D

Vitamin Deficiencies
and Therapies

Wernicke's Encephalopathy

Clinical Features

Wernicke's encephalopathy is an acute clinical syndrome consisting of mental changes, ocular movement abnormalities, and ataxia as the key features (Victor et al., 1971). The mental change is one of a generalized encephalopathy, usually with inattention, apathy, disorientation, inability to concentrate, and impaired cognition and memory. Often the patients are withdrawn and somnolent. Less commonly, an agitated confusional state may occur, especially in the alcoholic population where alcohol withdrawal may add to the picture. Stupor or coma, sometimes with hypothermia, may be the initial manifestation. A minority show an initial selective memory deficit, the sensorium otherwise being intact, features of Korsakoff's psychosis.

Ocular abnormalities offer the most specific clue to the diagnosis and consist of nystagmus, paresis of the lateral rectus on one or both sides, and a conjugate gaze palsy. These can be present separately or in any combination. The nystagmus can be either vertical or horizontal or both. The gaze palsy can vary from a gaze paretic nystagmus on looking to one side to a complete loss of eye movements in a particular direction or in all directions. Often there is reduced or absent response to caloric stimulation, which produces nystagmus in a normal, awake individual or tonic conjugate deviation of the eyes in a comatose patient with intact brainstem and eighth nerve function. Occasionally, ptosis and problems in convergence and accommodation may be seen, as may associated optic neuropathy.

The ataxia typically is one that affects stance and gait. It may be so severe that the patient cannot even stand without support. In milder cases, it may be brought out by testing tandem gait or with the heel-knee-shin test. The upper limbs and speech are, as a rule, less involved than the lower limbs and stance and gait.

Pathology and Pathogenesis

Patients dying with acute Wernicke's encephalopathy show characteristic, symmetrical lesions in mammillary bodies, walls of the third and fourth ventricles, gray matter surrounding the cerebral aqueduct, and cortex of the anterior superior vermis of the cerebellum. There is disruption of the neuropil with prominence of capillaries, sometimes with microscopic or macroscopic hemorrhages in the affected regions. The neurons in these regions are relatively preserved.

There is good evidence that Wernicke's encephalopathy is due to thiamine deficiency (Victor et al., 1971). Blass and Gibson (1977) described a genetic defect in Wernicke's encephalopathy in which patients' fibroblast transketolase bound thiamine pyrophosphate less than in control subjects. Thus, there may be a subpopulation of chronic renal failure patients who are more prone to develop Wernicke's encephalopathy. Sometimes a sudden carbohydrate load precipitates the condition. The ophthalmoplegia, nystagmus, and ataxia are usually fairly rapidly reversed by administration of thiamine alone. The impairment of level of consciousness, attention, and cognition also improve, but many patients are left with Korsakoff's psychosis. The latter is a profound memory disturbance consisting of the inability to lay down new memories and to recall past memories in proper sequence or context. Some patients may show florid confabulation, but this is not a necessary component, nor is the nutritional polyneuropathy that was described in some earlier cases. The enduring memory deficit appears to be due to structural changes in the medial dorsal nuclei of the thalamus.

In early days of dialysis treatment, cases of Wernicke's encephalopathy occurred in patients who did not receive supplemental thiamine to compensate for the loss through dialysis of this water-soluble vitamin (Lopez and Collins, 1968; Faris, 1972). Jagadha et al. (1987) have recently pointed out that thiamine deficiency in more recent times arises in uremic patients who are too ill to eat or who are subject to repeated vomiting and are then placed on intravenous therapy without added thiamine. (Ill patients with chronic renal failure and hyperkalemia may be especially at risk, as glucose boluses are sometimes given intravenously.) Furthermore, in the context of an acute illness such as sepsis, the signs of Wernicke's encephalopathy may be missed or masked. In some patients, the classic ocular findings may not appear (Jagadha et al., 1987); in such cases the diagnosis is made only at autopsy.

Prevention and Treatment

A corollary from the above is that the physician should have a high index of suspicion and keep in mind the possibility of Wernicke's encephalopathy in any patient with chronic renal failure who develops an unexplained confusional syndrome. Further, parenteral thiamine supplements should be given to any uremic patient who develops anorexia or vomiting.

Biotin Deficiency

Clinical Features

Yatzidis et al. (1984) described nine patients with peripheral neuropathy who had received hemodialysis treatment for two to 10 years. Four of these also had encephalopathic features. Following the administration of 10 mg/day of biotin by mouth, within three months there was a striking improvement in orientation, speech, and memory. Myoclonic jerks, asterixis, and gait disturbance all improved or subsided.

Yatzidis et al. (1984) argue that biotin deficiency could have caused the central and peripheral neurological problems in these patients. They note the similarity of the CNS manifestations to dialytic encephalopathy and suggest that biotin deficiency should be considered as a factor in that condition.

Role of Biotin in the Body

Biotin is a B vitamin that is water soluble and shows little protein binding in plasma. It is, therefore, probable that it may be lost from the body into the dialysate. Further, in uremia, there may be reduced formation of biotin by intestinal flora, and absorption across the intestinal mucosa may be impaired (Yatzidis et al., 1984). The estimated daily requirement for biotin in humans is about 10 μg.

Biotin serves as a prosthetic group in a number of enzyme reactions that fix carbon dioxide into organic linkage (Tanaka, 1981). Biotin-deficient animals show reduced CO_2 incorporation into oxaloacetate, urea, and purines, as well as diminished synthesis of fatty acids because of deficient acetyl coenzyme A formation. Propionyl coenzyme A, which is involved in propionate oxidation, and 3-methylcrotonyl coenzyme A, involved in leucine oxidation and pyruvate metabolism in gluconeogenesis, are also reduced. At least some of the carboxylase reactions involving biotin appear to be metal dependent.

Our main understanding of clinical manifestations of biotin deficiency comes from animal studies and the occurrence of a number of biotin-responsive carboxylase deficiencies in humans. Features described include retardation, irritability, lethargy, seizures, prostration, rash, and alopecia. In some, hyperammonemia and lactic acidosis occur (Hsia and Wolf, 1981). In adult humans and animals, biotin deficiency can be produced by feeding raw egg white, which contains a biotin-binding protein called avidin. Volunteers developed dermatitis, lassitude, somnolence, precordial pain, distress, hallucinations, anorexia, muscle pains, and anemia (Sydenstricker et al., 1942).

Implications for Treatment

The role of biotin deficiency in production of dialysis-associated neurological syndromes is unproven. Yatzidis et al. (1984) make some interesting observations and speculations, but they are very preliminary and need further investigation. Their study did not use a control group; it is uncertain whether other therapeutic variables were controlled. Furthermore, the dose of biotin used was 1,000 times greater than the usual oral maintenance dose. Could the vitamin have a pharmacological effect?

While waiting for more proof, the possibility of biotin deficiency in patients on long-term dialysis who develop peripheral neuropathy with or without encephalopathy should be considered. A trial of the vitamin would do no harm.

References

Blass JP, Gibson GE. Abnormality of a thiamine-requiring enzyme in patients with Wernicke-Korsakoff syndrome. N Engl J Med 1977;297:1367–1390.

Faris AA. Wernicke's encephalopathy in uremia. Neurology 1972;22:1293–1297.

Hsia YE, Wolf B. Disorders of amino acid metabolism. In: Siegel GJ, Albers RW, Agranoff BW, Karzman R, eds. Basic neurochemistry. 3rd ed. Boston: Little, Brown, 1981:566.

Jagadha V, Deck JHN, Halliday WC, Smyth HS. Wernicke's encephalopathy in patients on peritoneal dialysis or hemodialysis. Ann Neurol 1987;21:78–84.

Lopez RI, Collins GK. Wernicke's encephalopathy: a complication of chronic hemodialysis. Arch Neurol 1968;18:248–259.

Sydenstricker VP, Singal SA, Briggs AP, et al. Observation on "egg-white" injury in man and its cure. JAMA 1942;118:1199–1200.

Tanaka K. New light on biotin deficiency. N Engl J Med 1981;304:839–840.

Victor M, Adams RD, Collins GH. The Wernicke-Korsakoff syndrome. Philadelphia: FA Davis, 1971.

Yatzidis H, Koutsicos D, Agroyannis B, et al. Biotin in the management of uremic neurologic disorders. Nephron 1984;36:183–186.

E

Hemodialysis Headache

Incidence and Clinical Features

Bana et al. (1972) first clearly described a headache related to the dialysis procedure. This occurred in eight of 44 chronic hemodialysis patients. A larger study in the Boston area reported the incidence to be about 60 percent of hemodialysis patients (Yap and Graham, 1971a). In these affected individuals, 95 percent of the headaches occurred on dialysis days. The headache began most commonly between three and seven hours from the onset of dialysis, beginning as a mild bifrontal discomfort. The headache increased to severe, throbbing pain that was aggravated by lying flat. When severe, it was commonly associated with nausea and vomiting. No neurological symptoms such as visual disturbance that would suggest classical migraine occurred, however.

Individuals who experienced headache at the onset of their clinical renal disease were more likely to develop headache than those without this complaint. In those with dialysis headache, the intensity was greater with longer time between dialyses.

Factors that helped the headache included ergot drugs (tried in only two patients), pressure on scalp arteries, nephrectomy, and renal transplant. It should be emphasized that ergot-containing drugs are dangerous if hypertension is present.

There was no clear association with any of the following: headache (including migraine) prior to renal disease, hypertension (although the likelihood of other headaches—including migraine and muscle contraction headaches unrelated to dialysis—was increased, as was headache intensity for any type of headache), type of renal disease (although headaches in general were more common with chronic glomerulonephritis), and type of dialyzer (Kiil versus Kolff).

Pathogenesis of Dialysis Headache

Dialysis headache has features of a vascular headache: the throbbing nature and the relief with compression of the scalp arteries or with ergot drugs are very suggestive.

Dialysis headaches appear to be linked to a decrease in serum sodium and osmolality, a drop in arterial pressure, and the use of negative pressure to increase fluid washout during dialysis (Yap and Graham, 1971b). Bana and Graham (1976) found plasma renin levels to be low during dialysis headache, and Bana and Graham (1978) further showed that this was associated with low aldosterone levels during dialysis headache compared with controls without headache. It is still unclear how these hormonal changes might cause headache, but it is possible that reduced activity of the renin-angiotensin-aldosterone system might promote vascular headaches by producing vasodilation. This is further supported by the success of ergot drugs.

Hemodialysis with the Cuprophan membrane induces interleukin-1 activity (Yamagami et al., 1986). Interleukin-1 causes release of prostaglandin E_2 in various tissues and alters CNS neuropeptide release (Dinarello, 1984). It is possible that interleukin-1 could play a role in dialysis headache; the release of other substances such as bradykinin, serotonin, histamine, and substance P during dialysis also requires further study.

References

Bana DS, Graham JR. Renin response during hemodialysis headache. Headache 1976;16:168–172.

Bana DS, Graham JR. Renin-angiotensin-aldosterone system in vascular headache. In: Green R, ed. Current concepts in migraine research. New York: Raven Press, 1978:111–114.

Bana DS, Yap AU, Graham JR. Headache during hemodialysis. Headache 1972;12:1–14.

Dinarello CA. Interleukin-1. Rev Infect Dis 1984;6:51–95.

Yap AU, Graham JR. Headache and hemodialysis. Natural history and epidemiology (Part I). In: Dalessio DJ, Dalsgaard-Nielsen T, Diamond S, eds. Proceedings of the International Headache Symposium, Elsinore, Denmark, May 16–18, 1971. Basel: Sandoz, 1971a:79–84.

Yap AU, Graham JR. Headache and hemodialysis. Natural history and epidemiology (Part II). In: Dalessio DJ, Dalsgaard-Nielsen T, Diamond S, eds. Proceedings of the International Headache Symposium, Elsinore, Denmark, May 16–18, 1971. Basel: Sandoz, 1971b:85–90.

Yamagami S, Yoshihara H, Kishimoto T, et al. Cuprophan membrane induces interleukin-1 activity. Trans Am Soc Artif Intern Organs 1986;32:98–101.

Chapter 8

Neurological Complications of Renal Transplantation

Contents

Acronyms

AIDS	acquired immunodeficiency syndrome
CNS	central nervous system
CPM	central pontine myelinolysis
CSF	cerebral spinal fluid
CT	computed tomography
EEG	electroencephalogram
ELISA	enzyme-linked immunosorbent assay
HIV	human immunodeficiency virus
MRI	magnetic resonance imaging
RE	rejection encephalopathy

Survival following kidney transplantation has improved substantially in recent years. In the United States in 1977, 53 percent of patients who received a cadaveric renal transplant survived for one year, but in 1984 this incidence had improved to 68 percent (Eggers, 1988). The reasons are multifactorial, but certainly improved perioperative care and less vigorous immunosuppression, particularly the use of cyclosporine at least partly account for this good result. The continuing mortality, and morbidity in many of the remaining patients, are due to a wide variety of conditions that continue to complicate the posttransplant state and reduce survival to 45 percent at ten years (Fassbinder et al., 1987). The incidence of these complications remains relatively high, even into the second decade (Table 8.1).

In assessing the posttransplant patient, the diagnosis may be established by the typical symptoms and signs of the primary disease, e.g., a typical skin lesion such as herpes zoster. However, in many instances the history and physical findings will give no clue as to the nature of the condition, including central nervous system involvement. Thus, comprehensive investigations are almost always indicated, and admission to a hospital is required.

The nervous system is directly or indirectly affected in most of these conditions, perhaps not frequently in specific instances, although data on this is not available. Central nervous system involvement is probably common and usually presents a difficult differential diagnosis (Table 8.2). If the renal transplantation was recent, a medication effect such as complication of cyclosporine treatment, or the phenomenon of rejection encephalopathy, should be considered. Then, infection should be thoroughly investigated. Blood, urine, and if indicated, other specimens should be cultured for viruses, bacteria, and fungi. Serological studies should also be done for specific changes in antibody titer, including the human immunodeficiency virus (HIV). For example, the diagnosis of cytomegalovirus is established by a fourfold or greater seroconversion in cytomegalovirus antibody titers. It should be noted here that all types of infections—viral, bacterial, or fungal—if left unchecked will ultimately produce systemic symptoms not due to direct invasion of organisms, which has been recognized as a septic syndrome. This may ultimately be complicated by multiorgan failure. The systemic response often includes both encephalopathy and a critical illness polyneuropathy.

In launching specific tests of the central nervous system (CNS), the electroencephalogram (EEG) is often of great value. It may rule in or out organic disease, the EEG being normal in mental depression and nonorganic psychoses. The computed tomographic (CT) head scan is of even more value. It may reveal the relatively specific findings of subdural hematoma, infarction, or hemorrhage. The CT head scan may also aid in identifying lesions due to immunosuppression. *Toxoplasma gondii* and *Nocardia* species may produce ringenhancing lesions, although if immunosuppression has been great, such enhancement may be lost. Lymphomas tend to produce solidly enhancing lesions. Progressive multifocal leukoencephalopathy produces nonenhancing hypodense areas near the ventricles (Williams, 1985). However, such signs are not invariably specific, and brain biopsy is often necessary. At a minimum, the CT head scan will rule out a mass lesion, which would contraindicate the performance of a subsequent lumbar puncture. Lumbar puncture is also contraindicated in any bleeding tendency, i.e., low platelet levels, anticoagulant treatment, or aspergillosis. If a lumbar puncture is performed, adequate

Table 8.1. Complications and Clinical Results in the Second Decade of Renal Transplantation

Complications/Results	Number (N = 57)	(%)
Infection	24	(44)
Malignancy	9	(16)
Vascular disease	9	(16)
Hypertension	24	(42)
Aseptic necrosis	6	(11)
Cataracts	19	(33)
Death rate	7	(12)
Graft loss	7	(12)

Source: Rao (1987). Data from The University of Minnesota, with permission.

Table 8.2. Central Nervous System Features of Posttransplant Infection and Malignancy

Condition/Organism	Time after Transplant	Neurological Manifestations	Cerebrospinal Fluid	CT Head Scan	Treatment
Cyclosporin complications	0–3 mo	Tremor, ataxia, seizures, confusion, coma, paraplegia	Normal, or mild increase in protein and lymphocytic reaction	Normal, or white matter edema	Stop cyclosporin, give parenteral magnesium
Septic encephalopathy	0–3 mo	Diffuse encephalopathy, mild or severe	Normal, or mildly increased protein	Normal	Treat sepsis and multiple organ failure
Critical illness polyneuropathy	0–3 mo	Failed weaning from ventilator, axonal polyneuropathy	Normal, or mildly increased protein	Normal	Treat sepsis and multiple organ failure
Rejection encephalopathy	1–3 mo	Headache, confusion, and convulsions	Increased pressure	Normal or edema	Give steroids, manage hypertension and fluid balance
Cerebrovascular disease	Any time	Sudden onset of focal cerebral deficit	Normal, or signs of subarachnoid hemorrhage	Relatively specific for subdural hematoma, infarction, or hemorrhage	Conservative
Viruses					
Cytomegalovirus	1–4 mo	None	Normal	Normal	Prophylaxis only
Epstein-Barr	2–6 mo	None, or rare B-cell lymphoma	Normal	Normal, or rare B-cell lymphoma	Prophylaxis only
Herpes simplex	Any time	Encephalitis—rare	Increased WBC, RBC, and protein, normal or decreased glucose	Areas of decreased density, occasional small hemorrhages in frontal and temporal lobes	Acyclovir
Varicella zoster	Any time	Encephalitis—rare	Increased WBC and protein, normal glucose	?	Acyclovir
HIV	Any time	Encephalopathy, myelopathy, peripheral neuropathy	Variable	Variable, depending on type of infection or malignancy	None
JC virus	Any time	Progressive multifocal leukoencephalopathy	Normal	Areas of decreased density with no enhancement	None
Bacteria					
Listeria monocytogenes	1–3 mo(?)	Acute meningitis	Increased WBC (mainly neutrophils) and protein, decreased glucose	Normal, or generalized edema	Penicillin and tobramycin
Mycobacteria	Any time	Subacute and chronic meningitis or focal signs	Increased WBC (mainly lymphocytes) and protein, decreased glucose	Normal, or hydrocephalus	Isoniazid, rifampin
Fungi					
Cryptococci	1–8 mo	Mild, chronic meningitis	Increased WBC and protein, decreased glucose	Normal, or hydrocephalus	Amphotericin B
Coccidioides organisms	1–8 mo	Chronic meningitis	Increased WBC and protein, decreased glucose	Normal, or hydrocephalus	Amphotericin B

Table 8.2. *Continued*

Condition/Organism	Time after Transplant	Neurological Manifestations	Cerebrospinal Fluid	CT Head Scan	Treatment
Candida organisms	1–8 mo	Meningeal encephalitis	Normal or increased WBC and protein, decreased glucose	Normal, or focal lesions with ring enhancement	Amphotericin B
Aspergillus organisms	1–8 mo	Meningitis, focal or multifocal signs	Increased WBC and protein, decreased glucose	Normal, or focal lesions with poor enhancement	Amphotericin B
Mucoraceae organisms	0–18 mo	Sinus and orbital cellulitis to cerebral hemorrhagic infarction	Not tested	Sinusitis, proptosis, cerebral hemorrhagic infarction	Amphotericin B
Parasites					
Toxoplasma organisms	Any time	Diffuse or multifocal encephalopathy, meningitis	Increased WBC and protein, decreased glucose	Normal, or ring-enhancing lesion	Pyrimethamine and sulfadiazine
Neoplasms					
Lymphoma	1–50 mo	Focal cerebral signs	Pleocytosis, malignant cells	Solid, strongly enhancing lesion(s)	Radiation therapy

CT = computed tomography; WBC = white blood cells; RBC = red blood cells; HIV = human immunodeficiency virus.

amounts of fluid should be taken for all the tests that are necessary. Removal of such amounts is of no concern, since even after the needle is withdrawn, fluid will continue to leak for some hours from the puncture site. Cerebrospinal fluid (CSF) determinations of white blood cell count and differential and of glucose should be done immediately, since these elements deteriorate rapidly in the test tube. Fluid should be studied by a Gram stain for bacteria and by India ink stain for *Cryptococcus neoformans*. The fluid should then be subject to comprehensive culture for bacteria, including aerobic and anaerobic organisms, and for fungi. If mycobacterial infection is a possibility, it will be necessary to do an acid-fast stain for mycobacteria and to send the fluid for culture for *Mycobacterium tuberculosis*. Finally, CSF should be sent for identification of malignant cells.

In many instances, a precise diagnosis of central nervous system infection is not possible and empirical therapy should be started. *Listeria monocytogenes* is the most likely cause of bacterial meningitis and should be treated with penicillin and tobramycin. If there is a strong suspicion of a specific fungal, parasitic, or tubercular infection, therapy may have to be started empirically.

In a disturbing number of instances, the diagnosis may still be in doubt. For example, all microbiological studies may have initially been negative and no malignant cells found in the cerebrospinal fluid. A CT head scan may show single or multiple lesions of a nonspecific nature. In this case, brain biopsy may be necessary. The neuropathologist and microbiologist should be notified in advance of this procedure and be prepared to study the tissue comprehensively.

The remainder of this chapter deals with the various diseases that may involve the nervous system after renal transplantation.

Neurological Complications of Cyclosporine Medication

This topic is thoroughly discussed in Chapter 9; only a brief summary will be given here. Neurological complications of cyclosporine, an immunosuppressant, are mainly dose related and are most likely to occur in the first three months following transplantation, almost never occurring beyond one year posttransplantation. The commonest manifestation is a fine postural tremor of the hands, which occurs about 22 percent of the time. Generalized seizures occur in 5 percent. Patients may also experience burning paresthesias in the limbs. Examination may reveal evidence of cerebellar ataxia. A more severe encephalopathy rarely occurs, which may begin with confusion and quickly end in coma. It may be accompanied by decreased vision or visual hallucinations. CT head scans may show diffuse edema of the white matter and the CSF may reveal mild elevation in protein and a lymphocytic reaction of the white blood cells. In exceptionally rare circumstances, an acute spinal cord syndrome causes either a paraplegia or quadriplegia.

The diffuse encephalopathy and seizures may be due to a low magnesium level induced by the cyclosporine medication, which can be detected by measuring the magnesium blood level and corrected by giving parenteral magnesium. The precise mechanism by which cyclosporine itself may cause these neurological complications, including the more severe encephalopathy accompanied by white matter edema, is not known. However, the neurological signs and symptoms will reverse rapidly with discontinuation of cyclosporine.

Septic Encephalopathy and Critical Illness Polyneuropathy

Sepsis, the systemic response to invading organisms of all types, is most likely to occur within one month of renal transplantation, immunosuppression and the postsurgical state being important predisposing causes. Surgical wound infection and postoperative pneumonia are the usual primary causes of the septicemia. If left unchecked, multiple organ failure with a mortality rate of 60 percent results. Sepsis frequently causes an encephalopathy that produces a generalized disturbance in cerebral function and only occasionally causes focal signs (Young et al., 1986; Jackson et al., 1985; Young, 1986). It is, at times, severe and is presumably due to the same complex mechanisms, still poorly understood, that affect all body systems in the septic syndrome (Ayres,

1986). The CSF and CT head scans are unremarkable, but the EEG is invariably abnormal, showing several diffuse abnormalities that, in the main, reflect the severity of the encephalopathy. Complete recovery is possible with successful treatment of the sepsis: the use of appropriate antibiotics or surgical drainage of an abscess. However, if the sepsis extends beyond two weeks, requiring management in the critical care unit, a critical illness polyneuropathy may develop (Bolton et al., 1984; Zochodne et al., 1987), often in association with multiple organ failure. It is characterized by difficulty in weaning from the ventilator and a primary axonal degeneration of motor and sensory fibers that may be quite severe. However, it also resolves completely if the sepsis is successfully treated.

Rejection Encephalopathy

Gross et al. (1982) described 13 patients who developed an encephalopathy in association with acute rejection of a renal transplant. They termed the syndrome rejection encephalopathy (RE). The patients were relatively young: age range was 10 to 38 years; 11 patients were less than 18 years old. Twelve of the 15 episodes occurred within three months of transplantation, although the longest interval was two years. In each case, the encephalopathy was reversible.

The clinical neurological features included convulsions in each case. Of the 15 rejection episodes, 14 were associated with confusion and irritability, 11 with disorientation, 12 with headache, and one with papilledema. Features indicative of graft rejection included: fever, graft swelling and tenderness, weight gain, and hypertension.

EEGs during the rejection episode showed nonspecific, generalized slowing in most cases. Occasionally, some focal features were found. Eight patients had follow-up EEGs. These were abnormal but improving in most, although two showed epileptiform activity. It is unclear whether the abnormalities were related to the original encephalopathy, which had cleared, or to other active problems. CT head scans were obtained in four patients. Two were normal, and two showed white matter attenuation suggestive of edema. Follow-up scans showed resolution of the edema. Apart from elevated CSF pressure, lumbar puncture did not reveal any abnormality, except for elevated CSF protein in one patient.

In considering pathogenesis, comparing the RE patients with a control group of patients showing acute renal allograft rejection *without* encephalopathy, there was no significant difference in medication (only one dialysis encephalopathy patient was on cyclosporine; others received prednisolone and azathioprine), rate or degree of blood pressure elevation, or weight gain (fluid retention). Serum values for sodium, potassium, calcium, and phosphate were also similar. The percentage rise in serum creatinine was significantly higher in the RE than in the control patients, however. The degree of renal impairment and the associated features such as raised intracranial pressure suggest that the encephalopathy was not just an acute uremic encephalopathy. The cause is not known, but it is possible that a combination of factors or unrecognized, severe hypertensive episodes were involved.

The same considerations that applied to the differential diagnosis of cyclosporine-induced encephalopathy may be said to apply here: cyclosporine itself, infection inside or outside the CNS, CNS lymphoma, fluid and electrolyte disturbances, malignant hypertension, and stroke are the major ones.

Patients with rejection encephalopathy should be treated symptomatically with anticonvulsants, especially diazepam. Dilantin might be used only during the acute episode. Long-term anticonvulsants are not necessary. Patients may require emergency treatment of acute hypertension with parenteral drugs. The most definitive therapy is that of the renal graft rejection. The syndrome should resolve when the rejection is checked by the use of immunosuppressive therapy.

The outlook is favorable for full recovery with no clinical sequelae. Some patients may experience recurrence of RE with other rejection episodes, however.

Cerebrovascular Disease in the Renal Transplant Recipient

Next to infection, this is the commonest neurological complication following renal transplantation. It is comprehensively discussed in Chapter 6A.

Mahony et al. (1982) studied 119 renal transplant patients, of which 44 percent survived 10 years. Of these, 24 percent died of vascular disease. In half of these patients, the fatal disease was a cerebral infarct. Of the patients who survived, 30 percent had vascular disease, but in only one-quarter of these was it of cerebral origin, either strokes or transient cerebral ischemic attacks. Posttransplant strokes are predisposed to by pretransplant diabetes mellitus, atherosclerosis, or systemic lupus erythematosus. The tendency to hypertension is worsened if there is an associated renal artery stenosis or because of renal allograft rejection, recurrent nephritis, volume overload, or high dosages of corticosteroids. Cyclosporine may induce posttransplant hypertension, particularly in children. It has been shown that after transplantation, serum cholesterol, serum triglycerides, and cholesterol levels may become further elevated. Also, corticosteroids may further increase the serum glucose. As a result of all these factors, atherosclerosis is clearly accelerated following transplantation.

The various symptoms and signs will depend on the type and nature of the stroke. There may be signs of major infarction due to large vessel occlusion, or the effects of hypertension alone may cause lacunar infarction. Any bleeding tendency will further increase the risk of cerebral hemorrhage. However, cerebral infarction is the most likely cause of a stroke after transplantation, and in a significant number of patients it will be fatal. Salicylates have a significant effect in preventing both myocardial infarction and cerebral infarction in patients not suffering from renal failure. Perhaps this drug should be considered for routine use after transplantation. This, coupled with careful control of blood pressure and appropriate diet to control lipid abnormalities, might lessen these fairly common posttransplant complications.

Central Pontine Myelinolysis

Central pontine myelinolysis (CPM) was first described by Adams et al. (1959) in three alcoholic, malnourished patients. Although the authors emphasized the malnutrition as the common denominator, the more important association is with correction of hyponatremia. Because of this association, the terms osmotic demyelination syndrome (Sterns et al., 1986) and electrolyte-induced myelinolysis (Kleinschmidt-DeMasters and Norenberg, 1982) have been suggested. It has been reported following renal transplantation (Schneck, 1966), but it should be realized that CPM may result whenever dilutional hyponatremia is too vigorously corrected, whatever the association. In renal failure, hyponatremia is not uncommonly seen following excessive water intake, when the kidneys have reduced free water clearance. Hyponatremia is now increasingly recognized as a complication of diuretic therapy (Ashraf et al., 1981).

Clinical Features

The condition is mainly found in adults between 30 and 70 years of age, but Cadman and Rorke (1969) reported it in childhood and adolescence, with the youngest case being 3 years of age. All the cases have begun and evolved in a hospital setting (Norenberg, 1983). The onset is subacute, over a few days. Convulsive seizures, vomiting, clumsiness, or mental changes such as hallucinations, restlessness, confusion, or obtundation (Price and Mesulam, 1987)—probably related to extrapontine disease—often herald the more definitive features localized to the basis pontis. It should be noted, however, that these are often missed or not noted clinically. Sometimes the central pontine lesion is too small to interrupt the corticobulbar and corticospinal tracts. Alternatively, the patient may be in a deep coma from associated metabolic encephalopathy, and the neurological signs may be obscured.

The characteristic brainstem abnormalities include dysphagia, dysarthria, progressive weakness of the limbs, and incontinence. The pseudobulbar palsy is a supranuclear dysfunc-tion affecting lower cranial nerve function: inability to open or close the jaw and paralysis of voluntary facial, pharyngeal, laryngeal, neck, and tongue movements. Reflex swallowing and coughing and automatic breathing are preserved. There is often "emotional incontinence," with pathological, uncontrollable crying or laughter.

Ocular movements, facial sensation, and pupillary and corneal reflexes are spared, as a rule. However, we have seen CPM patients with bilateral sixth nerve palsies or with preservation of only vertical gaze, which, along with the quadriplegia and pseudobulbar palsy, produces a "locked-in syndrome."

Limb paralysis is typically flaccid quadriplegia, which becomes spastic if there is no significant associated neuropathy. Although sensation is usually spared (Adams et al., 1959), it is very difficult to test.

Dickoff et al. (1988) recently described parkinsonian features in a patient with CPM who had involvement of the striatum as well as the basis pontis on MRI. The patient also had mild corticobulbar and corticospinal dysfunction.

Investigations

There should be documentation of recent hyponatremia, with serum sodium below 116 mmol/L (Sterns et al., 1986) or a significant increase in serum sodium, regardless of the previous level (see Pathogenesis, below). Depending on the quality of the records, it may be possible to show that the serum sodium had been corrected at a rate of greater than 12 mmol/L/day (Sterns et al., 1986).

The principal electrophysiological test of value is brainstem auditory evoked potential (see section on Event-Related Potentials in Chapter 4B). There is an intrinsic brainstem conduction abnormality, with prolongation of the I–V interpeak latency (Stockard et al., 1976; Wiederholt et al., 1977, Dickoff et al., 1988). Clinical improvement is reflected in improvement in this latency (Stockard et al., 1976; Wiederholt et al., 1977). Dickoff et al. (1988) also reported absent visual evoked response from one eye in their patient, who had striking extrapontine involvement.

Advances in neuroimaging have contributed greatly to *in vivo* confirmation of the diagnosis. The central pontine lesion can occasionally be seen on CT scans (Tefler and Miller, 1979; Sterns et al., 1986). Because of difficulty in adequately visualizing the posterior fossa on CT scans, magnetic resonance imaging (MRI) has emerged as the premier diagnostic test (DeWitt et al., 1984; Brunner et al., 1988). The lesion in the pons shows abnormal T_1 and T_2 relaxation times (see Figure 8.1a and b). The MRI may reflect the true extent of the pathology in showing lesions beyond the pons (Dickoff et al., 1988) (see next section).

Pathology

The fundamental lesion is in the midline basis pontis. There is demyelination with sparing of axons. Descending, as well as crossing, fiber tracts are affected in an indiscriminant fashion (Adams et al., 1959). Occasionally, the oligodendroglia, the cells responsible for the formation and maintenance of myelin in the CNS, are reduced in number (McCormick and Daneel, 1967). Axons are usually preserved, but some may show segmental swellings or spheroid formation in the demyelinated region, sometimes to a striking degree (Schenck, 1966). Neurons in the involved area may undergo necrosis, especially in the center of larger lesions (Chason et al., 1964). Histopathologically, some authors have also noted hypertrophy of endothelial cells of capillaries (Adams et al., 1959; Klavins, 1963) and tissue edema (Powers and McKeever, 1976). There is some evidence that this may relate to increased blood-brain barrier permeability in that the demyelinated lesion has been noted to show bile staining in patients who were jaundiced (Chason et al., 1964).

Although some cases showed associated brain lesions related to other etiologies, such as Wernicke's encephalopathy in malnourished alcoholics (Adams et al., 1959), it has recently been recognized that myelinolysis can involve brain regions in addition to the basis pontis (McCormick and Daneel, 1967; Wright et al., 1979; Sterns et al., 1986; Boon and

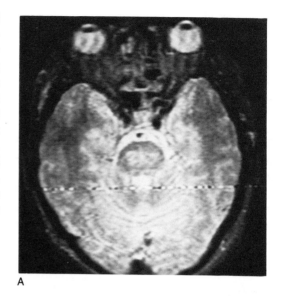

A

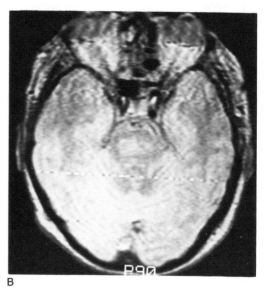

B

Figures 8.1. (A) and (B). These transverse magnetic resonance images of the head are heavily T_2 weighted (TR 2,500, TE 70). They show increased signal in the central pontine white matter and extrapontine sites. Less heavily weighted T_2 images and a CT head scan did not show the lesions.

Potter, 1987). In many cases, there are no other diseases or conditions; the extrapontine white matter lesions constitute a component of CPM. These extrapontine sites lie in the midbrain, cerebellum, and cerebral hemispheres, especially near the interfaces of deep gray matter structures with white matter

(Wright et al., 1979; Sterns et al., 1986; Boon and Potter, 1987). Within the brainstem, the pontine tegementum is variably involved. The midbrain has been reported to contain demyelination in the decussation of the brachia conjunctiva, medial lemnisci, and central tegmental tracts, as well as destructive change in the substantia nigra (Boon and Potter, 1987). The deep white matter of the cerebellum may be involved. In the cerebral hemispheres, the deep white matter of the parietal lobes, projection association and commissural fibers, internal and external capsules, and the subcortical white matter may be involved in various combinations (Wright et al., 1979; Boon and Potter, 1987). Some microcystic change and loss of myelinated fibers may occur within gray matter structures such as the thalamus (Finlayson et al., 1973; Tomlinson et al., 1976; Wright et al., 1979) including the lateral geniculate body (Goldman and Horoupian, 1981), putamen and globus pallidus (Tomlinson et al., 1976; Wright et al., 1979), subthalamus (Finlayson et al., 1973; Wright et al., 1979), amygdala (Wright et al., 1979), and even deeper layers of the cortex, as well as in the subjacent white matter (Wright et al., 1979). It is likely that some of the clinical features, such as epileptic seizures and obtundation, are due to disease in these extrapontine sites.

Pathogenesis

The common situation underlying CPM is a sudden, marked increase in serum osmolality. There is now fairly strong evidence that CPM occurs following overly rapid correction of hyponatremia, particularly to a normal or above normal serum sodium concentration. Hyponatremia has been a common factor, as has a rise in serum sodium of more than 20 to 30 mmol/L over three days (Leslie et al., 1980) or greater than 12 mmol/L/day (Sterns et al., 1986). Experimental studies have validated these clinical observations. Kleinschmidt-DeMasters and Norenberg (1982) produced CPM in rats by rendering them hyponatremic with dextrose and water plus antidiuretic hormone and then giving them hypertonic, followed by isotonic, saline. CPM developed in these animals, but not in groups of transiently hyponatremic or hypernatremic control animals.

McKee et al. (1988) recently described 10 burn patients with CPM, none of whom had documented hyponatremia. All had, however, a sustained, nonterminal period of marked *hyperosmolality* related to hypernatremia, hyperglycemia, azotemia, or a combination of these. Thus, hyponatremia appears not to be required, but a rapid increase in osmolality of any type may be the essential factor (i.e., a *relative* hypertonic insult.)

Just how overly rapid correction of hyponatremia (or any abrupt, fairly sustained rise in serum osmolality) might cause CPM is not known. It has been shown that with hyponatremia, the brain adapts by losing intracellular solute (Grantham and Linshaw, 1984). If the extracellular fluid sodium concentration is then raised, could the brain have difficulty adapting to the increased osmolality by attempting to quickly raise its idiogenetic osmols? If so, how would this affect myelin or oligodendroglia?

Norenberg (1983) proposed that there is osmotic damage to the capillary endothelium that results in the release of myelinotoxic factors and/or vasogenic edema. It has been suggested that edema in itself may produce demyelination (Feigin and Budzilovich, 1978). From this concept theories evolved that the white matter was "choked" by the gridlike arrangement in the pons (Messert et al., 1979) and lateral geniculate body (Goldman and Horoupian, 1981). Alternatively, Norenberg (1983) suggests that the richly vascular gray matter has a greater store of myelinotoxic substances that are released in the correction of hyponatremia. Norenberg (1983) suggests that these substances may activate plasminogen, which gets into the parenchyma through leaky blood vessels. The plasmin could hydrolyze myelin basic protein and further increase vascular permeability by activating the kininogen system (Christman et al., 1977). Lockwood (1975) showed that acute hyperosmolality (it might be argued that acute *relative* hyperosmolality occurs in abruptly corrected hyponatremia) was associated with reduced cerebral metabolic rates, even though stores of high-energy phosphate were maintained. He also showed an alteration of cerebral amino acids, notably an increase in glutamine and a decrease in N-acteylaspartic acid compared to the dry weight of the brain.

How the original association of malnutrition and CPM relates to the above theory is uncertain. Norenberg (1983) suggests that malnourished individuals may not be able to generate idiogenetic osmols (especially amino acids) to adjust to higher osmolality during treatment of hyponatremia. Patients with hypercatabolic states in association with burns or sepsis may also have this problem, as they have a net loss of nitrogenous compounds derived from proteins and amino acids (McKee et al., 1988). Amino acid alterations in relative hyperosmolality may rely on astrocytic metabolism. In hepatic disease, protoplasmic astrocyte function may be decreased, as evidenced by Alzheimer type II astrocytes, which are thought to be damaged cells (Norenberg, 1977).

It has also been our clinical impression that central pontine myelinolysis is found mainly in patients who are systemically ill, e.g., with sepsis, renal or hepatic failure, diabetes, and low-output cardiac failure. While systemic illness is not essential for CPM, we feel it plays a facilitative role when hyponatremia is corrected. This impression is confirmed by the autopsy study of McKee et al. (1988), who found CPM in seven percent of burn patients, yet in only 0.28 percent of the general autopsy population.

Treatment

From the above, it appears obvious that overly rapid correction of hyponatremia should be avoided. Sterns et al. (1986) suggest that serum sodium be corrected at a rate no faster than 12 mmol/L per day, primarily by water restriction and withdrawal of thiazide diuretics (Abramow and Cogan, 1984).

While it is usually possible to correct even symptomatic hyponatremia conservatively without neurological residua, severe hyponatremia with convulsions may be associated with a fatal outcome (Arieff, 1986). The issues of what constitutes too slow a correction and what is the maximum rate at which severe symptomatic hyponatremia should be corrected are unsettled. It appears that if severe dilutional hyponatremia requires prompt treatment with hypertonic saline, it is best to only *partly* correct it, i.e., to about 125 mmol/L or so, and allow further correction to proceed more slowly (Auys et al., 1987).

Central Nervous System Infection

Immunosuppression from the drugs used to prevent transplant rejection predisposes these patients to the development of opportunistic infections. Since the immunosuppressive agents tend to suppress cell-mediated immunity, the opportunistic organisms are those most able to take advantage of this type of immune failure. However, the incidence of such infections has decreased considerably in recent years, likely due to the use of cyclosporine and lower, alternate-day steroid dosages, which cause much less immunosuppression. Nonetheless, Morduchowicz et al. (1985) reported from Israel a 50 percent incidence of infection after transplantation. Moreover, Rao (1987) observed in 169 patients that in the second decade following renal transplantation, 25 percent had significant infection as a complication. In a recent multicenter European study (Fassbinder et al., 1987) of 9,873 renal transplant patients, the incidence of death from infection 10 years or more posttransplantation was 18 percent, less than half the incidence during the first two years after the transplant procedure.

As emphasized earlier, these conditions may be quite uncommon, but they are frequently involved in the differential diagnosis of fever, confusion, and other CNS signs. Moreover, there is considerable overlap in their time of occurrence following transplantation and in the various symptoms and signs of nervous system dysfunction that may occur (see Table 8.2). Thus, in the individual patient, the various infections, whether they be viral, fungal, etc., or whether the condition is a lymphoma induced by Epstein-Barr virus infection, may not be apparent even after intensive investigation with repeated CSF cell cultures and a CT head scan. Ultimately, brain biopsy and special studies of the brain tissue may be necessary before a correct diagnosis is made. Arriving at a precise diagnosis is important, since many of these conditions are treatable.

Viral Infections

Four herpes-type viruses are particularly likely to occur in the posttransplant period. These are cytomegalovirus, Epstein-Barr virus, herpes simplex virus, and varicella-zoster virus. All may produce a somewhat similar clinical picture and tend to occur within the first one to six months after renal transplantation.

Cytomegalovirus

This infection may occur in at least two-thirds of all patients who receive a renal transplant. It is often asymptomatic, but it may produce fever, pneumonia, and occasionally more widespread serious effects. The source of infection is likely the graft itself, the donor being seropositive. It is a common cause of prolonged and unexplained fever, and there are rarely focal clinical signs. In a recent study by Trachtman et al. (1985), it was present in approximately one-quarter of all children who had received a transplant. In addition to fever, there might be signs of hepatitis, leukopenia, and thrombocytopenia. It is probably uncommon for the CNS to be involved. As noted under Central Nervous System Neoplasms below, this virus will occasionally be the cause of Kaposi's sarcoma.

Epstein-Barr Virus

This virus is often confused with cytomegalovirus. However, it may produce an infectious mononucleosis–like syndrome in children and, in adults, leukopenia, fever, and pulmonary infiltrates (Charpentier, 1986). The only way the CNS becomes involved is if the virus induces a B-cell lymphoma, which may involve the CNS primarily (see Central Nervous System Neoplasms, below).

Herpes Simplex Virus

This virus may infect up to two-thirds of patients in the posttransplant period (Charpentier, 1986). It also may be difficult to distinguish from cytomegalovirus. In the series of children reported by Trachtman et al. (1985), it occurred in about 10 percent of the cases. The typical cutaneous and mucous membrane lesions might be present. The CNS was apparently not involved in any of these children, and it is presumably a rare complication in this situation.

Varicella-Zoster Virus

Infection with this virus occurs in less than 10 percent of patients (Charpentier, 1986). The typical rash, in a cutaneous dermatome, may or may not be present. While the CNS is rarely involved, either by encephalitis or meningitis, when it occurs it runs quite a fulminant course. Peterson and Anderson (1986) documented three such cases. All patients with varicella-zoster infection should be hospitalized and azathioprine medication should be reduced as much as possible. They should be treated with either vidarabine or acyclovir. The latter drug may be preferable, in dosages of 0.5 g/m² body surface area every eight hours, in children. The serum creatinine should be monitored during therapy. Adequate hydration is necessary to prevent drug crystallization in renal tubules (Centers for Disease Control, 1981b).

Progressive Multifocal Leukoencephalopathy (JC Virus)

This rare disorder usually develops in patients who are immunosuppressed due to chronic lymphocytic leukemia, lymphoma, acquired immunodeficiency syndrome (AIDS), and drugs, including those used after renal transplantation (Saxton et al., 1984). Symptoms and signs of multifocal involvement of the cerebral hemispheres develop over weeks or months. Seizures are rare. A CT head scan shows relatively characteristic circumscribed, low-density areas that enhance poorly. Brain biopsy will usually disclose the typical lesions of this demyelinating disorder. Electron microscopy reveals the crystalline arrays of particles resembling papovaviruses. These have been shown to be either JC or SV40 virus. Unfortunately, no treatment has been found effective and the disease ends fatally.

HIV Infection

The first cases of AIDS were reported in 1985 (Centers for Disease Control, 1981a; 1981b). It is now apparent that patients who have received an organ transplant and are immunosuppressed may be particularly susceptible to this infection (Rubin et al., 1987). They may receive the virus either as a result of blood transfusions or from the allograft itself, or the recipient of the transplant may have harbored the virus before this procedure, and it became manifest with immunosuppression afterwards. However, the incidence of positive reactors to enzyme-linked immunosorbent assay (ELISA) or to Western Blot analysis is less than one percent in transplant recipients (Kerman et al., 1987). Nonetheless, small numbers of such patients with what appear to be genuine AIDS infection are being reported from several centers around the world (Rubin et al., 1987).

The CNS manifestations of AIDS are remarkably complex and have consisted of the virus itself causing a subacute or chronic encephalopathy, myelopathy, and polyneuropathy. Opportunistic infection of the CNS, particularly toxoplasmosis or neoplasms such as a lymphoma, may also cause CNS signs. Diagnosis and management is remarkably complex (Sever and Gibbs, 1988), since the posttransplant state and AIDS are both associated with immunosuppression and the same tendency to and types of, opportunistic infection and neoplasm.

It is recommended (Rubin et al., 1987) that all potential transplant donors be screened for the presence of antibody to HIV and if donors prove to be positive they should be regarded as unacceptable. Since there is a small incidence of false-negative results in rapid screen for HIV antibody, all donors who are or have been homosexual or bisexual men, intravenous drug users, hemophiliacs, prisoners in correctional facilities, and immigrants from Central Africa or Haiti should not be considered as potential donors under most circumstances. An exception is a living related donor who proved negative for the more comprehensive ELISA and Western Blot analysis techniques. All potential recipients of organ transplants should be screened for antibody to HIV. Dialysis, rather than transplantation, in most circumstances is the method of choice in end-stage renal disease in patients who are seropositive for HIV. The issue is complex and for further discussion the reader is referred to the article by Rubin et al. (1987).

Bacterial Infections

Listeria Monocytogenes

Infection with *Listeria monocytogenes* occurs within one to six months of transplantation and is probably acquired as a nosocomial infection. These patients present with signs of acute bacterial meningitis. In rare circumstances, focal neurological signs with evidence of abscess on CT scans are present (Hoeprich, 1987). Early identification of the organism may, at times, be difficult, and an erroneous diagnosis of diptheroids or nonpathogens may initially be given. Thus, it is wise to consider all such cases as *Listeria monocytogenes* and treat them as such, usually with a combination of penicillin and tobramycin.

Mycobacteriosis

Mycobacterium tuberculosis, or atypical mycobacteria, infection may present from months to years after a transplant procedure and often is difficult to diagnose. It should always be considered a possible cause of unexplained posttransplant infection. It most commonly involves the lungs, skin, and joints. Occasionally the CNS is involved as meningitis, often accompanied by focal neurological signs due to a concomitant vasculitis. Tuberculous abscesses may also occur in various parts of the

CNS. If the sputum is negative for acid-fast stains, bronchoscopy should be done, and the aspirate subjected to repeat staining and culture for *Mycobacterium tuberculosis* or atypical mycobacteria. Especially in the case of suspected nervous system infection, treatment should be started before the organism has been identified. Treatment consists of administration of isoniazid and rifampin over a period of many months. If the patient is receiving cyclosporine, pyrazinamide should be substituted for rifampin (Peterson and Anderson, 1986).

Nocardiosis

Infection by *Nocardia asteroides* occurs within one to six months of the renal transplant and tends to produce soft-tissue abscesses and pneumonia. Occasionally, it will spread to the CNS as brain abscess and/or meningitis. The organism may be isolated from the CSF. In treatment, any abscess, including that of brain, should be drained surgically, and then there should be prolonged treatment with sulfisoxazole or trimethoprim-sulfamethoxazole. In one of the three transplant recipients reported by Baddour et al. (1986), the only patient to have CNS involvement, which comprised meningitis and brain abscess, ultimately died.

Legionellosis

After transplantation, infection by *Legionella pneumophila* usually presents as pneumonia, and the diagnosis is confirmed by the study of sputum, bronchoscopic specimens, or lung biopsy material for special immunofluorescent studies and culture (Peterson and Anderson, 1986). While there have been no reported cases of CNS involvement after renal transplantation, such involvement has been reported in other patients. A variety of clinical syndromes, a diffuse encephalopathy, or isolated cerebellar and brainstem involvement may occur. The results of CSF culture and CT head scans may be negative, causing diagnostic confusion. However, with prompt treatment by erythromycin, with or without rifampin, the CNS signs quickly resolve (Baddour et al., 1986).

Fungal Infections

All of these present within a period of approximately one to eight months following a transplant procedure. The organisms usually involved are *Cryptococcus neoformans*, *Histoplasma capsulatum*, *Coccidioides immitis*, *Aspergillus species*, *Candida albicans*, and the *Mucoraceae*. All may potentially involve the CNS, but this is most likely to occur with cryptococcosis, coccidioidomycosis, and aspergillosis.

Cryptococcosis

Cryptococcosis is a ubiquitous infection that affects the lung first, often asymptomatically, and then presents insidiously as chronic headache, less commonly with more severe or focal neurological signs. Hydrocephalus may ultimately develop. Repeated lumbar punctures are often necessary before the diagnosis of chronic meningitis is made and the organism (*Cryptococcus neoformans*) is finally cultured. Amphotericin B is used in treatment, but the complications of renal tubular acidosis should be watched for, and of course, the presence of renal failure dictates careful monitoring of dosage. Mortality is over 40 percent, even in patients who are not immunocompromised (Adams and Victor, 1985).

Watson et al. (1984; 1985) emphasized that cryptococcal infection can be successfully treated in a renal transplant patient. They report survival in 10 of 13 patients. They were able to maintain immunosuppressive therapy, and consequently renal function, during the prolonged period of treatment with antifungal therapy.

Coccidioidomycosis

Coccidioidomycosis is acquired only by living in the southwestern United States. It commonly begins with pulmonary involvement and more rarely becomes more widely disseminated, occasionally affecting the nervous system as meningitis. It most commonly mimics tuberculous meningitis. Again, treatment is with amphotericin B, which often needs to be administered intraventricularly through an Ommaya reservoir. Unfortunately, the mortality rate may be over 50 percent (Adams and Victor, 1985).

Candidiasis

Infection with *Candida albicans* arises by the nosocomial route and may occur at almost any time following renal transplantation. It may be manifest by the typical mucous membrane or cutaneous manifestations, but at other times, it may not have any localized findings. The nervous system is occasionally involved, either as meningitis or as single or multiple brain abscesses. In such instances, the treatment of choice is intravenous amphotericin B. Treatment must be vigorous since mortality is high in immunocompromised patients. A positive blood culture indicates dissemination and mandates emergency treatment (Adams and Victor, 1985).

Aspergillosis

This fungus infection usually occurs during the first six months of the posttransplant period. It initially causes fever and pulmonary infiltrates. It may occur as a secondary complication of cytomegalovirus disease (Bennett, 1987). In this setting, the neurological signs often occur suddenly and might be either those of meningitis, or those of focal or multifocal cerebral dysfunction. The CSF reveals a modest increase in protein concentration and white blood cells, but glucose is normal. The CT head scan shows areas of decreased density, with little mass effect. There may be no ring-enhancing lesions. In the series of 12 cases of nervous system aspergillosis reported by Beal et al. (1982), six occurred after renal transplant. The course was remarkably rapid, death occurring in a matter of a few days after neurological involvement. However, identification of the organism and treatment with amphotericin B was begun late.

Investigation of these patients by lumbar puncture or brain biopsy may be hampered by a bleeding diathesis (McClellan et al., 1985), which occasionally occurs in renal transplant recipients who have disseminated aspergillosis.

Mucormycosis

Infection by fungi belonging to the Mucoraceae family is most likely to occur in post-renal transplant patients who also have diabetes mellitus. In 1985, Carbone et al. reported two patients of their own and an additional 20 that they had gleaned from the world literature. The illness began within a few weeks of renal transplantation.

Mucormycosis characteristically infects the nose and paranasal sinuses to produce fever and bloody nasal discharge. The infection then spreads to one orbit, where signs of cellulitis, proptosis, chemosis, and restricted ocular movement are evident. In some cases, the hard palate becomes necrotic or the skin of the cheek inflamed. In two-thirds of the cases reported by Carbone and associates, the brain became involved. This usually occurs through direct inflammation of the carotid artery, where thrombosis produces unilateral blindness and cerebral infarction. A lumbar puncture is usually of little value, but the CT head scan will show clouding of the sinuses and edema of the orbit, with proptosis. If the brain is involved, there will be evidence of hemorrhagic infarction.

The diagnosis is established by biopsy of the nose and/or sinuses. A wet smear of the tissue usually provides a rapid diagnosis. Cultural confirmation should be attempted, but this may be delayed and is often negative for blood and cerebrospinal fluid. The organism may be isolated from the sputum.

Treatment is of an emergent nature and consists of a rapid lowering in the dosage of immunosuppressive agents and institution of intravenous amphotericin B. It is beneficial to control, as closely as possible, the associated diabetes mellitus. Recovery occurred in half of the 22 cases reported by Carbone et al. (1985).

Parasitic Infections

Pneumocystis carinii, a natural inhabitant of the lung, is particularly likely to be the cause of an opportunistic infection in immunocompromised patients. The clinical features are usually those of pneumonia. The nervous system is rarely involved.

A much more frequent occurrence is toxoplasmosis due to the organism *Toxoplasma gondii*. An obligate intracellular parasite, it may be acquired through the eating of raw beef, contact with cat feces, and the handling of uncooked mutton.

Of 39 patients gleaned from the world literature in 1975 who had acquired CNS toxoplasmosis (Townsend et al., 1975), half were immunosuppressed, two following renal transplantation. Moreover, toxoplasmosis infection is particularly common in patients who have AIDS (Levy et al., 1988).

The neurological manifestations are quite variable. They may occur in the setting of widespread infection with skin rash, encephalitis, myocarditis, and polymyositis. The neurological signs may suggest a diffuse encephalopathy, with asterixis, myoclonus, and seizures. Signs of meningeal irritation may be present, or there may be focal or multifocal signs. The CSF reveals increased cell and protein content. CT head scans may show multiple ring-enhancing lesions. A certain diagnosis can usually only be made by identification of the organisms in CSF sediment or by biopsy of an involved area of the body, such as the brain. However, diagnosis may be difficult, and if there is any suspicion of toxoplasmosis, it is recommended that therapy with pyrimethamine and sulfadiazine be instituted; this should result in prompt clinical and radiographic responses.

While infection with the parasite *Strongyloides stercoralis* is rare, Morgan et al. (1986) were able to report eight patients. The clinical manifestations were those of bacteremia, meningitis, urinary tract infection, and pneumonia. The diagnosis was made by identifying the larvae on direct microscopy of stool, upper intestinal fluids, sputum, urine, or biopsy specimens. Prolonged treatment with oral thiabendazole was recommended. The organism may or may not be isolated from the CSF.

Central Nervous System Neoplasms

The incidence of cancer in patients following renal transplantation has been reported from two to 13 percent, 100 times greater than is expected in the general population (Penn, 1981b; 1984). The mechanisms are postulated to be the result of loss or impairment of surveillance mechanisms for neoplastic cells, viral oncogenesis, failure of feedback immunoregulation, chronic antigenic stimulation by the allograft, and potentiating actions of immunosuppressive agents (Penn 1981a; 1984; Mattas et al., 1975). However, in recent years more details on the mechanism have been worked out, and the chain of events is becoming clearer. Infection by certain viruses, predisposed to by immunosuppression, would appear to be the main mechanism of tumor production in these patients. The subject has been reviewed by Purtilo et al. (1985) and by Charpentier (1986).

In some centers, cytomegalovirus infection may occur in almost all recent allograft recipients. The nervous system is rarely involved; however, it is now believed that the virus induces Kaposi's sarcoma, an indolent tumor most frequently involving the skin and occasionally other organ systems. However, in the immune-compromised individual, particularly a patient with AIDS, it may become remarkably aggressive. Kaposi's sarcoma is an occasional complication of renal transplantation (Sakellariou et al., 1986), but involvement of the CNS must be exceptionally rare.

Epstein-Barr virus plays a more prominent role in tumorigenesis in these patients. It selectively infects, and is latent in, B lymphocytes. In the general population it is responsible for infectious mononucleosis, Burkitt's lymphoma, and nasopharyngeal carcinoma. In renal allograft recipients it causes an infectious lymphoproliferative syndrome. In young patients, the condition is called polyclonal B-cell hyperplasia. It occurs soon after transplantation and is manifest as generalized lymphadenopathy with symptoms and signs similar to those of infectious mononucleosis. It may be easily confused with cytomegalovirus infection. In adults, it may be manifest as leukopenia, fever, and pulmonary infiltrates. Ultimately it may cause a B-cell lymphoma (Charpentier, 1986), formerly called reticulum cell sarcoma. The CNS, usually the brain, is involved in at least one-third of these patients (Hanto et al., 1983), possibly because of a relative immune deficiency within the CNS as compared to other organs (Brikeland, 1983). Thus, the tumor may arise primarily within the nervous system. Here, focal cerebral signs dominate the clinical picture. A CT head scan will show single or multiple solid, strongly enhancing lesions (Williams, 1985). The cerebrospinal fluid often shows a pleocytosis with abnormal lymphomatous cells, The diagnosis is made by craniotomy and biopsy, or in the case of spinal cord neoplasms, by MRI or possibly a myelogram and then laminectomy and biopsy. Radiation therapy is initially quite successful. Reduction or cessation of immunosuppressive therapy may also be worthwhile (Starzl et al., 1984).

Touraine et al. (in press) failed to observe the infectious lymphoproliferative syndrome in their first 680 renal transplants. However, 15 of their last 700 patients developed the syndrome. It was likely induced both by the presence of Epstein-Barr virus and immunosuppressive drugs, including cyclosporine. The syndrome is reversible by reduction of the immunosuppression. However, if allowed to continue, an irreversible malignant lymphoma is likely to develop.

Herpesvirus infection predisposes to carcinoma of the cervix and uterus, hepatitis B virus infection to primary liver carcinoma, and papilloma virus infection to squamous cell carcinoma of the skin. Involvement of the nervous system in these instances appears to be quite rare.

References

Abramow M, Cogan E. Clinical aspects and pathophysiology of diuretic-induced hyponatremia. Adv Nephrol 1984;13:1–28.

Adams RD, Victor M. Nonviral infections of the nervous system. In: Adams RD, Victor M, eds. Principles of neurology. 3rd ed. New York: McGraw-Hill, 1985:536–538.

Adams RD, Victor M, Mancall EL. Central pontine myelinolysis: a hitherto undescribed disease occurring in alcoholic and malnourished patients. Arch Neurol Psychiatry 1959;81:154–172.

Arieff AI. Hyponatremia, convulsions, respiratory arrest, and permanent brain damage after elective surgery in healthy women. N Engl J Med 1986;314:1529–1535.

Ashraf N, Locksley R, Arieff AI. Thiazide-induced hyponatremia associated with death or neurologic damage in outpatients. Am J Med 1981;70:1163–1168.

Auys JC, Krothapalli RK, Arieff AI. Treatment of symptomatic hyponatremia and its relation to brain damage. A prospective study. N Engl J Med 1987;317:1190–1195.

Ayres SM. Sepsis and septic shock—a synthesis of ideas and proposals for the direction of future research. In: Sibbald WJ, Sprung CL, eds. Perspectives on sepsis and septic shock. Fullerton: Society of Critical Care Medicine, 1986:375–392.

Baddour LM, Baselski VS, Herr MJ, et al. Nocardiosis in recipients of renal transplants: evidence for nosocomial acquisition. Am J Infect Control 1986;14:214–219.

Beal MF, O'Carroll CP, Kleinman GM, Grossman RI. Aspergillosis of the nervous system. Neurology 1982;32:473–479.

Bennett JE. Fungal infections. In: Braunwald E, Isselbacher KJ, Petersdorf RG, et al., eds., Harrison's principles of internal medicine. 11th ed. New York: McGraw-Hill, 1987:742.

Bolton CF, Gilbert JJ, Hahn AF, Sibbald WJ. Polyneuropathy in critically ill patients. J Neurol Neurosurg Psychiatry 1984;47:1223–1231.

Boon AP, Potter AE. Extensive extrapontine and central pontine myelinolysis associated with correction of profound hyponatremia. Neuropathol Appl Neurobiol 1987;13:1–9.

Brikeland SA. Cancer in transplanted patients—the Scandia transplant material. Transplant Proc 1983; 1:1071–1078.

Brunner JE, Redmond JM, Haggar AM, Elias SB. Central pontine myelinolysis after rapid correction of hyponatremia: a magnetic resonance imaging study. Ann Neurol 1988;23:389–391.

Cadman TE, Rorke LB. Central pontine myelinolysis in childhood and adolescence. Arch Dis Child 1969;44:342–350.

Carbone KM, Pennington LR, Gimenez LF, et al. Mucormycosis in renal transplant patients—a report of two cases and review of the literature. Q J Med [New Ser 57] 1985;2224:825–831.

Centers for Disease Control. Kaposi's sarcoma and pneumocystis pneumonia among homosexual men—New York and California. MMWR 1981a;30:305–308.

Centers for Disease Control. Pneumocystis pneumonia—Los Angeles. MMWR 1981b;30:250–252.

Charpentier B. Viral infections in renal transplant recipients: an evolutionary problem. Adv Nephrol 1986;15:353–378.

Chason JL, Landers JW, Gonzales JE. Central pontine myelinolysis. J Neurol Neurosurg Psychiatry 1964;27:317–325.

Christman JK, Silverstein SC, Aes G. Plasminogen activators. In: Barrett AJ, ed. Proteinases in mammalian cells and tissues. Amsterdam: North-Holland, 1977;91–149.

DeWitt LD, Buonanno FS, Kistler JP, et al. Central pontine myelinolysis: demonstration by nuclear magnetic resonance. Neurology (Cleveland) 1984;34:570–576.

Dickoff DJ, Raps M, Yahr MD. Striatal syndrome following hyponatremia and its rapid correction. A manifestation of extrapontine myelinolysis confirmed by magnetic resonance imaging. Arch Neurol 1988;45:112–114.

Eggers PW. Effect of transplantation on the Medicare end-stage renal disease program. N Engl J Med 1988;318:223–229.

Fassbinder W, Challah S, Brynger H. The long-term renal allograft recipient. Transplant Proc 1987;19:3754–3757.

Feigin I, Budzilovich GN. The role of edema in diffuse sclerosis and other leukoencephalopathies. J Neuropathol Exp Neurol 1978;32:326–357.

Finlayson M, Snider S, Oliva LA, Gault M. Cerebral and pontine myelinolysis. Two cases with fluid and electrolyte imbalance and hypotension. J Neurol Sci 1973;18:399–409.

Goldman JE, Horoupian DS. Demyelination of the lateral geniculate nucleus in central pontine myelinolysis. Ann Neurol 1981;9:185–189.

Grantham J, Linshaw M. The effect of hyponatremia on the regulation of intracellular volume and solute composition. Circ Res 1984;54:483–491.

Gross MLP, Sweny P, Pearson RM, et al. Rejection encephalopathy. J Neurol Sci 1982;56:23–34.

Hanto DW, Gajl-Peczalska JG, Frizzera G, et al. Epstein-Barr virus (EBV) induced polyclonal and monoclonal B-cell lymphoproliferative diseases occurring after renal transplantation. Ann Surg 1983;198:356–369.

Hoeprich PD. Infections caused by Listeria monocytogenes and Erysipelothrix rhusiopathiae. In: Braunwald E, Isselbacher KJ, Petersdorf RG, et al., eds. Harrison's principles of internal medicine. 11th ed. New York: McGraw-Hill, 1987:554–555.

Jackson AC, Gilbert JJ, Young GB, Bolton CF. The encephalopathy of sepsis. Can J Neurol Sci 1985;12:303–307.

Kerman RH, Flechner SM, Van Buren CT, et al. Investigation of human T-lymphotropic virus III serology in a renal transplant population. Transplant Proc 1987;19:2172–2175.

Klavins, JV. Central pontine myelinolysis. J Neuropathol Exp Neurol 1963;22:302–317.

Kleinschmidt-DeMasters BK, Norenberg MD. Neuropathologic observations in electrolyte-induced myelinolysis in the rat. J Neuropathol Exp Neurol 1982;41:67–80.

Leslie KO, Robertson AS, Norenberg MD. Central pontine myelinolysis: an osmotic gradient pathogenesis. J Neuropathol Exp Neurol 1980;39:370.

Levy RM, Bredesen DE, Rosenblum ML. Opportunistic central nervous system pathology in patients with AIDS. Ann Neurol 1988; S7–S12.

Lockwood AH. Acute and chronic hyperosmolality. Arch Neurol 1975;32:62–64.

Mahony JF, Sheil AGR, Etheridge SB, et al. Delayed complications of renal transplantation and their prevention. Med J Aust 1982;2:426–429.

Mattas AJ, Simmons RL, Najarian JC. Chronic antigenic stimulation, herpes virus infection and cancer in transplant recipients. Lancet 1975;1:1277–1280.

McClellan SL, Komorowski RA, Farmer SG, et al. Severe bleeding diathesis associated with invasive aspergillosis in transplant patients. Transplantation 1985;39:406–410.

McCormick WF, Daneel CM. Central pontine myelinolysis. Arch Intern Med 1967;119:444–477.

McKee AC, Winkelman MD, Banker BQ. Central pontine myelinolysis in severely burned patients: relation to serum osmolality. Neurology (Cleveland) 1988;38:1211–1217.

Messert B, Orrison WW, Hawkins MJ, Quaglieri CE. Central pontine myelinolysis. Considerations on etiology, diagnosis and treatment. Neurology 1979;29:147–160.

Morduchowicz G, Pitlik SD, Sharpira Z, et al. Infections in renal transplant recipients in Israel. Isr J Med Sci 1985;21:791–797.

Norenberg MD. A light and electron microscopic study of experimental portal-systemic (ammonia) encephalopathy: progression and reversal of the disorder. Lab Invest 1977;36:618–627.

Norenberg MD. A hypothesis of osmotic endothelial injury. Arch Neurol 1983;40:66–69.

Penn J. Depressed immunity and the development of cancer. Clin Exp Immunol 1981a;146:459–474.

Penn J. Renal transplantation and cancer. In: Zurukzoglu W, Papadimitriou M, Pyrpasopoulos M, et al., eds. Proceedings of the 8th International Congress on Nephrology, Athens, 1981. Basel: Karger, 1981b:527–538.

Penn J. Cancer in immunosuppressed patients. Transplant Proc 1984;2:492–494.

Peterson PK, Anderson RC. Infection in renal transplant recipients. Current approaches to diagnosis, therapy and prevention. Am J Med 1986;81:2–10.

Powers JM, McKeever PE. Central pontine myelinolysis: an ultrastructural and elemental study. J Neurol Sci 1976;29:65–81.

Price BH, Mesulam MM. Behavioral manifestations of central pontine myelinolysis. Arch Neurol 1987; 44:671–673.

Purtilo DT, Tatsumi E, Manolov G, et al. Epstein-Barr virus as an etiological agent in the pathogenesis of lymphoproliferative and aproliferative diseases in immune deficient patients. In: Richter GW, Epstein MA, eds. International review of experimental pathology, Vol 27. Cambridge, MA: Academic Press, 1985:113–183.

Rao KV. Renal transplantation: complications and results in the second decade. Transplant Proc 1987; 19:3758–3759.

Rubin RH, Jenkins RL, Shaw BW, et al. The acquired immunodeficiency syndrome and transplantation. Transplantation 1987;44:1–4.

Sakellariou G, Alexopoulos E, Sinakos Z, et al. Cancer in renal transplant recipients. Cancer Detect 1986;9:389–393.

Saxton CR, Gailunas P, Helderman JH, et al. Progressive multifocal leukoencephalopathy in a renal transplant recipient: increased diagnostic sensitivity of computed tomographic scanning by double-dose with delayed films. Am J Med 1984;77:333–337.

Schneck SA. Neuropathological features of human organ transplantation: II. Central pontine myelinolysis and neuroaxonal dystrophy. J Neuropathol Exp Neurol 1966;25:18–39.

Sever JL, Gibbs CJ, eds. Retroviruses in the nervous system. Proceedings of a symposium sponsored by the National Institutes of Health, Bethesda, Maryland, May 4–6, 1987. Ann Neurol 1988;3(Suppl).

Starzl RW, Porter KA, Iwatsuki S, et al. Reversibility of lymphomas and lymphoproliferative lesions developing under cyclosporine-steroid therapy. Lancet 1984;1:583–587.

Sterns RH, Riggs JE, Schochet SS Jr. Osmotic demyelination syndrome following correction of hyponatremia. N Engl J Med 1986;341:1535–1542.

Stockard JJ, Rossiter VS, Wiederholt WC, Kobayashi RM. Brain stem auditory-evoked responses in suspected central myelinolysis. Arch Neurol 1976;33:726–728.

Tefler RB, Miller EM. Central pontine myelinolysis following hyponatremia, demonstrated by computerized tomography. Ann Neurol 1979;6:455–456.

Tomlinson B, Peirides A, Bradley W. Central pontine myelinolysis. Two cases with associated electrolyte disturbance. Q J Med 1976;40:373–386.

Touraine JL, Bosi E, El Yafi MS, et al. The infectious lymphoproliferative syndrome in transplant patients under immunosuppressive treatment. Transplant Proc, in press.

Townsend JJ, Wolinsky JS, Baringer JR, Johnson PC. Acquired toxoplasmosis. Arch Neurol 1975;32:335–343.

Trachtman H, Weiss RA, Spigland I, Griefer I. Clinical manifestations of herpes virus infections in pediatric renal transplant recipients. Pediatr Infect Dis 1985;4:480–486.

Watson AJ, Russell RP, Cabreja RF, et al. Cure of cryptococcal infection during continued immunosuppressive therapy. Q J Med [New Ser 55] 1985;217:169–172.

Watson AJ, Whelton A, Russell RP. Cure of cryptococcemia and preservation of graft function in a renal transplant recipient. Arch Intern Med 1984;144:1877–1878.

Wiederholt WC, Kobayashi RM, Stockard JJ, Rossiter VS. Central pontine myelinolysis. A clinical reappraisal. Arch Neurol 1977;34:220–223.

Williams AL. Infectious diseases. In: Williams AL, Haughton VM, eds. Cranial computed tomography. A comprehensive text. St Louis: CV Mosby, 1985: 269–270.

Wright DG, Laureno R, Victor M. Pontine and extrapontine myelinolysis. Brain 1979;102:361–385.

Young GB. The encephalopathy associated with sepsis. Ann R Coll Physicians Surg Can 1986;19:279–282.

Young GB, Bolton CF, Austin TW, Archibald Y. The electroencephalogram (EEG) in sepsis. Can J Neurol Sci 1986;13:164.

Zochodne DW, Bolton CF, Wells GA, et al. Polyneuropathy associated with critical illness: a complication of sepsis and multiple organ failure. Brain 1987;110:819–842.

Chapter 9

The Nervous System, Drugs, and Uremia

Contents

Acronyms

CNS   central nervous system
CsA   cyclosporine
CSF   cerebrospinal fluid
CT   computed tomography
HPLC   high-performance liquid
chromatography
Vd   volume of distribution

A recent survey in a university hospital revealed that patients with chronic renal failure take an average of 12 medications (Muther and Bennett, 1981). Less than half are prescribed for the underlying renal disease. Since the kidney is the major organ for ultimate elimination of drugs and since renal failure affects other organ systems such as the liver and gastrointestinal tract, renal failure predisposes to accumulation of drugs and/or their metabolites. In addition, the polypharmacy predisposes to drug–drug interactions.

In this chapter, we shall review the general principles of altered drug handling in uremia, followed by the pharmacological treatment of neurological complications of renal failure. Finally, the neurological complications of other drugs used in the treatment of renal disease will be discussed.

General Principles of Pharmacokinetics

This section deals with altered pharmacokinetics in uremia, as well as the effects of dialysis. A number of problems exist with drugs in uremia: altered bioavailability; altered metabolism; impaired elimination, especially of unmetabolized drugs and active polar metabolites; decreased plasma protein binding; drug interactions; altered tissue responsiveness; and assay reliability problems. Some general suggestions regarding dosage regimens in uremia are made. Excellent discussions of these issues can be found in reviews by Muther and Bennett (1981) and Perucca et al. (1985).

Bioavailability

Bioavailability refers to the relative amount of a drug that reaches the systemic circulation unchanged and the rate at which this occurs (Atkinson and Kushner, 1979). Since more than 80 percent of drugs are administered orally, the term is largely applied to gastrointestinal absorption of the drug. Absorption may be active or passive. In general, drugs that have a smaller molecular weight and are lipid soluble and nonionized, cross the gastrointestinal mucosa more readily than larger molecular weight, ionized, lipid-insoluble compounds.

There is little information on the effects of renal failure on bioavailability. For the most part, the effect may be indirect (Muther and Bennett, 1981). Nausea and recurrent vomiting obviously can affect absorption of orally administered drugs. Gastrointestinal edema in uremia may play a role, but this is not adequately documented.

Most drugs are absorbed in the small intestine, and any factors that delay gastric emptying may decrease bioavailability and alter the timing of appearance of the drug in the blood. Gastric emptying and intestinal peristalsis are delayed in peritonitis associated with peritoneal dialysis (Nimmo, 1976). Rimer (1966) lists uremia among a number of metabolic conditions that, on their own, may produce delayed gastric emptying. Diabetics, who represent a significant proportion of patients with uremia, may have autonomic neuropathy (gastroparesis diabeticorum) (Rimer, 1966). Headache and psychological and psychiatric conditions may also delay gastric emptying (Nimmo, 1976). Aluminum, contained in many phosphate-binding antacids used in uremia, can delay gastric emptying, as can dioctyl sodium sulfosuccinate, the stool softener that is often used to counteract the constipating effect of the aluminum-containing antacids.

Antacids may also act in other ways to diminish bioavailability. They may form insoluble chelation products with a number of drugs, including digoxin and tetracycline (Hurwitz, 1977). The increased gastric pH from antacids may retard absorption of many compounds, such as phenytoin, phenobarbital, warfarin, and acetylsalicylic acid, by increasing the ionized form of the drug.

Since orally administered drugs go into the portal venous system to the liver, the effects of uremia on hepatic function (see Drug Elimination, below) may reduce the "first pass" metabolism of drugs by the liver.

Drug Distribution

Distribution of a drug in the body is dependent on lipid solubility and plasma protein binding.

The volume of distribution (Vd) is a pharmacological concept that assumes that the body acts as a single compartment in which the drug is distributed. Vd is equal to the amount of drug in the body divided by its plasma concentration. The more lipid soluble a drug is, the greater its Vd. The higher the plasma protein binding, the lower the Vd, or, the Vd more closely approximates the plasma volume.

Although little is known about uremia's effects on lipid solubility, there is considerable information on plasma protein binding. In general, most of the drugs that show abnormal protein binding in uremia are organic acids, while organic bases have normal protein binding (Muther and Bennett, 1981). Reidenberg and Affrime (1973) suggest that this is because most organic acids have only one binding site to albumin, while organic bases bind at multiple regions. For phenytoin, Reidenberg and Affrime (1973) showed that impairment in plasma protein binding was directly proportional to serum creatinine level (Figure 9.1).

Several mechanisms may account for the decreased plasma protein binding of drugs in uremia: hypoproteinemia, especially hypoalbuminemia; a posttranslational structural abnormality in serum albumin; and competitive displacement of binding sites by retained chemicals. Hypoalbuminemia may play a significant role only in certain circumstances, such as nephrotic syndrome. Altered albumin structure has been suggested by several authors. Boobis (1977) demonstrated abnormal amino acid composition of albumin in uremic plasma. Indirect evidence of a structural abnormality in albumin is the failure of *in vivo* or *in vitro* dialysis to improve drug binding by albumin (Reidenberg and Affrime, 1973; Shoeman and Azarnoff, 1972; Brewster and Muir, 1980). An explanation that has been put forward to explain the altered amino acid ratios and altered binding is the presence of two albumin bands on isoelectric focusing of normal and uremic plasma (Shoeman and Azarnoff, 1972). The relative proportions of the two bands differed in the uremic and normal samples. It may be that one of the bands more effectively binds acidic drugs and that the two bands differ in their amino acid composition. As Boobis (1977) pointed out, there may not be two structurally different molecules; one of the bands could contain a tightly bound endogenous ligand that was incorporated in the electrophoretic study and in the amino acid electrophoresis. Altered conformation of the albumin molecule could also affect drug binding in uremia (Perucca et al., 1985). However, Sjoholm et al. (1986) did not find any difference in secondary and tertiary structure of plasma proteins in their comparison of uremic and normal individuals. Changes in pH, acid-base balance, and electrolyte composition may play a minor role (Perucca et al., 1985).

Most authorities feel that the main mechanism for altered protein binding in uremia is the displacement of the drug from the binding site by retained compounds that become tightly bound to albumin. Supportive evidence is the increase in protein binding of phenytoin and warfarin when uremic plasma is diluted, showing a small component of dissociative, competitive binding (Sjoholm et al., 1976), and improvement in plasma protein binding by acidification followed by charcoal dialysis or anion-exchange resin perfusion (Depner et al., 1980). These two studies largely refute those quoted above that maintain that a permanent structural abnormality in albumin is responsible for the decreased binding. Renal transplantation also restores normal plasma protein binding to drugs that have an organic acid

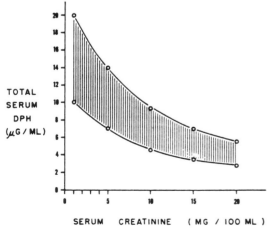

Figure 9.1. Calculated values of total serum phenytoin (DPH) concentration that will produce a DPH concentration of 0.7 to 1.4 μg/mL in plasma water. (Reprinted with permission from Reidenberg and Affrime, 1973.)

chemistry (Lyons et al., 1979). Gulyassy et al. (1986) have recently identified hippurate, β-(*m*-hydroxyphenyl)hydracrylate, and *p*-hydroxyphenylacetate as endogenous binding inhibitors in renal failure, using a rigorous series of purification and identification steps. Their work needs to be confirmed, and other ligands probably also remain to be identified.

The effect of uremia on plasma protein binding is to effectively increase the Vd of drugs that are ordinarily highly protein bound, such as phenytoin, valproate, salicylic acid, quinidine, and theophylline (Perucca et al., 1985). The free or unbound concentration of the drug may not be affected, but the total plasma or serum level of the drug is reduced. For accurate assessment of the adequacy of treatment, it is necessary to measure the free or unbound level.

Tissue binding of drugs is also affected by uremia but has not been extensively studied, except for the discovery of reduced binding of digoxin to the myocardium and reduced apparent Vd by Jusko and Weintraub (1974).

Increased end-organ sensitivity has been observed with certain drugs in uremia. Whether this is related to enhanced receptor binding, increased responsiveness once the drug is bound to receptors, synergism with unidentified chemicals, or other mechanisms is not known. Anecdotal reports of increased sensitivity of the brain to phenytoin (Reidenberg, 1977; Reynolds et al., 1976) have received indirect support from work on experimental uremic animals showing enhanced sensitivity to the central nervous system (CNS) depressant effect of phenobarbital (Danhof et al., 1983). With phenytoin, the increased CNS effect could result from an increased amount of the drug in the "central compartment" of a two-compartment pharmacokinetic model (Odar-Cederlof and Borga, 1974).

Drug Elimination (Metabolism and Excretion)

Once a drug reaches equilibrium in the plasma after absorption and distribution, its concentration declines progressively, depending on the type of kinetics involved in its metabolism.

An excellent discussion of pharmacokinetic principles is found in Browne (1983). The general rate of metabolism (V) is determined by the formula

$$V = \frac{V_{max}}{K_m + C} \times C$$

where V_{max} is the maximum velocity of the enzyme system, K_m is the Michaelis constant of the enzyme system, and C is the concentration of the drug. The term $V_{max}/(K_m + C)$ is referred to as the clearance of the drug.

The three types of enzyme kinetics are

1. Linear or first-order kinetics, in which C is small in relation to K_m. In this situation, $V_{max}/(K_m + C)$ is constant and V varies directly with C. The drug is cleared at a constant half-life (equal to 0.693 × Vd/clearance). An example of a drug cleared in this manner is phenobarbital.

2. Nonlinear (concentration-dependent) kinetics, in which C is large in comparison with K_m. Thus, the clearance varies inversely with C, and V changes in a nonlinear fashion with C. An example of a drug cleared by concentration-dependent kinetics is phenytoin.

3. Time-dependent kinetics, in which V_{max} and/or K_m changes with time, thus altering V. This is the concept of enzyme induction. Thus, the serum concentration at a constant dosage rate varies as enzyme induction (or V_{max} or K_m) varies. Eventually, a maximum or steady state of induction is reached, and the drug level stabilizes. The prototype of this kind of drug is carbamazepine.

In uremia, drug clearance is obviously most affected for those drugs that are largely excreted unchanged by the kidney, such as amantadine, 5-fluorocytosine, and penicillin. In this situation, accumulation of the drug in the plasma and in the body would directly relate to the increase in half-life, the dosage rate, and the degree of renal failure (Tozer, 1974).

Renal failure may also have a significant effect on certain drugs cleared by hepatic biotransformation. In general, oxidative metabolism is unaffected, but the oxidation of antipyrine (Lichter et al., 1973) and phenytoin (Odar-Cederlof and Borga, 1974) is increased. This probably relates to the increased free fraction of these drugs in uremic plasma, as a higher proportion of the serum concentration of the drug is immediately available to the liver. Also, it is possible that retained chemicals in uremia cause induction of hepatic enzymes in some patients. In general, however, the mean steady-state unbound level of drugs is not affected by the degree of protein binding, but peak levels achieved are higher and trough levels are lower in uremic patients than in individuals with normal protein levels and normal protein binding (Levy, 1976). Although clearance is increased, the Vd is also increased, and the half-life is relatively unaffected (Figure 9.2). Many drugs that require reduction and/or hydrolysis for elimination show slowed clearance in uremia. Acetylation rates may be decreased, but formation of glycine, sulfate, or glucuronide conjugates is unaffected for most drugs. For specific information on altered hepatic metabolism of drugs in uremia, see Reidenberg (1977) or Reidenberg and Drayer (1980).

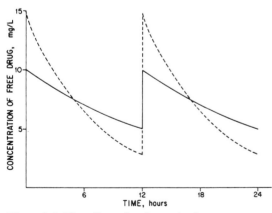

Figure 9.2. The effect of a change in the concentration of the free (unbound) drug when 100 mg/kg is given intravenously every 12 hours. The continuous line represents the free fraction at 0.01 and Vd of 0.20 L/kg. The dashed line shows the free fraction at 0.03. The Vd has increased to 0.25 L/kg. Note the more marked swings in concentration with the free fraction at 0.03. (Reprinted with permission from Levy, 1976.)

It should be remembered that renal excretion of various active metabolites, most of which are not routinely measured in hospital laboratories, would be expected to be markedly reduced in uremia. The following drugs all have active metabolites that accumulate in uremia: acebutolol, allopurinol, digoxin, methyldopa, meperidine, procainamide, and dextropropoxyphene (Verbeek et al., 1981). Primidone is a drug that has two metabolites with CNS side effects, phenobarbital and phenylethylmalonamide, both of which accumulate in renal failure. Asconapé and Penry (1982) reported two uremic patients who developed toxicity from phenylethylmalonamide when prescribed primidone.

Even biologically inactive metabolites may cause trouble. Sirgo et al. (1984) found that the accumulation of 5-(p-hydroxyphenyl)-5-phenylhydantoinglucuronide, a metabolite of phenytoin, interfered with homogenous enzyme immunoassays for phenytoin (EMIT and ACA) to give a falsely high concentration for both total phenytoin and its free fraction. The true level was determined with the more precise high-performance liquid chromatographic (HPLC) method. The patients' medications could then be properly adjusted for better seizure control. Another mechanism for inactive metabolites creating problems in renal failure is the regeneration of the active drug: enterohepatic recycling can remove the glucuronic moiety that is conjugated to the drug (Verbeek et al., 1981). This may happen with oxazepam, lorazepam, and propranolol (Verbeek et al., 1981).

Drugs that are not highly protein bound may be lost into the dialysate (Maher, 1977). Dialyzability with hemodialysis depends on molecular weight, protein binding, blood flow, and features of the dialysis machine. With peritoneal dialysis, the presence of vascular disease, peritoneal inflammation or scarring, and the influence of vasoactive hormones or chemicals are additional factors. Examples of some drugs that may require supplementation after dialysis are phenobarbital, salicylates, penicillins, cephalosporins, methotrexate, cyclophosphamide, and procainamide. A more complete list can be found in Maher (1977). Another complication of dialysis that may alter pharmacokinetics is the reduction of plasma protein binding after hemodialysis. This is thought to be due to the displacement of drugs from protein binding sites by free fatty acids that are liberated from fats by heparin-activated lipoprotein lipase (Dromgoole, 1973).

Approach to Drug Treatment in Uremia

Because of the complexities of drug handling in uremia, it is best to use drugs only when necessary, to use them in the lowest effective doses, and to monitor serum levels. In those that are normally highly protein bound (greater than 80 percent), the free (unbound) level should be measured. Further, to allow better absorption, oral drugs should not be given simultaneously with antacids unless this is necessary to prevent gastric irritation.

In general, drugs that are more than 50 percent dependent on renal elimination and do not have a low therapeutic ratio (ratio of toxic dose to therapeutic dose) can be adjusted roughly, using the following formula (Kreeft and Linton, 1985):

$$\text{New dose} = 2 \times \text{usual dose} \times \frac{\text{normal creatinine concentration}}{\text{new creatinine concentration}}$$

For a drug that has a therapeutic index of less than three, the two in the above formula is changed to one (Kreeft and Linton, 1985).

It is usually advisable to give the recommended loading dose of a drug in uremia, if it is acutely indicated. Subsequent dosage adjustments are often necessary (Muther and Bennett, 1981). These involve adjusting the frequency or dosage of maintenance therapy. In drugs with decreased clearance, one can lengthen the interdose interval without changing the dose. This is acceptable if the drug has a high therapeutic index, but such therapy may allow toxic peaks and subtherapeutic valleys to develop. Such toxic peaks and subtherapeutic valleys may also be seen with reduced protein binding in uremia or with hypoalbuminemia. Fluctuation in serum levels of the free fraction may be lessened by reducing the dose but giving the drug at the regular dosing intervals. Checks should always be made to assure that therapeutic serum levels are achieved. It should also be remembered that, in some patients, hypoalbuminemia may be a marker for impaired liver function and the potential for toxic effects (Lewis et al., 1971).

Nomograms have been well-developed for the use of a number of antibiotics in renal failure (Aranoff and Luft, 1979). The amount of drug lost in dialysis should also be estimated or serum levels can be measured after dialysis. Tozer (1974) has developed a nomogram for calculating the appropriate dose of any drug, provided the percent renal excretion and the degree of renal impairment are known. This can serve as a useful guide to modify dosage regimens for drugs for which guidelines for altered renal function are not available. The nomogram has a number of assumptions: linear kinetics; inactive, nontoxic metabolites; stable renal, hepatic, and cardiac function; and no alteration in distribution or metabolism caused by the renal failure. These assumptions may be more or less valid for different drugs. For example, they may not be valid for drugs with nonlinear kinetics such as phenytoin. It is almost always necessary to monitor the levels of such drugs in the blood.

Drugs that have active metabolites requiring renal excretion should be used with great caution in uremia. For example, diazepam is metabolized to oxazepam, which can accumulate and cause encephalopathy, as can flurazepam's metabolite, N-desallylflurazepam. A metabolite of meperidine, normeperidine, can cause myoclonus and seizures. If problems with enzyme assays are suspected because of interfering metabolites, drug levels can be most accurately determined using HPLC.

Pharmacological Treatment of Neurological Complications of Renal Failure

This section is devoted chiefly to the use of antiepileptic drugs in uremia. Benzodiazepines, which are used in the treatment of anxiety and dialytic encephalopathy as well as seizures, are also reviewed. Treatment of tetany, chemotherapy of CNS tumors, and vitamin supplements for treatment and prevention of nutritional disorders are dealt with elsewhere in this volume (see Chapter 7D) or in standard texts.

Antiepileptic Drugs

Seizures are not infrequent in uremia. They occur in acute and chronic renal failure, dialytic encephalopathy, dialysis dysequilibrium syndrome, hypertensive encephalopathy, as a consequence of ischemic or hemorrhagic stroke, and in the context of metabolic and toxic, septic and direct CNS infections and neoplasms. Thus, the use of antiepileptic drugs in patients with renal failure is not uncommon. An excellent review can be found in Asconapé and Penry (1982).

Concern was expressed by Wassner et al. (1976) that antiepileptic drugs, especially phenytoin and phenobarbital, were associated with decreased survival of renal allografts in children. Those children treated with antiepileptic drugs fared significantly worse than transplanted patients not on antiseizure medication. The authors proposed that this was because of decreased cortisol activity related to the drug use. We are not aware of any further work on this issue. However, with the advent of more effective immunosuppressive therapy such as cyclosporine, this concern may no longer be valid.

Phenytoin

Phenytoin is a first-line drug in treating partial or focally originating epilepsies. Its main mechanism of action is the inhibition of rapidly conducting sodium channels in neuronal membrane, but it has many other actions on membranes, synapses, and metabolic processes, which can play a role in preventing spread of epileptic discharges (Woodbury, 1982).

Phenytoin (5,5-diphenylhydantoin) is normally 90 percent protein bound, almost exclusively to albumin. It is metabolized by p-hydroxylation by the P-450 system in the liver to 5-p-hydroxyphenyl-5-phenylhydantoin, which is conjugated to glucuronide.

Although phenytoin is poorly soluble in the stomach fluid, its absorption is further reduced by the presence of alkali, i.e., antacid. It should not be given orally at the same time as antacids.

Renal failure is associated with a marked reduction in the protein binding of phenytoin. This results in an increase in the Vd. The absolute free concentration does not significantly change, although the ratio of the free to the total drug level is increased. Although nomograms have been constructed for phenytoin levels in renal failure, the most practical and reliable method is determination of the free or unbound level in the plasma or in tears (Bocher et al., 1974). The latter is, in essence, a filtrate containing phenytoin unbound to albumin. In measurements it is best to use HPLC or the TDX fluorescence polarization immunoassay methods, which give a more accurate measure of unmetabolized phenytoin (Sirgo et al., 1984). Only about 4.5 percent of phenytoin presented to the dialyzer is lost; it is usually not necessary to supplement the drug because of dialysis.

If the patient has associated liver disease, the half-life of phenytoin is prolonged, and less of the drug is bound to albumin. The latter may be in part due to displacement by elevated plasma bilirubin (Perucca, 1979). The degree of impairment in phenytoin metabolism is, however, seldom significant; doses do not usually need to be reduced (Asconapé and Penry, 1982).

In renal failure, phenytoin is a suitable drug to use in management of epileptic seizures, provided the above pharmacological considerations are kept in mind. Frequent determinations of the free serum level are usually advisable. Because swings in concentration of the free fraction are enhanced, it is best to administer the drug in three divided doses during the day. Another point not mentioned previously is the tendency for phenytoin to aggravate osteomalacia by causing increased metabolism of 25-hydroxyvitamin D_3 (Richens, 1979). Thus, additional vitamin D supplementation may be necessary.

Valproic Acid

Valproate has a wide spectrum of efficacy in epilepsy, but is best suited for primary generalized seizures: absence, generalized tonic-clonic, and myoclonic seizures. It can be used as an additional drug or as a second-line drug in the treatment of partial seizures. The mechanism of action is uncertain. It was originally thought to act by increasing levels of γ-aminobutyric acid, an inhibitory neurotransmitter, but its main mode of antiepileptic action may not be dissimilar to that of phenytoin.

Valproic acid (2-propylpentanoic acid) is available in the acid form or as the sodium salt. The latter has fewer gastrointestinal side effects. Like phenytoin, valproate is about 90 percent protein bound and is almost entirely metabolized in the liver, although by a variety of pathways to various compounds some of which may be active metabolites.

Like phenytoin, valproate's plasma protein binding is reduced in renal disease. The degree of impaired binding has been found to correlate with serum creatinine and to be largely independent of albumin and total protein concentration (Gugler and Mueller, 1978). Brewster and Muir (1980) showed that normal protein binding could be achieved by treating uremic plasma with activated charcoal. This gives support to the concept that binding sites on protein may be occupied by high-affinity endogenous chemicals in uremia. Interestingly, protein binding of valproate is reduced after hemodialysis (Bruni et al., 1980); perhaps the same explanation as for phenytoin applies (see previous section). The free fraction of valproate in plasma or serum, as with phenytoin, remains fairly constant.

The effect of uremia on the metabolism of valproate is not clear. The drug normally has a fairly short half-life of 10 to 16 hours on monotherapy and as short as six hours with polypharmacy.

Valproic acid may be valuable in treating or preventing myoclonic and generalized tonic-clonic seizures occurring with uremia and related conditions such as dialytic encephalopathy. Furthermore, valproate does not have strong enzyme-inducing properties (Asconapé and Penry, 1982). Adjustment of dose is usually not necessary in renal failure, but the drug should be given in at least three or four divided doses. Free levels are probably the best, but

serum levels of the total drug can be used if the clinician remembers that patients should be controlled at levels less than those for non-uremic patients. Caution should be used if the patient also has hepatic disease, because of the known hepatic toxicity of the drug.

Phenobarbital

Phenobarbital is used for partial seizures, whether they remain focal or become secondary generalized seizures. Its use is limited because of sedative side effects in adults and hyperactivity with impaired attention span in children.

Phenobarbital is 40 to 60 percent protein bound. It has a long half-life, ranging from 50 to 140 hours, which varies with polypharmacy, pH, and urine flow. About 25 percent is normally excreted in the urine; the rest is metabolized by the mixed oxidase system of the liver, conjugated, and excreted in the urine. Its metabolites are not biologically active.

Accumulation of phenobarbital is expected in chronic use in uremia. Serum levels need to be followed to check for accumulation of the drug. Lower maintenance doses are often necessary to prevent the development of toxicity. Reduced protein binding can affect serum levels, but not as much as for more highly protein-bound drugs such as phenytoin or valproate.

Primidone

Primidone, 2-deoxyphenobarbital, is closely related to phenobarbital. Primidone itself is not significantly bound to plasma proteins. Primidone's half-life is three to 12 hours. About 28 percent is converted to phenobarbital; 20 percent is excreted in the urine and the remainder is metabolized in the liver to phenylethylmalonamide. Its antiepileptic uses are similar to those of phenobarbital.

Caution is advised in the use of primidone in uremia. Although phenylethylmalonamide may not be an effective antiepileptic drug, it probably has CNS side effects and can accumulate in renal failure (Asconapé and Penry, 1982). This chemical, unlike the primidone and phenobarbital that may also accumulate, is not routinely measured in hospital laboratories.

Carbamazepine

Carbamazepine, 5H-dibenz[b,f]azepine-5-carboxamide, is effective in treating partial seizures while producing a minimum of cognitive side effects. Some older individuals do not tolerate the drug well. It must always be introduced gradually to avoid or minimize gastrointestinal and CNS side effects.

Carbamazepine shows about 80 percent protein binding in nonuremics. It is hydroxylated in the liver; one of its metabolites, 10,11-carbamazepine epoxide, is pharmacologically active. The half-life is highly variable among individuals, but the drug induces its own metabolism, often reducing the elimination half-life to about eight hours.

Because it can induce a syndrome of inappropriate antidiuretic hormone secretion, the risk of fluid retention should be borne in mind when the drug is used in patients with compromised renal function (Morselli and Bossi, 1982). It is unlikely that carbamazepine or its metabolites would, however, accumulate to any significant degree in renal failure. Dosage adjustment in uremia is usually unnecessary (Asconapé and Penry, 1982).

Benzodiazepines

Nitrazepam, clorazepate, and clonazepam are the main benzodiazepines in use as maintenance antiepileptic drugs, while diazepam and lorazepam are used as parenteral drugs in treating status epilepticus. While the latter are highly effective in this limited use, long-term benzodiazepines present several problems when used as monotherapy maintenance drugs for epilepsy. They have sedating properties, strongly potentiated by concomitant use of barbiturates. In addition, they have active metabolites, especially desmethyldiazepam, which has a half-life of three to four days, and oxazepam, an active, sedating chemical.

The drugs are used for primary generalized seizures and sometimes as add-on drugs in treating partial seizures. Unfortunately, tolerance often develops to their antiepileptic action. They are second-line maintenance antiepileptic drugs. Their use in renal failure is extremely limited. A reduction in dose and lengthening of interdose intervals are necessary steps. The main role in uremia is in treating status epilepticus and myoclonus. Diazepam has temporary beneficial effect on the clinical and electroencephalographic features of dialytic encephalopathy.

Other Drugs and Their Complications

In this section we shall deal with immunosuppressive drugs, chelating agents, opiates, antibiotics, and antihypertensive drugs.

Immunosuppressive Drugs

This section is devoted to cyclosporine, the most promising of the immunosuppressive drugs for renal transplantation. Discussion of other immunosuppressants such as corticosteroids and azathioprine can be found in standard texts; only brief mention of them is given in this volume.

Cyclosporine (cyclosporine A, CsA) is a cyclic endecapeptide with a molecular weight of 1,202 daltons. It was first isolated from two strains of fungi imperfecti of the species *Tolypocladium inflatum*. Because of the complex structure, it is still produced by a fermentation process and is chromatographically refined (Kahan, 1985). The use of CsA has been a major advance in the transplantation of solid organs (kidney, heart, liver) as well as bone marrow.

The effect of CsA on the immune system is twofold. First, CsA inhibits the production by macrophages of interleukin-1, a peptide that is necessary for T cell activation. Second, at concentrations of 10 to 100 ng/mL, T helper cells are inhibited from producing lymphokines, including interleukin-2, interleukin-3, B cell growth factor, macrophage-activating factor, monocyte/macrophage procoagulant activity, migration inhibition factor, lymphocyte-derived macrophage-chemotactic factor, gamma interferon, and colony-stimulating factor (Kahan, 1985; Kahan et al., 1986). At the same time, the non–T cell-dependent, B cell–mediated immunity is maintained. In doses of 10 to 15 mg/kg, even when used with corticosteroids, CsA results in a lower incidence of opportunistic infections than other immunosuppressive agents such as the azathioprine-prednisone combination. The risk of malignancy with CsA is probably no greater than with other agents: lymphomas have an incidence of 0.5 percent, in contrast to the 2 to 11 percent with previous conventional immunosuppressive agents (Atkinson et al., 1984a).

The gastrointestinal absorption is highly variable, and there may be an enterohepatic cycle, necessitating individual monitoring of serum levels. Ideal serum trough levels are 100 to 400 ng/mL. The drug is highly protein bound in plasma and is metabolized by the P-450 system of the liver.

Neurological Complications of Cyclosporine

The mildest neurological complication of CsA is fine postural action tremors of the upper limbs, which occur in about 22 percent of patients (Kahan et al., 1986). Tremors appear within the first three months of therapy and are rarely seen beyond 12 months. They are dose-dependent, subsiding with dose reduction. Occasionally, intention tremors, indicating dysfunction of cerebellar connections, may occur, often combined with other signs of CNS dysfunction (Atkinson et al., 1984b). Burning paresthesias in the palms and soles also tend to occur in the first few months after surgery and respond to reduction of dosage (Kahan et al., 1986).

Cerebral seizures occurred in 1.5 to 5.5 percent of patients on CsA therapy in the series compiled by O'Sullivan (1985), but in 11 of 43 (25 percent) of patients in the cardiac transplant group of Hardesty et al. (1983). There were some additional factors in this group: high-risk surgery with chance of embolization

to brain and increased blood-brain barrier penetration, and high-dose CsA and concomitant use of high-dose corticosteroids. CsA-related seizures are usually generalized tonic-clonic or grand mal seizures (Thompson et al., 1984; Polson et al., 1985), which may proceed to fatal status epilepticus (Velu et al., 1985). Some may show myoclonus; absencelike spells have also been described (Kahan et al., 1986). We have noted generalized epileptiform activity on electroencephalograms of such encephalopathic patients who have had seizures near the time of recording. Cerebellar ataxia may also occur, often combined with a drowsy or confusional (encephalopathic) state and tremor (Thompson et al., 1984; Atkinson et al., 1984a; 1985). This situation is reversible.

Thompson et al. (1985) reported two patients on CsA with a transient, expressive aphasic syndrome that subsided with magnesium replacement. Both patients had had long periods of hypomagnesemia (11 and 40 days). Electroencephalograms, computed tomographic (CT) scans and cerebrospinal fluid (CSF) analyses were unremarkable.

Complex visual hallucinations, as well as loss of visual acuity, have been reported as toxic encephalopathic effects of CsA (Noll and Kulkarni, 1984). A syndrome consisting of visual changes and a variety of other clinical features, along with white-matter alteration on CT head scans, has been described in CsA-treated patients. Berden et al. (1985) reported CsA-induced coma associated with white-matter hypodensity on CT scan in a patient after renal transplantation. Rubin and Kang (1987) described a patient with a similar CT scan who developed acute cerebral blindness (with preserved pupillary reflexes), global encephalopathy, and right occipital seizures following bone marrow transplantation and CsA therapy. A similar syndrome occurred in a patient 149 days after bone marrow transplant (López Mezza et al., 1986). De Groen et al. (1987) reported three patients with liver transplantation who suffered CNS symptoms 3 to 8 days after initiation of intravenous CsA therapy. Two patients had anorexia or nausea just before the encephalopathy. Inattention, disorientation, and confusion were followed by cerebral blindness in all patients. One patient became comatose with associated hyperventilation; the other showed lesser degrees of obtundation. One patient had receptive aphasia and delusional and inappropriate behavior. One developed quadriplegia and hyperreflexic upper limb reflexes. In each case: (1) CT scans revealed white-matter hypodensity, maximal posteriorly; this was associated with prolonged T_2 relaxation time on magnetic resonance imaging, indicative of increased water content; (2) serum cholesterol levels were significantly lower than in similarly treated patients without symptoms; (3) the syndrome was reversible when CsA was discontinued. One patient showed a recurrence of encephalopathy and white-matter changes on CT scan when CsA was restarted after a second liver transplant; she improved again when the drug was stopped.

Wilczek et al. (1985) reported one patient who developed advanced toxicity with CsA. Improvement followed stopping the drug, but reinstitution of low-dose CsA evoked immediate return of the previous toxic features.

A spinal cord syndrome with either quadri- or paraparesis, urinary retention, and in some, extensor plantar responses may occur from 30 to 195 days after initiation of CsA (Atkinson et al., 1984a; 1984b; 1985). The neurological features were uniformly completely reversible. Findings are predominantly motor, although one patient (Atkinson et al., 1984b) had a sensory deficit below the mid-thoracic region. Some patients showed other evidence of CNS involvement, such as confusion, memory disturbance, ataxia, and intention tremor (Atkinson et al., 1984b). Some were hyperreflexic, but most had depressed or absent deep tendon reflexes. (The reports did not mention electrophysiological studies to exclude a peripheral neuropathic component). CSF protein levels were mildly elevated, in the range of 600 mg/L, and showed a very mild, predominantly lymphocytic pleocytosis.

Papa et al. (1985) described a single case of bilateral deltoid paralysis in a patient on CsA after bone marrow transplantation for chronic myelogenous leukemia. The paralysis was painful and neurogenic, fitting into the syndrome of neuralgic amyotrophy (Tsairis et al., 1972), but it was unusual in being bilateral. The condition improved when the dosage of drug was reduced. It is unclear whether there is a causal relationship between CsA and the acute dysfunction of the circumflex nerves in this patient; in more than one-third of patients with neuralgic amyotrophy, there is no antecedent factor and improvement is spontaneous. This patient had a mild, asymptomatic polyneuropathy on nerve conduction studies. De Groen et al. (1987) had one patient with a peripheral neuropathy showing features of both axonal degeneration and demyelination, which improved when CsA was stopped. There was an associated reversible encephalopathy. Clearly, more clinical and electrophysiological surveys of CsA-treated patients are needed.

Pathogenesis of the Neurological Complications

There is good evidence that in most cases reported, the neurological signs and symptoms were related to the use of CsA. The symptoms and signs occurred while on the drug, subsided with dose reduction or withdrawal, and recurred when the original dose was resumed. Furthermore, there was no other adequate explanation for the condition in most cases. The question is, by what mechanism does CsA cause neurological problems?

The most obvious explanation is the drug itself. Cyclosporine is lipophilic and, therefore, can cross the blood-brain barrier. Boland et al. (1984) administered CsA to mice; those on 12.5 mg/kg/day remained well; all mice given 50 or more mg/kg/day were lethargic; 31 of 32 given 200 mg/kg/day showed imbalance, loss of coordination, and generalized tremor, and terminally there was usually hindlimb paralysis with severe, generalized convulsions and respiratory distress. The brains of those mice given 50 to 100 mg/kg/day showed large vacuoles in the white matter of brain and spinal cord. Penetration into brain was less than for other organs. Brain concentration approached that of serum only at 200 mg/kg/day; in other organs, the tissue concentration was on the order of tenfold greater than that of serum. The values showed considerable interindividual variability. Atkinson et al. (1982; 1983) found CsA in the human brain at autopsy, even when the drug had been discontinued 16 days before death. The tissue concentration was much lower in brain than in other organs: 0.24 ng of CsA/mg of tissue compared with 1.7 to 7.7 for other systemic organs (Atkinson et al., 1983). Only one of three humans studied by Atkinson et al. in 1983 showed any detectable CsA in the brain.

Penetration into the brain is likely to depend on blood level of the drug, especially the free fraction. In the series of De Groen et al. (1987) the low serum cholesterol may have allowed the free fraction of the drug to achieve higher levels, since CsA is lipophilic and likely associated with plasma lipids. Intravenous administration of the drug is more likely to cause higher peak plasma concentrations than oral dosing. Since CsA likely exerts its lymphocytic effect on the cell membrane (Kahan, 1985), it may do the same in the brain. Whether the drug interferes with synaptic activity by blocking receptors (e.g., by multimeric attachment or receptor cross-linking) is not known. It appears that there is no interference with membrane potential, calcium influx, phospholipid methylation, or second messenger physiology, at least in lymphocytes (Kahan, 1985).

The reversible white-matter changes noted on CT scans in some patients with encephalopathy are almost certainly associated with vasogenic edema, as shown by magnetic resonance imaging. Whether there is actual myelin damage is uncertain. The dysfunction in the patients reported by De Groen et al. (1987) and others with this syndrome, seems to be more than would be expected from edema alone; in several there was no evidence of significant mass effect or raised intracranial pressure. Whether the dysfunction is due to a toxic effect on the nervous system associated with structural changes has yet to be settled. The rapidity and completeness of clinical recovery in most patients suggests the dysfunction is not associated with serious structural changes in CNS tissue.

Wilczek et al. (1985) showed that in a patient with meningitis from cytomegalovirus, the symptoms of toxicity were temporaly related to CsA. Presumably, the inflamed meninges allowed greater penetration into the brain and CSF.

Hypomagnesemia is a common complication of CsA therapy. It occurs because of increased renal clearance, as a result of CsA's nephrotoxicity (Stiller and Keown, 1984). Thompson et al. (1984) found an association of cerebral seizures, cerebellar ataxia, and transient aphasia with hypomagnesemia. Symptoms and signs resolved promptly when magnesium was administered. Only one of the seven patients with seizures had a raised CsA serum level. It was not stated whether doses of CsA were reduced or withheld in these patients. All the patients received anticonvulsants (phenytoin and phenobarbital) in addition to the CsA. Among the three patients with cerebellar ataxia, tremor, and depression, CsA was withheld in two. All patients received magnesium supplementation and improved, including the one who was maintained on the same dose of CsA. In the two patients with aphasia, the speech problem cleared with replacement of magnesium; they remained on the same regimen of CsA.

There has been conflicting evidence and opinion regarding the role of hypomagnesemia as the pathogenic mechanism for CsA's neurotoxicity. Allen et al. (1985) described a patient on CsA who had seizures with hypomagnesemia. The seizures were more related to an elevated plasma CsA level than to the serum magnesium level, in that they stopped promptly with reduction of CsA, even though the magnesium level continued to fall. O'Connor et al. (1985) found the magnesium level with prednisone and azathioprine to be about the same as those with CsA; patients on the former regimen did not have the neurological complications. Furthermore, patients on CsA may have convulsions with normal levels of magnesium. Thus, the issue is unsettled. Probably, some patients, similar to some of those described by Thompson et al. (1984), do have seizures and other problems related to hypomagnesemia, while in others the hypomagnesemia occurs as an epiphenomenon.

Nordal et al. (1985) found that seizure activity in renal transplant patients treated with

CsA was associated with aluminum deposition in 21 to 78 percent of the trabecular bone surfaces of this group. They proposed that somehow CsA promoted release of the massive aluminum stores and that this produced the seizures. This theory requires substantiation with serum aluminum levels. Against a role for aluminum is the neurotoxicity in CsA-treated patients who have hematological or hepatic disorders rather than renal failure.

The above discussion relates to CsA itself. The intravenous preparation is mixed with a surfactant, polyoxyethylated castor oil (Cremophor EL), and this could play a role in the acute syndrome with cerebral edema. Against that possibility is the fact that encephalopathy recurred in one patient after being started on the oral preparation, which does not contain Cremophor EL.

Indirect Complications of Cyclosporine Therapy

Other complications of CsA therapy could, in some cases, cause neurological problems. Hypertension is a common complication of CsA therapy. It may be secondary to nephrotoxicity, as it is associated with elevated renin levels (Baxter et al., 1982; Siegl and Ruffel, 1982; Siegl et al., 1983). Both the nephrotoxicity and hypertension are dose-related and almost always improve after reduction of the dose of CsA (Klintmalm et al., 1983; Thompson et al., 1983). If severe, seizures may result from hypertensive encephalopathy or stroke (Joss et al., 1982).

Hepatic, pulmonary (Bacigalupo et al., 1985), or renal toxicity (Klintmalm et al., 1983) and a diabetogenic effect related to suppressed C peptide concentrations (Bending et al., 1987) may produce neurological complications of their own.

In children on CsA, the addition of high-dose methylprednisolone has been associated with convulsions (Durrant et al., 1982). Those children who convulsed had higher blood pressures than those who did not; the pathogenesis may relate to hypertension plus increased sodium and fluid retention.

CNS infections (see Chapter 8) should al-ways be considered in any immunosuppressed patient. For example, cytomegalovirus is especially common in immunosuppressed renal transplant patients and has been reported to produce a chorioretinitis in adults (DeVenecia et al., 1971). This can improve, as can cytomegalovirus encephalitis.

Thromboembolic complications of CsA therapy have been reported. A case of retinal emboli was reported by Choudhury et al. (1985). Vanrenterghem et al. (1985) found that CsA enhanced adenosine-5'-diphosphate–induced platelet aggregation. This effect was directly dependent on concentration of CsA.

Treatment

The development of CNS complications in conjunction with CsA should prompt checking the CsA plasma level as well as the serum magnesium, in addition to blood pressure measurement, neurological examination, CT, and CSF analysis when indicated. If the complication is related to CsA itself, particularly if the plasma level is elevated, the CsA should be reduced or stopped. Magnesium supplements should be given if the serum level is low.

Patients with seizures usually require an antiepileptic drug. Because phenobarbital, phenytoin, and carbamazepine also use the P-450 oxidase system of the liver for their metabolism, levels of CsA and the particular antiepileptic drug require close monitoring because of the interference, especially increased metabolism (Kahan et al., 1986).

Deferoxamine

Deferoxamine is a long, linear molecule with carbon and nitrogen in the chain to which double-bonded oxygen atoms and amino groups are attached. It is isolated as the iron chelate from *Streptomyces pilosus* and is treated to produce the iron-free ligand. Deferoxamine is a superior chelating agent and is used most extensively to treat iron overload. It is also used to reduce the body burden of aluminum in dialysis patients with dialytic encephalopathy, bone disease, and/or anemia (see Chapter 7).

Olivieri et al. (1986) reported visual and/or auditory neurotoxicity in 13 of 89 patients receiving subcutaneous deferoxamine therapy for thalassemia major or Diamond-Blackfan anemia. Duration of treatment was four months to six years, and doses ranged from 40 to 150 mg/kg/day. The visual loss was central, often with an afferent pupillary light defect and swelling of the optic disk. Visual acuity improved when the deferoxamine was discontinued, but some patients were left with impaired acuity and various degrees of optic atrophy and pigmentary change in the macula.

High-frequency hearing loss was present in the 13 cases mentioned, but auditory-evoked responses disclosed abnormalities in nine others. Hearing improved when the drug was stopped, but six patients required hearing aids.

Opiates

Ball et al. (1985) reported accumulation of morphine in patients treated in intensive care units. Those who showed this had impaired renal function. About 10 percent of the drug is normally excreted in the urine, probably accounting for the accumulation in these patients. Normeperidine, a metabolite of meperidine, can accumulate in renal failure and cause CNS excitation as tremor, individual or multifocal myoclonus, or seizures (Kaiko et al., 1983). There is some evidence that there are different receptors for the convulsant and analgesic properties of normeperidine (Umans and Inturrisi, 1982). Opioid antagonists such as naloxone block the convulsant effects of normeperidine in mice (Jaffe and Martin, 1985), but it is usually more appropriate to substitute morphine for meperidine, if an analgesic is still required, and to use diazepam or other anticonvulsants if further seizures occur (Kaiko et al., 1983). Respiratory function may require support.

Antibiotics

In patients with anuria and no dialysis the half-life of penicillin G is increased from 0.5 to about 10 hours (Mandell and Sande, 1985). Penicillins and cephalosporins may accumulate in uremia and cause encephalopathy, including impaired consciousness, myoclonus, asterixis, and refractory focal or generalized convulsive seizures, even in patients on hemodialysis (Schwankaus et al., 1987; Josse et al., 1987). Petit mal (absence) status epilepticus with impaired consciousness has also been reported (Vignaendra et al., 1976). This might occur because of an effect of these drugs on inhibition in the brain (Schwartzkroin, 1983) or because of these drugs causing a competitive inhibition of transport of other organic acids out of the CNS in uremia (Fishman, 1966).

The aminoglycoside drugs tobramycin, gentamicin, streptomycin, neomycin, and kanamycin rely on renal excretion as a major mechanism of elimination (Reidenberg and Drayer, 1980). They accumulate in renal failure and can cause ototoxicity, especially irreversible damage to hair cells in the membranous labyrinth and cochlea, with resultant loss of vestibular and auditory function (Brummet and Fox, 1982). Peripheral neuropathy has also been associated, although rarely, with aminoglycoside toxicity. This is initially a primarily sensory, reversible neuropathy characterized by paresthesias in the extremities and around the mouth (Sande and Mandell, 1985). This should be clearly differentiated from the neuromuscular blockade that can be an idiosyncratic effect of aminoglycosides (Sande and Mandell, 1985).

Antihypertensive Drugs

β-Blockers with low lipophilicity, such as nadolol and atenolol, tend to be poorly metabolized and are excreted unchanged in the urine. These drugs also have longer half-lives than other β-blockers. Thus, their dose has to be reduced in renal failure. The latter also applies to propranolol because it has active metabolites that are excreted in the urine (Wilkinson, 1982). Because of their low lipid solubility, atenolol and nadolol do not cross the blood-brain barrier to any great extent and are sometimes preferable to propranolol and other β-blockers in treating hypertension because of fewer CNS side effects. The latter are largely anecdotal but include light-headedness, lethargy, drowsiness, insomnia, anorexia, poor concentration, reversible memory problems and catatonia, vivid dreams, hallucinations, paresthesias, and incoordination.

Active metabolites having long half-lives, which accumulate in renal failure, are produced from acebutolol and metoprolol. The former drug may need dosage adjustment in uremia (Verbeek et al., 1981).

β-Blockers may rarely significantly diminish renal function in uremic patients. This is likely due to blockade of β$_2$-receptors in the kidney, reducing renal blood flow (Wilkinson, 1982).

References

Allen RD, Hunnisett AG, Morris PJ. Cyclosporine and magnesium. Lancet 1985;1:1283–1284.

Aranoff GR, Luft FC. Antimicrobial therapy in patients with impaired renal function. Dial Transplant 1979;8:14.

Asconapé JJ, Penry JK. Use of antiepileptic drugs in the presence of liver and kidney diseases: a review. Epilepsia 1982;23(Suppl 1):565–579.

Atkinson AJ, Kushner W. Clinical pharmacokinetics. Annu Rev Pharmacol Toxicol 1979;19:105–127.

Atkinson K, Biggs JC, Britton K. Distribution and persistence of cyclosporin in human tissues. Lancet 1982;2:1196.

Atkinson K, Biggs JC, Karveniza P, et al. Cyclosporine-associated central nervous system toxicity after allogenic bone marrow transplantation. Transplantation 1984;38:34–37.

Atkinson K, Biggs JC, Karveniza P, et al. Spinal cord cerebellar-like syndromes associated with the use of cyclosporine in human recipients of allogenic marrow transplants. Transplant Proc 1985;17:1673–1675.

Atkinson K, Britton K, Boland J, Biggs JC. Blood and tissue distribution of cyclosporine in humans and mice. Transplant Proc 1983;15:2430–2433.

Bacigalupo A, Frassoni F, van Lint MT, et al. Cyclosporin A in marrow transplantation for leukemia and aplastic anemia. Exp Hematol 1985;13:244–248.

Ball M, Moore RA, Fisher A, et al. Renal failure and the use of morphine in intensive care. Lancet 1985;1:784–786.

Baxter CR, Duggin GG, Willis NS, et al. Cyclosporin A induced increases in renin storage and release. Res Commun Chem Pathol Pharmacol 1982;37:305–311.

Berden JHM, Goitsma AJ, Merx JL, Keyser A. Severe central-nervous-system toxicity associated with cyclosporin. Lancet 1985;1:219–220.

Boland J, Atkinson K, Britton K, et al. Tissue distribution and toxicity of cyclosporin A in the mouse. Pathology 1984;16:117–123.

Boobis SW. The alteration in plasma albumin in relation to decreased drug binding in uremia. Clin Pharmacol Ther 1977;22:147–153.

Brewster D, Muir NC. Valproate plasma protein binding in the uremic condition. Clin Pharmacol Ther 1980;27:76–82.

Browne TR. Pharmacological principles of antiepileptic drug administration. In: Browne TR, Feldman RG, eds. Epilepsy: diagnosis and management. Boston: Little, Brown, 1983:145–160.

Brummet RE, Fox KE. Studies of aminoglycoside ototoxicity in animal models. In: Wheton A, Neu HC, eds. The aminoglycosides: microbiology, clinical use and toxicity. New York: Marcel Dekker, 1982:419–451.

Bruni J, Wang LH, Marbury TC, et al. Protein binding of valproic acid in uremic patients. Neurology 1980;30:557–559.

Choudhury N, Neild GH, Brown Z, Cameron JS. Thromboembolic complications in cyclosporin-treated kidney allograft recipients. Lancet 1985;2:606.

Danhof M, Hisaoka M, Levy G. Effect of experimental renal failure on the relationship between phenobarbital concentration and pharmacologic activity. II World conference on clinical pharmacology and therapeutics. Washington, DC, 1983:138.

De Groen PC, Aksamit AJ, Rakela J, et al. Central nervous system toxicity after liver transplantation. The role of cyclosporine and cholesterol. N Engl J Med 1987;317:861–866.

Depner TA, Stanfel LA, Jarrard EA, Gulyassy PF. Impaired plasma phenytoin binding in uremia: effect of in-vitro acidification and ion-exchange resin. Nephron 1980;25:231–237.

DeVenecia G, Zu Rhein GM, Pratt M, Kisken W. Cytomegalic inclusion retinitis in an adult. Arch Ophthalmol 1971;86:44–57.

Dromgoole SH. The effect of haemodialysis on the binding capacity of albumin. Clin Chim Acta 1973;46:469–472.

Durrant S, Chipping PM, Palmer S, Gordon-Smith EC. Cyclosporin A, methylprednisolone and convulsions. Lancet 1982;2:829–830.

Fishman RA. Blood-brain and CSF barriers to penicillin and related organic acids. Arch Neurol 1966;15:113–124.

Gugler R, Mueller G. Plasma protein binding of valproic acid in healthy subjects and in patients with renal disease. Br J Clin Pharmacol 1978;5:441–446.

Gulyassy PF, Bottini AT, Stanfel LA, et al. Isolation and chemical identification of plasma ligand binding. Kidney Int 1986;30:391–398.

Hardesty RL, Griffith BP, Debski RF, Bahnson HT. Experience with cyclosporine in cardiac transplantation. Transplant Proc 1983;15:2553–2558.

Hurwitz A. Antacid therapy and drug kinetics. Clin Pharmacokinet 1977;2:269–280.

Jaffe JH, Martin WR. Opioid analgesics and antagonists. In: Gilman AG, Goodman LS, Rall TW, Murad F, eds. Goodman and Gilman's the pharmacological basis of therapeutics. 7th ed. New York: Macmillan, 1985:499–531.

Joss DV, Barrett AJ, Kendra JR, et al. Hypertension and convulsions in children receiving cyclosporin A. Lancet 1982;1:906.

Josse S, Godin M, Fillastre JP. Cefazolin-induced encephalopathy in a uraemic patient. Nephron 1987; 45:72.

Jusko WJ, Weintraub M. Myocardial distribution of digoxin and renal function. Clin Pharmacol Ther 1974;16:449–454.

Kahan BD. Cyclosporine: the agent and its actions. Transplant Proc 1985;27:5–18.

Kahan BD, Flechner SM, Lorber MI, et al. Complication of cyclosporine therapy. World J Surg 1986; 10:348–360.

Kaiko RF, Foley KM, Krabinski PY, et al. Central nervous system excitatory effects of meperidine in cancer patients. Ann Neurol 1983;13:180–185.

Klintmalm G, Ringden O, Groth CG. Clinical and laboratory signs in nephrotoxicity and rejection in cyclosporine-treated renal allograft recipients. Transplant Proc 1983;15(Suppl 1):2815–2820.

Kreeft JH, Linton AL. Renal dysfunction and drug dosage. Medicine 1985;28:3854–3862.

Levy G. Effect of plasma protein binding of drugs on duration and intensity of pharmacological activity. J Pharm Sci 1976;65:1264–1265.

Lewis GP, Jusko WJ, Burke CW, et al. Prednisone side-effects and serum-protein levels. Lancet 1971; 2:778–780.

Lichter M, Black M, Arias JM. The metabolism of antipyrine in patients with chronic renal failure. J Pharmacol Exp Ther 1973;187:612.

López Mezza JB, González Gómez N, Alonso Alonso P, et al. Convulsiones y hipertensión arterial en tres patientes sometidos a trasplante de medula ósea y en tratamiento con ciclosporina A. Rev Clin Esp 1986;178:186–188.

Lyons PJ, Affrime MB, Blecker DL, et al. The effect of renal transplantation on plasma protein binding. Clin Pharmacol Ther 1979;25:235.

Maher JF. Principles of dialysis and dialysis of drugs. Am J Med 1977;62:475–481.

Mandell GL, Sande MA. Antimicrobial agents: penicillins, cephalosporins, and other beta-lactam antibiotics. In: Gilman AG, Goodman LS, Rall TW, Murad F, eds. Goodman and Gilman's the pharmacological basis of therapeutics. 7th ed. New York: Macmillan, 1985:1115–1149.

Morselli PL, Bossi L. Carbamazepine: absorption, distribution and excretion. In: Woodbury DM, Penry

JK, Pippenger CW, eds. Antiepileptic drugs, 2nd ed. New York: Raven Press, 1982:465–482.

Muther RS, Bennett WM. Drug metabolism in renal failure. In: Brenner BM, Stein JH, eds. Chronic renal failure. New York: Churchill-Livingstone, 1981:287–323.

Nimmo WS. Drugs, diseases and altered gastric emptying. Clin Pharmacokinet 1976;1:189–203.

Noll RB, Kulkarni R. Complex visual hallucinations and cyclosporine. Arch Neurol 1984;41:329–330.

Nordal KP, Talseth T, Dahl E, et al. Aluminum overload: a predisposing condition for epileptic seizures in renal-transplant patients treated with cyclosporine? Lancet 1985;1:153–154.

O'Connor JP, Kleinman DS, Kunze HE. Hypomagnesemia and cyclosporine toxicity. Lancet 1985;1:103–104.

Odar-Cederlof I, Borga O. Kinetics of diphenylhydantoin in uremic patients: consequences of decreased plasma protein binding. Eur J Clin Pharmacol 1974;7:31–37.

Olivieri NF, Buncic JR, Chew E, et al. Visual and auditory neurotoxicity in patients receiving subcutaneous deferoxamine infusions. N Engl J Med 1986;314:869–873.

O'Sullivan DP. Convulsions associated with cyclosporin A. Br Med J 1985;290:858.

Papa G, Arcese W, Bianchi A, et al. Cyclosporine-associated bilateral deltoid paralysis after allogenic bone marrow transplantation for chronic myelogenous leukemia. Haematologica (Pavia) 1985;70:273–274.

Penn I. Lymphomas complicating organ transplantation. Transplant Proc 1983;15(Suppl 1):2790–2797.

Perucca E. Plasma protein binding of phenytoin. Clin Pharmacokinet 1979;4:153–169.

Perucca E, Grimaldi R, Crema A. Interpretation of drug levels in acute and chronic disease states. Clin Pharmacokinet 1985;10:498–513.

Polson RJ, Powell-Jackson PR, Williams R. Convulsions associated with cyclosporin A in transplant recipients. Br Med J 1985;290:1003.

Reidenberg MM. The binding of drugs to plasma proteins and the interpretation of measurements of plasma concentrations of drugs in patients with poor renal function. Am J Med 1977;62:466–469.

Reidenberg MM, Affrime M. Influence of disease on binding of drugs to plasma proteins. Ann NY Acad Sci 1973;226:115–126.

Reidenberg MM, Drayer DE. Drug therapy in renal failure. Annu Rev Pharmacol Toxicol 1980;20:45–54.

Reynolds F, Ziroyanis PN, Jones N, Smith SE. Salivary phenytoin concentrations in epilepsy and in chronic renal failure. Lancet 1976;2:384–386.

Richens A. Clinical pharmacokinetics of phenytoin. Clin Pharmacokinet 1979;4:153–169.

Rimer DG. Gastric retention without mechanical obstruction. Arch Intern Med 1966;117:287–299.

Rubin AM, Kang H. Cerebral blindness and encephalopathy with cyclosporin A toxicity. Neurology 1987;37:1072–1076.

Sande MA, Mandell GL. Antimicrobial agents: the aminoglycosides. In: Gilman AG, Goodman LS, Rall TW, Murad F, eds. Goodman and Gilman's the pharmacological basis of therapeutics. 7th ed. New York: Macmillan, 1985;51:1150–1169.

Schwankaus JD, Masucci EF, Kurtzke JF. Cefazolin-induced encephalopathy in a uremic patient. Nephron 1987;45:72.

Schwartzkroin PA. Local circuit considerations and intrinsic neuronal properties involved in hyperexcitability and cell synchronization. In: Jasper HH, van Gelder NM, eds. Basic mechanisms of neuronal excitability. New York: Alan R. Liss, 1983:75–108.

Shoeman DW, Azarnoff DL. The alteration in plasma proteins in uremia as reflected in their ability to bind digitoxin and diphenylhydantoin. Pharmacology 1972;7:169–177.

Siegl H, Ruffel B, Petric R, et al. Cyclosporine, the renin-angiotensin-aldosterone system and renal adverse reactions. Transplant Proc 1983;15:2719–2725.

Sirgo MA, Green PJ, Rocci ML Jr, Vlasses PH. Interpretation of serum phenytoin concentrations in uremia is assay-dependent. Neurology 1984;34:1250–1251.

Sjoholm I, Kober A, Odar-Cederlof I, Borga O. Protein binding of drugs in uremia and normal serum. The role of endogenous binding inhibitors. Biochem Pharmacol 1976;25:1205–1213.

Stiller CR, Keown PA. Cyclosporine therapy in perspective. In: Morris PJ, Tilney NL, eds. Progress in transplantation. Edinburgh: Churchill-Livingstone, 1984:11–45.

Thompson CB, Sullivan KM, Junk CH, Thomas ED. Association between cyclosporin neurotoxicity and hypomagnesemia. Lancet 1984;2:1116–1120.

Thompson ME, Shapiro AP, Johnsen AM, et al. New onset of hypertension following cardiac transplantation: a preliminary report and analysis. Transplant Proc 1983;15(Suppl 1):2573–2577.

Tozer TN. Nomogram for adjustment of dosage regimens in patients with chronic renal impairment. J Pharmacokinet Biopharmacol 1974;2:13–28.

Tsairis P, Dyck PJ, Mulder DW. Natural history of brachial plexus neuropathy. Arch Neurol 1972; 27:109–117.

Umans JG, Inturrisi CE. Antinociceptive activity and toxicity of meperidine and normeperidine in mice. J Pharmacol Exp Ther 1982;223:203–206.

Vanrenterghem Y, Lerut T, Roels L, et al. Thromboembolic complications and haemostatic changes in cyclosporine-treated cadaveric kidney allograft recipients. Lancet 1985;2:999–1002.

Velu T, Debusscher L, Stryckmans PA. Cyclosporin-associated fatal convulsions. Lancet 1985;1:219.

Verbeek RK, Branch RA, Wilkinson GA. Drug metabolites in renal failure: pharmacokinetic and clinical implications. Clin Pharmacokinet 1981;6:329–345.

Vignaendra V, Ghee LT, Lee LC. Petit mal status in a patient with chronic renal failure. Med J Aust 1976;2:258–259.

Wilczek H, Ringden O, Tyden G. Cyclosporine-associated central nervous system toxicity after renal transplantation. Transplantation 1985;39:110.

Wilkinson R. Beta-blockers and renal function. Drugs 1982;23:195–206.

Woodbury DM. Phenytoin: mechanisms of action. In: Woodbury DM, Penry JK, Pippenger CE, eds. Antiepileptic drugs, 2nd ed. New York: Raven Press, 1982:269–281.

Index

Abel JJ, 4
Abscesses, 148
Acebutolol, 231, 241
Acetylcholinesterase, 187
Acetylsalicylic acid, 228
Acid-base balance
  acidosis and. *See* Acidosis
  uremia and, 23–25
Acidosis, 23–25
  dialysis dysequilibrium syndrome and, 199–200
  encephalopathy of acute renal
    failure and, 46
Acids, aromatic, 16
Acquired immunodeficiency syndrome, 223
Action potentials, 81–83
Acute renal failure, 44–48. *See
  also* Neurotoxins
Adams F, 6
Addison T, 6
Adenine, 23
Adenine diphosphate, 23
Adenine monophosphate, 23
Adenosine diphosphate, 95
Adenosine triphosphatase
  aluminum toxicity and, 187
  uremia and, 23, 87
Adenylate cyclase, 187
Alcohol
  encephalopathy of acute renal
    failure and, 46
  myoglobinuria and, 158
Aldosterone, 207
Aliphatic amines, 16–17
Allergic granulomatosis, 130
Allopurinol, 231
Aluminum
  bioavailability and, 228

deposition of
  cerebral, 183–184
  cyclosporine and, 239
  dialysis osteomalacia and, 185
  encephalopathy and, 175–176
  levels of
    dialysate, 188–189
    serum, 189
  phosphate-binding agents and,
    190
  toxicity of, 25, 186–188
    deferoxamine in, 191–192
    dialytic encephalopathy and,
      183–185
    withdrawal from sources of, 191
Alzheimer type of senile dementia, 180
Amantadine, 230
Amaurosis, renal failure and
  acute, 45
  chronic, 54–55
American Rheumatism Association Criteria for systemic
  lupus erythematosus, 134
Amines, 16–17
Amino acids, 20–22
  septic encephalopathy and, 148
γ-Aminobutyric acid, 16, 21
  aluminum toxicity and, 187, 188
  binding sites for, 186
Aminoglycoside toxicity, 114, 156
3,4-Aminopyridine, 156
Amyloid
  carpal tunnel syndrome and, 36
  classification of, 113
  myeloma and, 145
  nerve biopsy and, 38
  role of, 110, 111–112
Amyotrophy, diabetic, 155

Angiitis, cerebral, 126
Angiography, cerebral, 35–36
Angiothrombosis, thrombotic, 141
Animal models
  encephalopathy and, 52
  uremic myoclonus and, 56
Ankle jerks after transplantation,
  99, 100
AN-69 polyacrylonitrile membrane, 93, 95, 112
Antacids
  bioavailability and, 228
  dietary phosphate and, 190
Antibiotics
  pharmacokinetics of, 240
  in renal failure, 232
  toxicity of, 156
Anticardiolipin levels, 137
Anticoagulants. *See also* Heparin
  peripheral nerve damage and,
    116
  stroke and, 123, 124
  subdural hematomas and, 201
Antiepileptic drugs, 233
Antihypertensives
  hypertensive encephalopathy
    and, 129
  pharmacokinetics of, 240–241
Antinuclear antibodies, 136
Antiplatelet drugs
  peripheral nerve damage and,
    116
  thrombotic thrombocytopenic
    purpura and, 142
Antipyrine, 231
Apnea, dialytic encephalopathy
  and, 175
Approaches in renal disease, 34–
  39

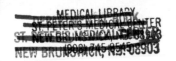